AF598071

Upper Tract Urothelial Carcinoma

Shahrokh F. Shariat • Evanguelos Xylinas
Editors

Upper Tract Urothelial Carcinoma

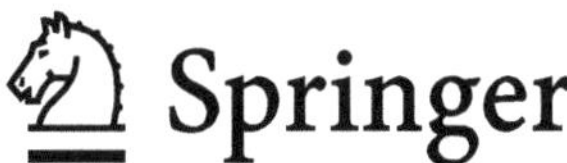

Editors
Shahrokh F. Shariat
Department of Urology and Comprehensive Cancer Center
Medical University of Vienna
Vienna, Austria

Evanguelos Xylinas
Department of Urology
Paris Descartes University
Paris, France

ISBN 978-1-4939-1500-2 ISBN 978-1-4939-1501-9 (eBook)
DOI 10.1007/978-1-4939-1501-9
Springer New York Heidelberg Dordrecht London

Library of Congress Control Number: 2014948335

© Springer Science+Business Media New York 2015
This work is subject to copyright. All rights are reserved by the Publisher, whether the whole or part of the material is concerned, specifically the rights of translation, reprinting, reuse of illustrations, recitation, broadcasting, reproduction on microfilms or in any other physical way, and transmission or information storage and retrieval, electronic adaptation, computer software, or by similar or dissimilar methodology now known or hereafter developed. Exempted from this legal reservation are brief excerpts in connection with reviews or scholarly analysis or material supplied specifically for the purpose of being entered and executed on a computer system, for exclusive use by the purchaser of the work. Duplication of this publication or parts thereof is permitted only under the provisions of the Copyright Law of the Publisher's location, in its current version, and permission for use must always be obtained from Springer. Permissions for use may be obtained through RightsLink at the Copyright Clearance Center. Violations are liable to prosecution under the respective Copyright Law.
The use of general descriptive names, registered names, trademarks, service marks, etc. in this publication does not imply, even in the absence of a specific statement, that such names are exempt from the relevant protective laws and regulations and therefore free for general use.
While the advice and information in this book are believed to be true and accurate at the date of publication, neither the authors nor the editors nor the publisher can accept any legal responsibility for any errors or omissions that may be made. The publisher makes no warranty, express or implied, with respect to the material contained herein.

Printed on acid-free paper

Springer is part of Springer Science+Business Media (www.springer.com)

Preface

In 2014, urothelial carcinoma of the bladder (UCB) is the fifth most common malignancy and the ninth most common cause of cancer death in the United States [1]. Conversely, upper tract urothelial carcinoma (UTUC) accounts for only 5–10% of all urothelial carcinomas. Largely due to the relative preponderance of UCB, much of the clinical decision-making surrounding UTUC is extrapolated from evidence that is based on UCB patients [2]. In fact, a recent review found 238 randomized controlled trials in bladder cancer [3], while a systematic search of the best evidence for the management of UTUC yielded only three such trials which are all very recent [4]. Notably only one major urological or oncologic association, the EAU (European Association of Urology), has published guidelines specific to UTUC [5]. Another professional organization, the International Consultation on Urological Diseases (ICUD), is now developing UTUC-specific guidelines, while others are including UTUC still as a subset of UCB guidelines or simply do not address UTUC in a guideline statement.

While significant similarities exist between UCB and UTUC, ignoring the important differences may be preventing us from optimizing therapy in patients with UTUC. Urothelial carcinomas of the lower and upper tract represent, indeed, two distinct yet related diseases. There are practical, anatomical, biological, and molecular differences that warrant consideration when risk stratifying and treating patients with these disparate twin diseases. This is specifically the reason for this book which is the "first" to specifically address this important, yet rare, disease.

As mentioned, there is, unfortunately, little evidence-based data to guide clinical decision-making in UTUC management. Recently, the tools available for the diagnosis and management of UTUC have improved significantly, complementing a growing understanding of the biology of this disease. To overcome the challenges that impede progress toward evidence-based medicine in UTUC, focused efforts based on multicenter collaborative research have augmented our understanding of this disease promising to improve the care we deliver to our patients.

UTUC requires appropriate management at all stages, since both the cure rate and morbidity are very sensitive to nuances of treatment. Yet proper risk stratification remains a challenge owing to the difficulty of clinical staging. This book will address contemporary concepts and controversies, including the timely and accurate diagnosis of UTUC, emphasizing the integration of pathologic and radiographic variables for appropriate risk stratification. Important features regarding the natural history of UTUC will also be emphasized; the role of imaging and endoscopy in clinical decision-making, diagnosis, staging, and follow-up; and common pathways of metastatic spread. Up-to-date information regarding boundaries of surgical resection, indication and extent of lymphadenectomy, clinical staging of UTUC, the role of perioperative chemotherapy, and optimal management of metastatic disease will be detailed.

This "first" textbook on UTUC is such organized to give clinicians, healthcare professionals, researchers, opinion leaders, and patients state-of-the art information on epidemiologic, basic science, and clinical aspects of UTUC. A group of superb experts in various aspects of UTUC was assembled all over the world to critically evaluate the literature and report their experience. We were privileged to work closely with each contributor and are immensely grateful to them for their time and dedication. We believe this book will serve as a comprehensive reference on this important disease that deserves more awareness.

Vienna, Austria Shahrokh F. Shariat, MD
Paris, France Evanguelos Xylinas, MD

References

1. Siegel R, Ma J, Zou Z, Jemal A. Cancer statistics, 2014. CA Cancer J Clin. 2014;64(1):9–29.
2. Green DA, Rink M, Xylinas E, et al. Urothelial carcinoma of the bladder and the upper tract: disparate twins. J Urol. 2013;189(4):1214–21.
3. Bachir BG, Shariat SF, Zlotta A, et al. Demographic analysis of randomized controlled trials in bladder cancer. BJU Int. 2013;111(3):419–26.
4. Matin SF, Shariat SF, Milowsky MI, et al. Highlights from the first symposium on upper tract urothelial carcinoma. Urol Oncol. 2014;32(3):309–16.
5. Roupret M, Babjuk M, Comperat E, et al. European guidelines on upper tract urothelial carcinomas: 2013 update. Eur Urol. 2013;63(6):1059–71.

Contents

Contributors

Mahul B. Amin, MD Department of Pathology and Laboratory Medicine, Cedars-Sinai Medical Center, Los Angeles, CA, USA

Arjun Vasant Balar, MD Division of Hematology and Medical Oncology, NYU Perlmutter Cancer Center, New York, NY, USA

Langone Medical Center, New York University, New York, NY, USA

Bernard H. Bochner, MD, FACS Urology Service, Department of Surgery, Kimmel Center for Prostate and Urologic Cancers, Memorial Sloan Kettering Cancer Center, New York, NY, USA

James Catto, MB, ChB, PhD, FRCS(Urol) Academic Urology Unit, University of Sheffield, The Medical School, Sheffield, UK

Department of Urology, Sheffield Teaching Hospitals, Sheffield Cancer Research Centre, The Medical School, Sheffield, Yorkshire, UK

Pierre Colin, MD, PhD Department of Urology, Hôpital Privé de La Louvière, Générale de Santé, Lille, Lille, France

Siamak Daneshmand, MD Department of Urology, Keck/USC School of Medicine, Los Angeles, CA, USA

Kathleen G. Dickman, PhD Departments of Pharmacological Sciences and Medicine/Nephrology, Stony Brook University, Stonybrook, NY, USA

Hans-Martin Fritsche, MD, PhD, FEBU Department of Urology, Caritas St. Josef Medical Center, University of Regensburg, Regensburg, Germany

Georgios Gakis, MD, FEBU Department of Urology, University Hospital Tübingen, Tübingen, Germany

Matthew D. Galsky, MD Mount Sinai School of Medicine, Tisch Cancer Institute, New York, NY, USA

Arthur P. Grollman, MD Department of Pharmacological Sciences, Stony Brook University, Stony Brook, NY, USA

Fatima Z. Husain, MD, MPH Department of Urology, Mount Sinai Hospital, New York, NY, USA

Ashish M. Kamat, MD Department of Urology, MD Anderson Cancer Center, Houston, TX, USA

Pierre Karakiewicz, MD Department of Urology, St. Luc Hospital, Montreal, Quebec, Canada

Wassim Kassouf, MD, CM, FRCS(C) Department of Surgery (Urology), McGill University Health Center, Montreal, Quebec, Canada

Tsunenori Kondo, MD Department of Urology, Tokyo Women's Medical University, Tokyo, Japan

Badrinath R. Konety, MD, MBA Department of Urology, Dougherty Family Chair in Prostate Cancer, Institute for Prostate and Urologic Cancers, University of Minnesota, Minneapolis, MN, USA

Seth P. Lerner, MD Scott Department of Urology, Baylor College of Medicine, Houston, TX, USA

Yair Lotan, MD Department of urology, University of Texas Southwestern Medical Center, Dallas, TX, USA

Vitaly Margulis, MD Department of Urology, UT MD Anderson Cancer Center, Houston, TX, USA

Surena F. Matin, MD Department of Urology, University of Texas MD Anderson Cancer Center, Houston, TX, USA

Matthew I. Milowsky, MD Department of Medicine, Division of Hematology/Oncology, University of North Carolina at Chapel Hill Lineberger Comprehensive Cancer Center, Chapel Hill, NC, USA

Giacomo Novara, MD Department of Surgical, Oncological and Gastroenterologic Sciences, Urology Clinic, University of Padua, Padua, Italy

Premal Patel, MD, BHSc Department of Pathology and Laboratory Medicine, University of Calgary and Calgary Laboratory Services, Calgary, AB, Canada

Sima P. Porten, MD, MPH Department of Urology, MD Anderson Cancer Center, University of Texas, Houston, TX, USA

Mesut Remzi, MD Department of Urology, Landeskrankenhaus Korneuburg, Korneuburg, Austria

Morgan Roupret, MD, PhD Academic Urology Department, Pitie Salpetriere Hospital (Assistance Publique Hopitaux de Paris), Paris, France

Shahrokh F. Shariat, MD Department of Urology, Weill Cornell Medical College, New York-Presbyterian Hospital, New York, NY, USA

Department of Urology, Medical University of Vienna, Wien, Austria

Arlene O. Siefker-Radtke, MD Department of Genitourinary Medical Oncology, The University of Texas MD Anderson Cancer Center, Houston, TX, USA

Steven Christopher Smith, MD, PhD Department of Pathology and Laboratory Medicine, Cedars-Sinai Medical Center, Los Angeles, CA, USA

Arnulf Stenzl Department of Urology, University Hospital Tuebingen, Tuebingen, Germany

Scott T. Tagawa, MD, MS Division of Hematology and Medical Oncology, Weill Cornell Medical College, New York, NY, USA

George N. Thalmann, MD Department of Urology, University Hospital Bern, Bern, Switzerland

Kiril Trpkov, MD, FRCPC Department of Pathology and Laboratory Medicine, University of Calgary, Calgary Laboratory Services, Rockyview General Hospital, Calgary, AB, Canada

Evanguelos Xylinas, MD Department of Urology, Weill Cornell Medical College, New York-Presbyterian Hospital, New York, NY, USA

Department of Urology, Cochin Hospital, Paris Descartes University, Paris, France

Alexandre R. Zlotta, MD, PhD, FRCSC Department of Surgery, Division of Urology, Mount Sinai Hospital, Toronto, ON, Canada

Department of Surgical Oncology, Division of Urology, University Health Network, Mount Sinai Hospital, Toronto, ON, Canada

Chapter 1
Epidemiology and Risk Factors for Upper Urinary Urothelial Cancers

Kathleen G. Dickman, Hans-Martin Fritsche, Arthur P. Grollman, George N. Thalmann, and James Catto

Abstract Urothelial carcinoma is a disease characterized by multiplicity, recurrence, and multifocality. Whilst around 5 % of tumors are in the upper tract, as with other human cancers, the study of unusual tumors within a spectrum can reveal insights into disease etiology and biology. Here we review genetic and acquired factors involved in the formation of upper tract urothelial carcinoma. This tumor is the main urological cancer found in Lynch syndrome. Around 10 % of sporadic tumors have similar molecular mechanisms to cancers arising within this most common cancer syndrome. With regard to acquired factors, we report data implicating aristolochic acid ingestion (through contaminated wheat or Chinese medicines) and tobacco smoking. Finally, we review risk factors for developing upper tract urothelial tumors, following treatment for bladder cancer.

K.G. Dickman, PhD
Departments of Pharmacological Sciences and Medicine/Nephrology, Stony Brook University, BST8-152, Stonybrook, NY 11794, USA
e-mail: kathleen.dickman@stonybrook.edu

H.-M. Fritsche, MD, PhD, FEBU
Department of Urology, Caritas St. Josef Medical Center, University of Regensburg, Landshuter Str. 65, Regensburg 93053, Germany
e-mail: hans-martin.fritsche@ukr.de; hans-martin.fritsche@klinik.uni-regensburg.de

A.P. Grollman, MD
Department of Pharmacological Sciences, Stony Brook University, Health Science Center BST 8-160, Stonybrook, NY 11733, USA
e-mail: Arthur.Grollman@stonybrook.edu

G.N. Thalmann, MD
Department of Urology, University Hospital Bern, Inselspital, Bern 3010, Switzerland
e-mail: george.thalmann@insel.ch

J. Catto, Mb, ChB, PhD, FRCS(Urol) (✉)
Academic Urology Unit, University of Sheffield, G Floor, The Medical School, Beech Hill Road, S10 2RX Sheffield, UK

Department of Urology, Sheffield Teaching Hospitals, Sheffield Cancer Research Centre, The Medical School, Beech Hill Road, Sheffield, Yorkshire S10 2RX, UK
e-mail: j.catto@sheffield.ac.uk

© Springer Science+Business Media New York 2015

S.F. Shariat, E. Xylinas (eds.), *Upper Tract Urothelial Carcinoma*,
DOI 10.1007/978-1-4939-1501-9_1

Keywords Urothelial cancer • Aristolochic acid • Lynch syndrome • Smoking • Ureter • Renal pelvis • Microsatellite instability • Mismatch repair • Bladder cancer • Transitional cell carcinoma • Balkan endemic nephropathy • Chinese herbs nephropathy • Phenacetin

Disease Demographics: Clues to Etiology

Urothelial carcinoma (UC) is predominantly a disease of industrialized nations with high cigarette smoking prevalence [1]. The vast majority of tumors arise following exogenous carcinogen exposure. Thus, whilst most UC occur in males, aged 60–80 years, who have often had manual occupations in heavy industry, the incidence in females is rising (given changes in work and smoking trends). Atypical demographic features related to gender balance, geographic clustering, and associations with other diseases often provide clues to the etiology of cancers, and more specifically to upper urinary tract urothelial carcinoma (UTUC). This is exemplified by upper tract tumors caused by exposure to specific drugs, including phenacetin, and toxins such as aristolochic acid (AA), a potent urothelial carcinogen and nephrotoxin produced by *Aristolochia* plants. Important insights into the association between AA and UTUC were derived from a landmark study of otherwise healthy young women in Belgium who, following ingestion of Chinese herbs, rapidly developed chronic kidney disease (CKD) requiring dialysis or renal transplantation [2, 3]. Ultimately, nearly half of these women with so-called Chinese herbs nephropathy (CHN) developed UC located primarily in the upper urinary tract.

The prevalence of UTUC in geographic hotspots is highlighted in Southern Europe by the syndrome known as Balkan endemic nephropathy (BEN). Here, the unusually high incidence of CKD and UTUC among both male and female residents of certain farming villages has been traced to dietary exposure to AA. Most recently, UTUC in Taiwan, where the incidence of this disease is the highest in the world, has been linked to the widespread use of *Aristolochia* herbs for medicinal purposes. These recently reported associations are discussed in more detail in this chapter.

Genetic Factors in Upper Tract Urothelial Carcinogenesis

All human tumors arise from a combination of hereditary/genetic factors and environmental/acquired exposures. The balance of these two varies between cancers and can be used to unlock the molecular biology of a disease. For example, insights into the genetics of hereditary colon and breast cancers lead to major breakthroughs in the understanding of sporadic disease. UC occurs in a few hereditary cancer syndromes. There are no known hereditary cancer syndromes in which UC is the only or majority tumor seen [4].

Hereditary Upper Tract Urothelial Cell Carcinoma

Hereditary factors increasing disease risk are mostly genetic events (although a few inherited epigenetic events are reported). These may produce gene mutations/truncations, leading to loss of function, or single base changes (so called single nucleotide polymorphisms (SNP)), leading to a modest modification in gene function. The latter are common and vital to produce genetic diversity. Epidemiologically these produce two distinctive patterns of disease risk: high penetrance and low penetrance.

High Penetrance Genetic Events

Classical Mendelian inherited diseases arise through the hereditary transference of rare, high-risk alleles. The commonest example in colorectal cancer and upper tract UC is Lynch syndrome (LS). Other examples involving upper urinary tract UC include Muir-Torre syndrome [5] (which is related to LS and may be caused by DNA Mismatch repair (MMR) gene mutation [6]), familial retinoblastoma (through Rb mutation), Li-Fraumeni (p53 mutation), Costello (H-Ras mutation), and Apert (FGFR2 mutation) syndrome (reviewed in [4]).

Lynch Syndrome

In 1895, Aldred Warthin found his seamstress crying with despair because of the certainty that she, like many of her family, would die at a young age from cancer [7]. Whilst his seamstress died of endometrial cancer, the predominant tumor type within her family was Gastric adenocarcinoma, leading Dr Warthin to describe the first family cancer syndrome, "Family G" [8]. In 1966, the description of two similar kindred suggested that Family G was not unique [7]. Lynch syndrome (also known as Hereditary Non-polyposis Colon Cancer: HNPCC) is now recognized as one of the commonest familial cancer syndromes.

LS arises through inherited loss of one member of the MMR system. MMR proteins are a complex of six or more members, highly conserved between unicellular organisms. In *E. coli*, the MutS protein binds preferentially to mismatched DNA bases forming a homodimer with another MutS molecule. The MutS homodimer translocates away from the DNA helix, to create a loop of DNA with the mismatch at its apex. The MutS/DNA complex then binds with a MutL homodimer and the MutH protein. The MutH protein ensures the strand specificity of this repair by binding to unmethylated adenine residues in a GATC complex [9]. Our knowledge of mammalian and human MMR is heavily based upon yeast and bacterial models [10]. The MutS and MutL mammalian equivalents are named according to their yeast homologues, MLH1p (called hMLH1 in humans), PMS1p (hPMS2), and MLH2p (hPMS1), and MutS homologues, MSH2p (hMSH2), MSH3p (hMSH3), and MSH6p (hMSH6) [11]. Mammalian MMR appears similar to that in yeast, with mismatch recognition by the MutS homologues, heterodimers of hMSH2 and either hMSH3 or hMSH6, and the initiation of mismatch repair by MutL, heterodimers of hMLH1 and hPMS2 or hPMS1. As with yeast, the duplicity of binding partners for hMSH2 and hMLH1 implies the process is complex, with redundancy of hMSH3 and possibly hPMS1. It is believed that the MutSβ and MutLβ (MLH1/PMS1) complexes repair insertion/deletion loops and not single base mutations. hMLH3 is located on chromosome 14q24.3 [12]. It interacts with MLH1, in addition to PMS2 and PMS1, suggesting a similar redundancy as seen with the three MutS homologues. hMLH1 and hMSH2 are key to MMR and so represent the most common mutant genes in Lynch syndrome.

Loss of MMR occurs in LS kindred when a second event, such as chromosomal deletion or DNA hypermethylation, removes the single remaining gene (as described by Knudson's with retinoblastoma). This allows DNA mutations to persist and sequentially knock out key tumor suppressor events. At the DNA level, these alterations may be seen as microsatellite instability (alterations in length of the highly repetitive microsatellites) [13, 14] (Fig. 1.1).

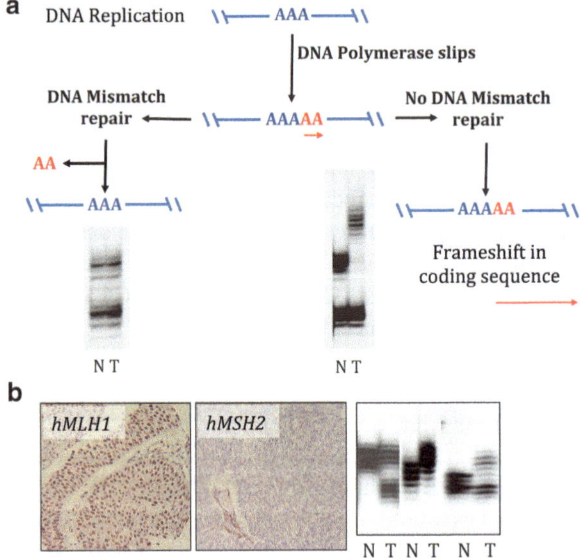

Fig. 1.1 Molecular biology of Lynch syndrome. During replication, DNA polymerase slips on highly repetitive microsatellites. Proficient MMR repairs these slips in normal cells, but they persist in those without MMR. These alterations lead to frameshifts in coding of gene with subsequent loss of gene function. Yates D and Catto J. Distinct patterns and behavior of urothelial carcinoma with respect to anatomical location: How molecular biomarkers can augment clinico-pathological predictors in upper urinary tract tumours. World J Urol 2013; 31(1): 21–9. With kind permission of Springer Science+Business Media

Tumor Spectrum Within Lynch Syndrome

Two patterns of tumor distribution in LS may exist [15]: Type I is characterized by the early onset of right-sided colorectal cancer [16], and type II by extra-colonic tumors, especially within the endometrium and upper urinary tracts (in addition to colorectal cancer). Watson and Lynch [17] reported 23 North American families, with over 7,500 persons, annotated into low and high risk, depending upon their germ line relationship to those affected by cancer. In the high-risk group ($n = 1{,}317$), an excess of tumors within the stomach, small bowel, hepatobiliary system, UTUC, and ovary was seen (Table 1.1). In low-risk persons ($n = 6{,}089$) no significant excesses of tumors were seen. Heterogeneity was seen with respect to the number of tumors of the upper urinary tract and endometrium, and to a lesser extent ovarian cancer, whilst stomach, small bowel, and hepatobiliary cancers were distributed evenly in all 23 families. Watson and Lynch concluded that whilst endometrial, ovarian, and UTUC were seen in some LS kindred, their evidence did not support the specific existence of two different Lynch syndromes [17]. However, subsequent correlations with MMR mutations have shown differences in tumor distribution, supporting a two-LS model [18]. Currently, kindred are best classified according to the presence of extra-colonic tumors and by the presence and type of MMR mutation.

It has been long recognized that UTUC occurs within LS [19–21]. In 1990, Vasen et al. described the tumor spectrum within 24 Dutch families, including 8 UC

Table 1.1 Incidence of tumors within 23 unrelated North American HNPCC kindreds (adapted from [17])

Tumor site	Observed	Expected	Poisson test *p* value
Colorectum	287		
Endometrium	53		
Stomach	17	4.1	<0.001
Small intestine	10	0.4	<0.001
Hepatobiliary	7	1.4	<0.05
Bladder	5	4.6	No sig diff
Kidney	3	2.8	No sig diff
Renal pelvis	7	0.4	<0.001
Ureter	5	0.2	<0.001
Ovary	13	3.6	<0.001
Lung/bronchus	5	12	<0.05*
Pancreas	6	4.1	No sig diff
Breast	19	22	No sig diff
Hematological	5	7.9	No sig diff
Skin	2	2	No sig diff
Larynx	1	2.2	No sig diff
Brain	3	1.9	No sig diff

*The observed incidence of carcinoma of the lung/bronchus was less than expected

in 4 kindred [22]. Whilst each of these reports described upper tract UC, there were also cases of bladder and renal cancer within these families. In 1998 Sijmons et al. used the Dutch LS registry to report 50 families (1,321 individuals) [23]. They observed 7 patients with upper tract UC, showing the relative risk of developing these tumors was increased 14-fold when compared to the general population (cumulative lifetime risk of an upper tract UC was 2.6 % with Lynch syndrome, versus 0.25 % (men) and 0.1 % (women) lifetime risk for the general Dutch population). The risks of bladder UC (95 % CI 0.63–3.66) and renal adenocarcinoma (95 % CI 0.85–4.89) were not increased within kindreds. Vasen et al. identified the largest increase in risk of developing kidney, renal pelvis, and ureteric cancer (combined) when they studied 210 proven LS gene mutation carriers, in 19 families [24]. They found that those families with hMSH2 mutations had a relative risk of 75.3 (95 % CI 31.3–180.9) for developing a renal or ureteric malignancy, unlike hMLH1 carriers that showed no increased risk, when compared with the general population. This corresponds to a lifetime's cumulative risk of 12 % for 70-year-old hMSH2 mutation carriers versus 1.3 % for hMLH1 [18]. Aarnio et al. studied 50 Finnish LS families with proven MMR gene mutations [25]. They also found an increased risk of UC, with a standardized incidence rate (SIR) of 7.6 (95 % CI of 2.5–18). When converted to a cumulative lifetime risk, in agreement with Sijmons et al., this represents a 2–4 % of developing uroepithelial cancer by 70 years of age. Most recently, Skeldon et al. reported an increase risk for bladder UC (as well as upper tract UC) in Canadian LS families [26].

Overall, the risk of developing an UTUC by the age of 70 in LS is between 2 and 4 %, which is around 8- to 16-fold higher than the general population. Urothelial tumors occur in younger patients; for example, the average age at diagnosis is around 56 years old [17] and 58 years old [23], compared to the general population (peak age is between 60 and 80 years old).

Detecting Lynch Syndrome

Clinicians may care for patients with undiagnosed LS [27]. Consensus criteria (Table 1.2) have been defined to aid identification of these patients. As urologists, the typical presentation may be an upper tract UC (of which the distal ureter seems more common) in a young patient (affecting females more commonly than sporadic tumors), without a risk factor for UC (such as a nonsmoker) and with either a family or personal history of cancers within LS [14]. Pathologically, UC within LS have an

Table 1.2 Amsterdam criteria for the identification of HNPCC [28]

After the exclusion of familial adenomatous polyposis
1) At least three family members with colorectal cancer, two of whom are first-degree relatives.
2) At least two generations represented.
3) At least one individual younger than 50 years old at diagnosis.

inverted growth pattern [13] that may be used to suggest the syndrome, and are typically diploid rather than aneuploid.

In patients suspected to have Lynch syndrome, loss of MMR may be detected by using either immunohistochemistry for MMR proteins (start with hMLH1 and hMSH2), DNA microsatellite analysis, or the detection of MMR mutation by DNA sequencing (Fig. 1.1) [29–31].

Clinical Implications of Loss of Mismatch Repair

MMR proteins are key to DNA repair. Tumors without MMR generate a larger number of DNA mutations than MMR-proficient cancers. As a consequence, MMR-deficient tumors lose control of many cellular processes, and the consequential tumors are more indolent than expected by their pathological appearance [32, 33]. In addition, the MMR proteins recognize DNA damage induced by certain chemotherapeutic agents, such as alkylating agents (MNNG), base analogues (6-thioguanine), adduct forming agents (cisplatin family), double strand break agents (doxorubicin (adriamycin)), and the fluoropyrimidine anti-metabolites (5-fluorouracil and 5-fluoro-2′-deoxyuridine) [34, 35]. Tumors without MMR fail to recognize DNA damage (from cisplatin) and do not respond by apoptosis. Thus these tumors do not respond to chemotherapy, as well as MMR-proficient cancers [36, 37]. In contrast, MMR-deficient cells are more sensitive to topoisomerase inhibitors, such as camptothecin and etoposide [38].

Implications for Sporadic Upper Tract Urothelial Carcinoma

In colorectal cancer, LS is estimated to account for around 5 % of all cancers. In the remaining 95 % of cancers, around 10 % share molecular features with MMR-deficient tumors, typically by losing MMR through DNA hypermethylation of hMLH1. The prevalence of LS in upper tract UC is unknown, but it is reasonable to assume a similar proportion to colorectal cancer (around 5 %). Between 10 and 15 % of sporadic upper tract UC also lose MMR expression by epigenetic means (also DNA hypermethylation of hMLH1) [13, 39, 40]. It is likely that these tumors will have a similar phenotype to LS cancers, in terms of prognosis and drug resistance.

Low Penetrance Genetic Events

Variation is necessary for the health of a population. This variation may arise at a number of molecular levels, including differences in DNA sequence. Sequence changes are extremely common and affect single DNA bases. SNPs may or may not alter the expression (if the SNP is within a promoter region) or amino acid coding (if exonic) of a protein. Changes in protein sequence may affect the structure and activity of that molecule. In UC, several important variations in gene efficacy have been identified, especially in detoxification and DNA repair pathways. More recently, technological advances allow the comparison of large numbers of SNPs between cases and controls. These experiments have yielded new knowledge into the biology of UC.

Detoxification Pathways

UC mostly arise following exposure to carcinogens, such as those from cigarette smoke or occupational tasks. Protein coding SNPs that affect the abundance and activity of detoxification proteins will prolong or reduce the duration of carcinogen exposure (Fig. 1.2). The two enzymes most implicated in UC carcinogenesis are N-acetyltransferase 2 (NAT2) and glutathione S-transferase M1 (GSTM1) [41]. Carcinogens may be detoxified by NAT2 or GSTM1 in the liver epithelium, before excretion of nonreactive (noncarcinogenic) products. Failure of this detoxification leads to CYP1A2 hydroxylation in the liver and transportation to the urine. In the urinary tract, NAT1 acetylation creates active carcinogenic metabolites. Thus, persons with slow or low NAT2 activity, reduced GSTM1 alleles, or fast/high NAT1 activity will create more urothelial carcinogens than the general population. Several authors have confirmed these effects in the bladder. For example, Garcia-Closas et al. investigated SNPs or deletions in NAT2, NAT1, GSTM1, GSTT1, GSTM3, and GSTP1 in 1,150 Caucasian Spanish patients with bladder UC and 1,149 controls. They identified elevated risks of UC for individuals with deletion of one or both copies of GSTM1 (odds ratio 1.2- and 1.9-fold, respectively) and for NAT2 slow acetylators (1.4 [1.2–1.7]). These SNPs appeared more

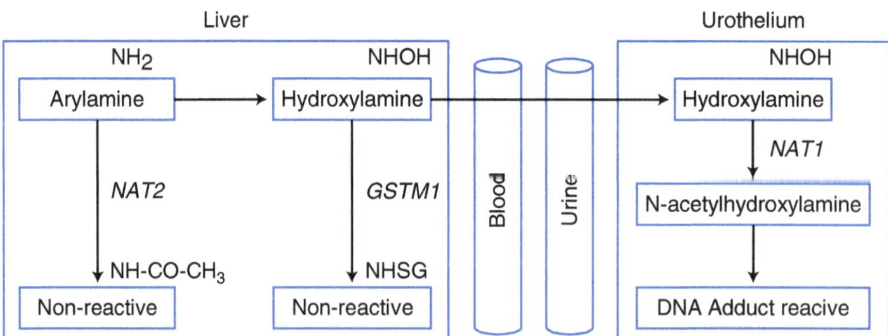

Fig. 1.2 Detoxification of arylamine and UCC carcinogenesis. Arylamines can be detoxified by acetylation (NAT2) in the liver, or hydroxylated by CYP1A2 and transported to the urinary tract. Here they undergo acetylation by NAT1, to form a highly reactive species. Genetic variants that reduce NAT2 activity and increase NAT1 activity increase UCC risk following arylamine exposure (adapted from Jung I, Messing E. Molecular Mechanisms and Pathways in Bladder Cancer Development and Progression. Cancer Control 2000: 7(4):pages 325–334)

important in cigarette smokers than never smokers (especially for NAT2), in keeping with their detoxification role.

While reports regarding bladder UC and detoxification enzyme SNPs are numerous, there are few examining UTUC. Bringuier et al. genotyped CYP1A1/NAT1 SNPs and GSTT1/GSTM1 deletions in 105 patients with renal pelvic UC, and compared to a history of analgesic ingestion or tobacco smoking [42]. Variants SNPs were detected in 6 % for CYP1A1 and 23 % for NAT1, and absent GSTT1 and GSTM1 were found in 12 % and 39 %, respectively. These proportions were similar to general population estimates, and so no association was found with these SNPs, carcinogen exposure, and renal pelvic UC. The authors concluded this may indicate that urinary mutagenicity is less important in renal pelvic than in bladder tumor development, though the sample size of this study does not allow definite conclusions. Katoh et al. examined deletion of GSTM1 and CYP1A1 polymorphisms in 83 UC patients (including 18 with upper tract UC) [43]. They identified an increased risk of UC, but were underpowered for an anatomical subgroup analysis. The same group examined GSTM1 and GSTT1 in 145 UC patients, of which 33 had upper tract disease (10 cases of renal pelvis cancer, 12 cases of ureter cancer, and 11 overlapping cases) [44]. An increased risk of UC was seen for bladder cancer (Odds ratio 1.78 [1.05–3.02]), and perhaps for ureteric cancer (2.00 [0.38–10.41]), but not renal pelvic disease (0.44 [0.07–2.66]). However, the low sample size prevented sufficiently powerful analysis to determine any true associations.

Other workers have focused on cytosolic sulfotransferases (SULT) [45], which detoxify environmental chemicals and activate mutagens through the conjugation of sulfo groups. There are two major families of sulfotransferases (phenol (SULT1A1) and hydroxysteroid (SULT2A)). *SULT1A1* is expressed in liver, lung, and kidney and has a polymorphism (SULT1A1*2) in exon 7 producing a histidine substitution of an arginine residue, which decreases enzymatic activity (to alter the rate of mutagen and pro-carcinogen detoxification/bioactivation rates). Rourpet et al. genotyped 268 patients with upper tract UC and 268 healthy matched controls. The SULT1A1*2 polymorphism was significantly more common in patients than controls (37 % versus 29 %) and conferred a higher risk of UC (odds ratio = 2.18 [1.28–3.69]).

Genome-Wide SNP Analysis in UC

Most recently, technological breakthroughs have enabled massive parallel SNP analysis in single experiments. This has allowed large studies to examine millions of coding SNPS in well-powered cohorts. Collaborative consortia have analyzed 11,914 UC bladder cancer cases and 53,395 matched controls for up to 591,637 SNPs [46]. Several key regions and SNPs have been identified, including 3q28, 4p16.3, 8q24.21, 8q24.3, 22q13.1, 19q12, and 2q37.1. With regard to UC in the upper tract, Roupret et al. analyzed rs9642880 on chromosome 8q24 in 261 patients with upper urinary tract UC and 261 matched controls [47]. They identified the T/T genotype increased the risk of UC (odds ratio = 1.72 (1.1–2.8) was associated with aggressive tumors when stratified by stage and grade G2 ($p = 0.04$).

Acquired Exposures and Upper Tract Urothelial Carcinogenesis

Exposures Shared by Urothelial Carcinoma in the Bladder and Upper Tracts

Regardless of genetic predisposition, most UC arise following exogenous carcinogen exposure. As detailed, a gene/environmental interaction occurs between carcinogens and an individual's ability to detoxify these chemicals. The vast majority of carcinogens for UC are thought to be derived from either tobacco smoke or occupational exposures.

Cigarette Smoking

It is estimated that cigarette smoking is the major carcinogenic exposure for around 50 % of UC [48]. Tobacco smoke contains aromatic amines, such as beta-naphthylamine and 4-aminobiphenyl, and polycyclic aromatic hydrocarbons known to cause UC [49]. Exposure to these chemicals varies with proximity (direct smokers versus passive inhalation of environmental tobacco smoke (ETS)), dose and chronicity (combined as pack years), tobacco type (dark (higher concentrations of N-nitrosamine and 2-napthylamine) versus blonde tobacco [49, 50]), inhalation into the mouth or chest [48], and current behavior (ex versus current smokers).

Cigarette smoke inhalation increases the risk of developing an UTUC by three- to sevenfold, compared to the general population [51–53]. As with bladder UC, this risk is dose adjusted, and doubles from 2.4-fold (history of <20 cigarettes per day) to 4.8-fold (>40 cigarettes per day) with increasing exposures [52]. This risk is halved with cessation of smoking for more than 10 years. Due to gender-specific smoking patterns, the same authors estimated that 7 of 10 cancers of the renal pelvis and ureter in men, and almost 4 of 10 among women were caused by smoking.

Occupational Carcinogen Exposure

It is estimated that between 5 and 15 % of UC arise following occupation carcinogen exposure and that there is a male predominance [54, 55]. Occupational carcinogens are best divided by chemical structure into aromatic amines, polycyclic aromatic hydrocarbons (PAHs), and tobacco smoke/combustion products (such as firefighters and bar staff). Exposure to aromatic amines occurs in printers, painters, rubber and dye workers, hairdresser, and the textile industry. Exposure to PAHs occurs in aluminum refining, diesel fumes (drivers, seamen, miners, etc.), metal workers, and medical staff (such as nurses).

As with other aspects of UC biology, most data exist for bladder cancer, rather than for UTUC. Wilson et al. surveyed 4.2 million Swedish persons, including

1,374 with renal pelvic and 21,567 with bladder UC for occupational history [56]. Most (80 %) has stayed in the same occupational group over the 16 years follow-up, including 16 % of those with upper tract UC were involved in metal work. When bladder and upper tract UC were compared there were many similarities. However, several occupations appeared more specific to the renal pelvices, including pharmacists, journalists, business executives, food-related workers, food process workers, and chemical workers for females, and insurance clerks, butchers, cleaners and pulp grinding, metal manufacturing, scientific/surgical instruments, insurance, and legal industries for males. McCredie et al. reported occupation risks for kidney cancer and renal pelvic UC in New South Wales [57]. When compared, an increased risk of only UC was seen in the dry cleaning (relative risk = 4.68 [1.32–16.56]) and Iron and Steel industries (2.13 [1.04–4.39]).

Acquired Exposures more Specific to UTUC

Aristolochic Acid

The *Aristolochiaceae* family of herbaceous plants, in particular, members of the genus *Aristolochia*, has been used for medicinal purposes for more than 2,500 years [58, 59]. *Aristolochia* species contain a family of structurally related nitrophenanthrene carboxylic acids, principally aristolochic acid I (AA-I) and aristolochic acid II (AA-II) [60] (Fig. 1.3). More than a century ago, Pohl noted the nephrotoxic effects of these compounds by administering to rabbits extracts prepared from seeds and roots of *Aristolochia clematitis* [61]. More recently, Mengs further documented in rodents the acute and chronic toxicities of purified AAs [62], including their carcinogenic effects [63, 64].

Less than 20 years have passed since exposure to AA was identified as a risk factor for UTUC in humans [65]. This association, manifested as an iatrogenic disease in Europe and Asia and as an environmental disease in the Balkans, resulted in AAs being classified formally as Group I human carcinogens [66, 67].

Fig 1.3 Chemical structures of aristolochic acids (AA)-I and -II, and phenacetin, carcinogens associated with upper tract urothelial cancers

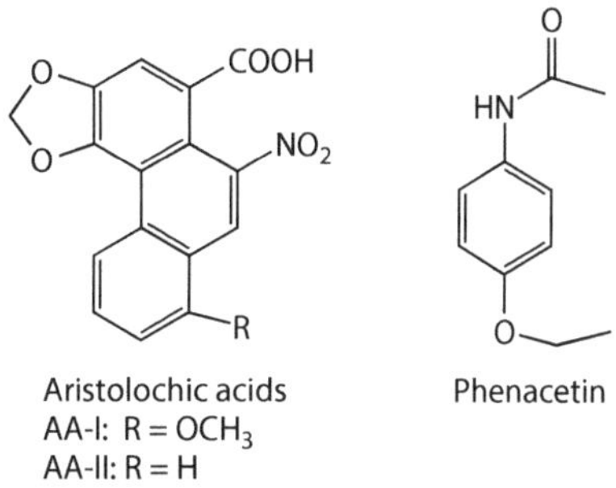

Chinese Herbs Nephropathy in Belgium

In the early 1990s, a direct connection was established between AA exposure and human disease, made possible by studies of a cohort of Belgian women exposed inadvertently to AA [2, 3]. This group was identified initially as a cluster of young women in Brussels with end-stage renal disease (ESRD) of unknown origin [68]. A shared etiology was suspected due to demographic features and grouping of cases. Further investigation revealed that all of these women participated in a weight-loss regimen that included the use of various drugs and Chinese herbs. Suspicions fell on *Stephania tetrandra*, an herb introduced into the formulation in May 1990 and used through July 1992. However, as *S. tetrandra* was known not to be toxic, the cause of the renal disease affecting the Belgian women remained a mystery until it was shown that this herb had been replaced with AA-containing *Aristolochia fangchi*. Proof of exposure to AA was subsequently validated by the (1) chemical identification of AA in the herbs imported from China [69] and (2) detection of unique AA metabolites bound covalently to DNA in tissues obtained from these patients [65, 70]. Based on prescription data and the AA content of the herb, the average dose of AA was estimated as 0.025 mg/kg body weight per day, consumed over 13 months [2]. Despite comparable dosing, nephropathy developed in only 5 % of the 1,500–2,000 Belgians who were exposed to AA, suggesting a significant role for gene variants in determining individual susceptibility to disease.

The renal disease affecting the Belgian patients was originally named Chinese herbs nephropathy (CHN) and later retitled aristolochic acid nephropathy (AAN) to more accurately reflect the etiology of this disease [71]. AAN is a chronic, progressive, and irreversible tubulointerstitial disease characterized by renal insufficiency, pronounced and early anemia, low molecular weight (tubular) proteinuria, and variable glycosuria [72, 73]. The histopathology of AAN has several defining features including (1) widespread atrophy of proximal tubules, with a gradient of injury decreasing in severity from outer to inner cortex; (2) interstitial fibrosis, mostly confined to the cortex; (3) absence of significant inflammation; and (4) relative sparing of glomeruli [72, 74].

The initial connection between AA exposure and urothelial malignancies arose from observations of three Belgian AAN patients who underwent kidney transplantation for ESRD [72]. All had used the AA-containing herbal product for 1–1.5 years and had discontinued its use 3–5 months prior to surgery. Histopathological review of the native upper urinary tract revealed the widespread presence of mild-to-moderate urothelial atypia and focal squamous metaplasia. Over the following year, one patient developed UC affecting the bladder, remnant ureter, and the contralateral ureter and renal pelvis [75].

The carcinogenic potential of AA was appreciated more fully as similar upper tract lesions were observed in other Belgian patients with AAN [65, 73, 76]. Concerns regarding the high risk of developing UTUC prompted the recommendation of prophylactic bilateral nephroureterectomy in this population [65, 76]. This strategy proved effective as renal pelvic and/or ureteral tumors were detected in over 40 % of the patients who opted for this surgery [77]. In one group of ten patients who received transplants 9–67 months after discontinuing use of the herbal remedy (mean use duration of 20 months), four had developed carcinoma in situ, present in three patients in both the ureter and renal pelvis, along with papillary upper tract UC in one case [76]. Atypia of the papillary collecting ducts and urothelium was noted in all ten patients.

In a second set of 39 patients with AAN, UC was present in 18, all confined to the upper urinary tract except for one incidence of bladder cancer; 19 of the remaining cases showed mild-to-moderate dysplasia, while no lesions were found in 2 patients [65]. Aristolactam–DNA adducts, products of AA metabolism, were detected in renal cortex and tumor tissues, providing irrefutable evidence of prior exposure to AA [65]. Retrospective analyses of exposure data for this cohort revealed a correlation between the risk of developing UTUC with cumulative dose of AA.

Although UTUC is the primary cancer caused by AA in humans, long-term follow-up studies of the Belgian cohort revealed a heightened risk of UC of the bladder, which developed in 15/38 AAN patients within 15 years following bilateral nephroureterectomy and renal transplant [77, 78]. As 80 % of these bladder cancer patients were diagnosed with UTUC at the time of surgery, these tumors may have originated from malignant cells shed from upper tract tumors and seeded in the bladder. However, 20 % of these tumors occurred in patients with no history of UTUC, suggesting that bladder malignancies may arise from a direct carcinogenic effect of AA on the bladder urothelium. Given its long-term carcinogenic potential, vigilant screening of the entire urinary tract is considered prudent practice for follow-up of patients with known or suspected exposure to AA [77].

Balkan Endemic Nephropathy

Balkan endemic nephropathy (BEN) is an acronym applied to a chronic, progressive, tubulointerstitial renal disease, limited to residents of rural villages located near tributaries of the Danube River in Bosnia and Herzogovina, Bulgaria, Croatia, Romania, and Serbia [79]. First reported in the late 1950s, BEN is estimated to affect at least 25,000 men and women in countries harboring this disease; a far larger number of individuals are believed to be at risk [80].

UTUC eventually develop in approximately half of all patients diagnosed with BEN. The prevalence of this cancer in certain endemic regions can be as much as 100-fold greater than in the country as a whole [81]. Data from a review of BEN-associated UTUC were used to explore the epidemiology of this otherwise rare cancer over the past 50 years [82, 83]. Until recently, the etiology of UTUC associated with BEN remained obscure. A variety of environmental mutagens, including mycotoxins and heavy metals, have been systematically investigated as potential causative agents of BEN/UTUC [84]. Ochratoxin A (OTA) had been the principal focus of this research. However, solid epidemiologic evidence supporting an association between exposure to OTA and the prevalence of BEN/UTUC in endemic regions is lacking [85]. In contrast, the studies summarized below support strongly the hypothesis that chronic, low-dose dietary poisoning by AA accounts for all of the important characteristics of BEN, including its geographical distribution, and the increased risk of developing UTUC.

The pathophysiology of BEN bears a striking resemblance to that observed in Belgian women with CHN/AAN; however, residents of endemic villages in Croatia deny the use of herbs containing *Aristolochia* [86]. An alternative route of exposure, first suggested by Ivić [87], is based on the frequent occurrence of *Aristolochia clematitis* as a weed growing in local wheat fields. Ivić observed that the traditional methods used for harvesting and milling of wheat permitted seeds of *A. clematitis* to comingle with the wheat grain used to prepare home-baked bread, a dietary staple among residents of all endemic regions. Thirty-five years later, these astute field observations were confirmed by Hranjeć et al. [88].

Molecular epidemiologic evidence that patients with BEN/UTUC had been previously exposed to aristolochic acid was provided by Grollman, Jelaković, and their colleagues [89, 90], who detected aristolactam (AL)–DNA adducts in the renal cortex of 70 % of these individuals. Their presence in renal tissue reflects active transport of AAs by the renal proximal tubule [91]. Enzymatic nitroreduction of AA yields a product that undergoes sulfonation [92], generating reactive intermediates that form covalent aristolactam (AL) adducts with dA and dG residues in DNA. Lower levels of these adducts are found in the urothelium. The steady-state level of AL-dA adducts in target tissues represents an integration of external exposure with interindividual variability in metabolism and other cellular processes, providing a link between exposure to AA and its cytotoxic and carcinogenic effects. Moreover, AL-dA adducts are highly resistant to global genomic nucleotide excision repair [93], leading to their persistence in target tissues, enhancing their usefulness as biomarkers of exposure. Thus, among Belgian women with CHN, AL-DNA adducts could be detected in the renal cortex 36–89 months following their last exposure to AA [65].

A:T-to-T:A transversions, predicted by the miscoding properties of AL-dA adducts in mammalian cells [94], represent only 5 % of somatic *TP53* mutations in all types of cancers combined [95], yet they dominate the *TP53* mutation spectrum in AA-induced UTUC [90, 96]. A-to-T transversions constitute 58 % of *TP53* sequence changes in UTUC linked to AA exposure but less than 2 % in UTUC of patients with no apparent exposure to AA [97]. Thus, the proportion of A:T-to-T:A mutations in UTUC, coupled with their predominance at splice sites and strong bias for the non-transcribed strand [96], was established as a mutational signature for exposure to AA [97].

Taken together, these molecular epidemiologic studies document a *causal* relationship between AA and BEN/UTUC. In commenting on this research, DeBroe proposed that BEN/UTUC and CHN should be considered a single clinical entity, namely AAN [98].

Herbal Medicine Use in Taiwan

The earliest mention of *Aristolochia* in China dates to the fifth century AD; references to various species of this herb appear in virtually all major treatises of traditional Chinese medicine that have appeared since that time [99]. Remarkably, descriptions of the medicinal use of *Aristolochia* rarely mention intrinsic toxicity, although the doses employed are similar to those in the Belgian cohort. To address this enigma, the molecular epidemiologic approach used to explore the etiology of BEN [90] was adopted for studies in Taiwan, where the incidence of UTUC is reported to be the highest of any country in the world [100]. Moreover, the demographics of UTUC in Taiwan mimic that in the endemic regions of the Balkans.

In Taiwan, a systematic analysis of the national prescription reimbursement database between 1997 and 2003 suggested that approximately one-third of the entire country's population had been exposed to herbs containing, or likely to contain, AA [101]. Additionally, a linear dose–response relationship has been demonstrated between the consumption of herbal remedies containing AA and the risk of developing UC [100].

Subjects of the study [102, 103], selected from among 212 consecutive Taiwanese UTUC patients who received nephroureterectomies between 1999 and 2011, included 151 patients with UTUC, and 25 cases of renal cell carcinoma (RCC) to serve as controls. Unequivocal evidence of exposure of this cohort to AA is reflected by the observation that 60 % of all cases of UTUC and 84 % of patients with A:T-to-T:A mutations in *TP53* contained AL-dA adducts in their renal cortex. AL-dA adducts also were present in 60 % of patients with RCC; however, in this group, A:T-to-T:A mutations were not detected in *TP53*. In the Taiwanese cohort, 60 % of women and 50 % of men with *TP53* mutations displayed signature A:T-to-T:A mutations. Remarkably, despite significant differences in the dose, frequency, and timing of exposure to AA, the overall distribution and positions of A:T-to-T:A transversions in the *TP53* gene of patients with UTUC were almost identical to those observed in the Balkan cohort [103].

An unusually large number of splice-site mutations are observed in AA-associated UTUC. And, when *TP53* mutational data derived from 97 patients with UTUC/BEN [96] are combined with data with 151 UTUC patients from Taiwan [103], all 5′-AG acceptor sites in *TP53* were found to be mutated at least once, with introns 6 and 8 identified as prominent hotspots. This unusual finding is consistent with the preferential targeting of adenine residues in DNA by AA [104].

In the Taiwanese cohort, the oncogenes, *FGFR3* and *HRAS*, appear to be activated by mutations induced by AA. As in *TP53*, adenine residues mutated in *FGFR3* codon 373 and *HRAS* codon 61 are found invariably on the non-transcribed strand. The majority of this subgroup of cases had been exposed to AA.

In conclusion, AA, an intrinsic component of all *Aristolochia* herbal remedies, contributes significantly to the incidence of UTUC in Taiwan. As the practice of traditional Chinese herbal medicine in Taiwan mirrors that of mainland China and the carcinogenic effects of AA do not manifest themselves until 30 years after exposure, this finding, as discussed below, has implications for public health in China, India, and other countries where *Aristolochia* herbs have been traditionally used for the treatment and prevention of disease in recent years [105].

Global Prevalence of AA-Induced UTUC

Aristolochia plants are components of herbal remedies used in the practice of (1) Traditional Chinese Medicine (TCM) in China and other Asian countries; (2) Kampo medicine in Japan; and (3) Ayurvedic medicine in India and South Asia. These practices, along with the traditional use of *Aristolochia* sp. for medicinal purposes in various regions of Africa and in South and Central America, pose a significant global health threat [58, 103, 106, 107]. Furthermore, the growing popularity of alternative medicine in Western countries has led to sporadic cases of nephropathy and/or UTUC related to *Aristolochia* use. Although many governments, including the US, have banned the importation of *Aristolochia* products, while others prohibit the use of this herb for medicinal purposes, over-the-counter formulations containing AA remain available for purchase in local herb shops and via the Internet [108]. Some suppliers fail to disclose that *Aristolochia* is a component of their herbal product, posing a hidden danger to consumers [109, 110].

Worldwide, more than 300 cases of UTUC related to AA exposure via herbal medicines have been reported [111–113]. Many cases go unrecognized due to the long (20–40 year) latency period between AA exposure and detection of cancer, resulting in underestimation of true prevalence. Sporadic cases of UTUC linked to the medicinal use of *Aristolochia* plants have been reported from Hong Kong, Japan, Australia, UK, and the United States, and there is documented evidence of widespread disease in China and Taiwan (see section above), countries with long histories of *Aristolochia* use. In China, renal transplant or chronic hemodialysis patients with a prior history of *Aristolochia* use have a greater risk of developing urothelial malignancies [111, 114, 115]. AA exposure also is associated with an increased incidence of contralateral metachronous UTUC in China [116].

Phenacetin and Analgesic Nephropathy

Phenacetin (*p*-ethoxyacetanilide; Fig. 1.3), a pro-drug for acetaminophen, is a synthetic analgesic antipyretic agent that was first introduced into the pharmaceutical market in 1897. The original formulations, sold over-the-counter under various trade names, such as Anacin® and Bex®, typically contained phenacetin in combination with other drugs including caffeine, aspirin, or phenazone. Due to their widespread availability and efficacy, phenacetin-containing analgesic mixtures were highly popular in Europe, Australia, and North America for much of the twentieth century. However, in the 1950s, safety concerns emerged when the habitual use of phenacetin was linked to renal insufficiency and tubulointerstitial disease [117–119], a condition known as analgesic nephropathy. Renal papillary necrosis is a frequent and distinctive feature of this disease. In the 1960s, Hultengren made the etiologic connection between abuse of phenacetin-containing analgesics and the development of UTUC through a study of six Swedish patients diagnosed with both papillary necrosis and UC of the renal pelvis [120]. All but one of the patients had a history of phenacetin addiction, with reported cumulative doses ranging up to 10 kg. Reports of similar cases soon followed, so that by 1983 more than 400 patients with UTUC worldwide, particularly in Australia, Switzerland, Belgium, Denmark, and Sweden, had been linked to excessive habitual use of phenacetin [118, 119]. The geographic distribution of many cases aligned closely with known sites of phenacetin hyperconsumption and analgesic nephropathy [118, 119, 121].

An estimated 8–10 % of patients diagnosed with nephropathy due to phenacetin abuse eventually develop urothelial malignancies [122]. The upper urinary tract appears to be the preferred target tissue, as UC rates are 77 and 89 times higher in the renal pelvis and the ureter, respectively, compared to only seven times higher in the bladder, among patients who consume excessive amounts of phenacetin [118]. These tumors are often multifocal, can be bilateral, and are more common in females since this gender appears to be more likely to abuse phenacetin-containing analgesics. The majority of patients with phenacetin-linked UTUC have renal insufficiency and renal papillary necrosis at the time of clinical presentation. The incidence of UTUC is associated with an average cumulative consumption of 9 kg phenacetin, a mean exposure duration of 17 years, and a mean induction period of 22 years [118].

Concerns regarding the high incidence of ESRD and UTUC associated with the prolonged and excessive use of phenacetin compelled both public health officials and pharmaceutical companies to ensure its removal from drug markets around the world. These efforts, which varied considerably among countries, began in the 1970s and continued throughout the 1980s [123]. In Australia, the incidence rate for renal disease related to analgesic use declined significantly within 10 years following withdrawal of phenacetin from analgesic mixtures [124], whereas no change occurred in the cancer incidence. This finding reflects the long latency period (20 years) associated with this type of malignancy, as the incidence did decline in subsequent years [125]. Retrospective review of over 600 autopsy samples collected between 2000 and 2002 in Switzerland revealed a tenfold decrease in the frequency of analgesic nephropathy, and a normal incidence of urothelial cell cancer, some 20 years after phenacetin was removed from the Swiss market [126]. Of concern, some countries, such as Hungary, where the drug was still available as of 2008, have lagged behind in efforts to remove phenacetin from the market [123].

Based on their association with UTUC, both phenacetin and analgesic mixtures that contain phenacetin are designated by IARC as a Group 1 carcinogen in humans [123]. Mutations in the tumor suppressor gene *TP53* are detected in 45 % of phenacetin-linked tumors [42], although neither the frequency nor the type of mutation differs from those found in UTUC of unknown etiology. The molecular mechanism underlying the carcinogenic action of phenacetin has not been resolved. Phase I N-hydroxylation products of this aromatic amide may undergo Phase II bioactivation to generate reactive metabolites that are directly mutagenic [127]. Alternatively, the chronic inflammation that accompanies renal papillary necrosis may promote malignant transformation in conjunction with chemical carcinogens [42, 128]. However, as UTUC is not associated with high intake of other analgesics that cause renal papillary disease [122], a role for phenacetin metabolites cannot be excluded.

Previous Urothelial Cancer in the Bladder or Contralateral Upper Tract

The frequent development of metachronous lesions throughout the entire urinary tract is a characteristic of UC. Metachronous bladder recurrence after UTUC occurs in up to 50 % of cases [129], while the secondary development of UTUC after UC of the bladder (UCB) occurs in 2–9 % of patients. Wright et al. reported these events in almost 100,000 patients from the Surveillance, Epidemiology and End Results (SEER) registry [130]. Of 56,271 patients with a Ta bladder tumor at diagnosis, 0.3 % were subsequently diagnosed with an UTUC. These findings are especially significant as they reflect the risk of recurrence in patients in community practice, rather than from tertiary centers alone. Risk of UTUC varies with UCB tumor stage and grade. Around 20 % of recurrences after radical cystectomy (for invasive UCB) are UTUCs [131]. Picozzi et al. evaluated the frequency of secondary UTUC after radical cystectomy. They conducted a meta-analysis covering a 40-year period with a total of 13,185 participants in 27 studies. The overall prevalence of UTUC after radical cystectomy ranged from 0.75 % to 6.4 % [132], supporting other reports [133, 134].

While numerous studies have reported UTUC after radical cystectomy, few data examine the risk of contralateral UTUC following a previous UTUC. In a population of 231 patients with primary UTUC, Novara et al. found a contralateral upper tract recurrence rate of 6 % [129]. Even scarcer are data on recurrences after organ-sparing approaches. Nearly all the published series included only patients with radical nephroureterectomy. The question as to whether terminal ureterectomy and ureteric reimplantation elevate the risk of metachronous bladder recurrence or contralateral recurrence cannot be answered based on the current literature.

Risk Over Time

Metachronous UTUC recurrences are considered late oncological events as they have been reported to occur after a time range of 24–41 months after radical cystectomy [135]. According to the analysis of the SEER database, about 71 % of all UTUC cases following primary UCB occur within the first 5 years from the diagnosis, with the median time to recurrence 33 months [130]. Tran and colleagues showed that the cumulative risk of upper urinary tract recurrence nearly doubles between 3 and 5 years after radical cystectomy from 4 % to 7 % [136]. Picozzi reported ureteral recurrences 13 years after curative surgery, which underlines the importance of long-term surveillance [132].

Prognostic Risk Factors for Upper Tract Recurrence

Tumor Grade at Cystectomy

Within the last 30 years, about 30 retrospective studies reported on prognostic factors for UTUC recurrence after radical cystectomy. The meta-analysis by Picozzi et al. included all these studies to identify the predictive capacity of different risk factors [132]. It was shown that patients with G1 tumors have eightfold greater probability of UTUC recurrence compared to those with G2 cancer, increasing to tenfold when compared to patients with G3 disease. This surprising relation between low-grade disease and late upper tract recurrence is explained by the hypothesis that improved survival rates in invasive bladder cancer put patients at a higher long-term risk for tumor recurrence in the upper urinary tract.

Tumor Stage at Radical Cystectomy

Most recurrences occur in patients with organ-confined bladder cancer (pT2b N0 M0 or lower stage disease) [133, 137], which led to primary tumor stage being described as a possible risk factor for secondary UTUC. Meissner reported a 1.8- to 3.8-fold higher risk of UTUC recurrence in patients with pTa-T1 UCB compared to patients with muscle-invasive disease [138]. The meta-analysis by Picozzi showed that patients who underwent cystectomy for superficial tumors had twice the risk of developing metachronous UTUC compared to those with invasive lesions [132]. These data may reflect selection bias, given that many patients with more advanced disease succumbed to their bladder disease [139]. Patients with nodal involvement potentially only have a short-term follow-up due to their high mortality rate and therefore show a lower risk of secondary UTUC. Picozzi et al. calculated an eight-fold higher risk for patients with negative lymph nodes [132].

Carcinoma In Situ

Hurle et al. postulated a higher risk for developing UTUC after radical cystectomy for UCB [140]. Volkmer et al. identified an increased risk of 2.3-fold for patients with CIS compared to patients without this [141]. Picozzi et al. reported that patients with CIS have a twofold higher probability of metachronous UTUC than those with noninvasive cancer, and four times as high as those with invasive disease [132].

Compared to other patients, those with CIS only at radical cystectomy exhibit a higher risk of UTUC recurrence [142]. Conversely, in patients with muscle-invasive disease, concomitant CIS was not found to be independently associated with upper tract recurrence [143]. According to the findings regarding tumor grading and tumor stage, the data favoring CIS as a risk factor may actually have been artificially shifted towards the patient cohort with low-stage disease at cystectomy, as one must assume that the survival differences between different tumor stages had a confounding effect. For patients with a history of CIS or concomitant presence of CIS, Picozzi et al. come to the conclusion that the available data are not sufficient to establish a statistically significant difference regarding recurrence in patients with or without CIS [132].

Recurrent UCB and Focality

Multifocality of the initial UCB was found to independently contribute to a higher risk of ureteral involvement at radical cystectomy and subsequent upper tract recurrence [144]. Picozzi et al. confirmed this finding. They showed that the risk of secondary recurrence within the upper urinary tract was three times higher for multifocal UCB. Furthermore, there is a statistically significant difference in metachronous upper tract recurrence in patients with a history of multiple urothelial recurrences (2–4 times) compared to those with radical cystectomy after initial UCB diagnosis [132].

Ureteral Margin and Frozen Section Analysis

It has been shown that tumor involvement of the distal ureter at radical cystectomy is an independent risk factor for secondary UTUC [136], with a relative risk of approximately 2.6 [141]. Ureteral tumor involvement upon the final pathological analysis of radical cystectomy specimens is a frequent event, occurring in up to 13 % of patients [145–147]. There is substantial evidence to suggest that intraoperatively frozen section analysis is a reliable tool when performing a radical cystectomy. Gakis et al. found the overall accuracy of this method for the detection of malignant ureteral margins to be 98 % [144]. Sequential resection of malignant ureteral margins can be advocated to reduce the risk of a malignant anastomotic margin at cystectomy. Patients with initially positive but ultimately negative margins have a 4.4-fold higher risk of recurrence compared to patients with initially negative margins, but their risk decreases after surgical conversion to a final negative ureteral margin, since those patients with positive anastomotic margins had an even higher (7.4-fold) risk of recurrence. This was confirmed by Picozzi et al. who found a relative risk of 7.1 for metachronous UTUC in patients with positive ureteral margins [132].

History of UTUC

UTUC itself is a risk factor for subsequent further UTUC. Patients with a history of UTUC have a sevenfold higher risk of metachronous secondary UTUC [132].

Upper Tract Surveillance

Who to Screen for UTUC After UCB

Most UTUC recurrences after radical cystectomy for UCB are detected when patients present with symptoms, such as hematuria or flank pain. Sanderson et al. reported that 78 % of all UTUC recurrences in 27 patients in a cohort of 1,359 patients who underwent radical cystectomy for UCB were detected after the development of symptoms [148]. These symptoms are often associated with locally advanced disease and with poor outcomes following subsequent radical nephroureterectomy (RNU). Patients diagnosed with asymptomatic upper tract recurrence during routine follow-ups have a significantly higher survival advantage than those with symptomatic recurrences. This emphasizes the importance of early detection of secondary UTUC for the timely initiation of a curative treatment. Thus, strategies for the earlier detection of upper tract recurrences while still localized are necessary for effective treatment in the form of an RNU. Identification of risk factors and subsequent creation of subgroups of patients at different risks for recurrence could help to develop follow-up strategies. Risk-tailored schedules would also reduce unnecessary follow-up examinations and surveillance costs for low-risk patients.

Current guidelines do not recommend surveillance for patients with a low-grade primary bladder tumor and only recommend periodic surveillance for patients with a high-grade tumor based on a risk-tailored strategy [149, 150]. That said, a risk-adapted schedule for surveillance of the upper urinary tract with imaging techniques and cytology has not yet been established. Efforts have nonetheless been made to define a threshold at which surveillance should be initiated: Volkmer et al. performed a large retrospective analysis of long-term risk of secondary UTUC in 1,420 patients after radical cystectomy, and identified four risk factors including history of CIS, recurrent UCB, non-muscle-invasive UCB and tumor involvement of the distal ureter [141]. Interestingly, patients with none of these risk factors showed UTUC recurrence in only 1 % of cases within 15 years, patients with 1 or 2 risk factors recurred in 8 %, and patients with 3 and 4 risk factors in even 14 %. The consequence is that if patients do not have a risk factor (CIS, recurrent bladder cancer, distal ureteral involvement, multifocality, history of UTUC) they simply do not require routine upper tract monitoring. The more risk factors that are present, the more important surveillance of the upper tract becomes. Future work must be aimed at identifying patients at the greatest risk of a metachronous UTUC, a group that requires thorough follow-up examinations of the upper tract.

How to Screen for UTUC After UCB

Using current evidence it is not possible to define a uniform follow-up schedule for upper tract surveillance after radical cystectomy. This is reflected by the wide variance found in the practice of community urologists [151]. It is even less possible to define a specific follow-up schedule for patients after primary UTUC treated with a kidney-sparing approach. Nevertheless, it is possible to look at every single available surveillance measure in an evidence-based manner, with the goal of establishing a rough overview of the topic as a whole.

Following the ALARA principle ("as low as reasonable achievable"), routine radiologic imaging of the upper tract should be avoided whenever possible. Ultrasound examination of the kidneys should form the front line of every surveillance strategy, because it is not harmful and, ignoring initial acquisition costs, is relatively cheap. Ureteral disease such as UTUC can reveal its presence through sonographically detectable hydronephrosis long before other symptoms occur. The optimal interval cannot be determined from the literature, but in patients with medium to high risk of upper tract recurrence, a trimonthly ultrasound examination of the kidneys seems reasonable.

A second measure that can be undertaken in order to limit the risks of exposure to ionizing radiation and potentially nephrotoxic intravenous contrast material is urine cytology. However, for a rare event like metachronous UTUC after UCB, urine cytology fails to be a well-weighted surveillance examination due to its extremely low sensitivity. Picozzi et al. calculated that approximately 2,000 urine cytologies must be performed to identify 1 patient with UTUC recurrence [132]. This figure might appear a little friendlier within a series of patients with primary UTUC and organ-sparing approach, as urine cytology remains more reliable without diverted urinary tract. Nevertheless, routine urine cytology should be restricted to high-risk cases with the potential for long survival periods, e.g., young patients after radical cystectomy due to CIS-only and positive or intraoperatively converted negative ureteral margins.

The available imaging techniques are excretory urography, computed tomography (CT), and magnetic resonance imaging (MRI). Meissner et al. focused on excretory urography to detect metachronous UTUC [138]. Only 50 % of UTUC recurrences were detected by routine examination, while the remaining 50 % were detected as a result of symptoms between routine follow-up examinations. Also here, a risk-adapted usage of excretory urography is the reasonable consequence. For several decades, intravenous urography remained the standard for exploring the upper urinary tract, but multislice-detector CT urography has since become the new gold standard [152]. Near-isotropic high-quality multiplanar image reconstruction enables the functional and oncological examination of the upper urinary tract, and even enables the detection of flat lesions of the renal pelvis or ureter. However, despite meta-analyses of sensitivities and specificities of excretory urography and computed tomography across the literature, no randomized prospective comparing data have been published to date. Furthermore, any X-ray examination should be performed with the minimum radiation dose, in keeping with the ALARA principle. For these reasons, the diagnostic quality of CT urography still does not preclude the application of excretory urography. MRI without contrast medium is less helpful in diagnosing UTUC compared to CT urography due to its lower diagnostic accuracy, higher costs, and lower patient acceptability. Furthermore, MRI urography suffers from the limitation of poorer spatial resolution when compared to CT urography, as well as various artefacts, including motion artefacts from breathing and peristalsis, limit its current clinical importance in the detection of UTUC.

Ureterorenoscopy with biopsy is the diagnostic procedure of choice for the final diagnosis of metachronous UTUC after radical cystectomy, especially when suspicious findings are detected during imaging and/or urine cytology.

In conclusion, an individual risk-tailored follow-up must be undertaken to detect secondary UTUC earlier. Risk stratification models like the one presented by Volkmer et al. help to determine the risk of recurrence [141]. In low-risk patients, routine surveillance is not necessary, an approach which is in line with current guidelines. Patients with a high risk of recurrence should receive a closely meshed net of surveillance examinations, including ultrasound of the kidneys, urine examination (including urine cytology in selected cases), excretory urography, or CT urography. For patients with a medium risk of metachronous UTUC, a sound solution for surveillance must be found on an individual basis.

Executive Summary

- UTUC is a rare tumor with some specific etiological factors.
- More specific genetic factors include involvement in one hereditary cancer syndrome (Lynch Syndrome).
- More specific acquired exposures include aristolochic acid ingestion, through herbal medication, and the analgesic phenacetin.
- Pathological epidemiology suggests that aristolochic acid ingestion is a continuing global problem that leads to a large number of UTUC worldwide.
- The time between ingestion and UTUC is estimated to be 20–30 years.
- The etiological specificities of UTUC can be used to gain insights into the biology of UC as a whole.
- UTUC is a key event in the biology of UC, given the multiplicity and multifocality of this malignancy.
- While the overall risk of UTUC following bladder cancer is between 2 and 9 %, this varies in extent with the nature of the bladder tumor.
- Future work needs to define more specific predictive features for this disease to allow screening of at risk individuals.

References

1. Chavan S, Bray F, Lortet-Teulent J, Goodman MM, Jemal A. International variations in bladder cancer incidence and mortality. Eur Urol. 2014;66(1):59–73.
2. Cosyns JP. Aristolochic acid and 'Chinese herbs nephropathy': a review of the evidence to date. Drug Saf. 2003;26(1):33–48.
3. Nortier JL, Vanherweghem JL. Renal interstitial fibrosis and urothelial carcinoma associated with the use of a Chinese herb (Aristolochia fangchi). Toxicology. 2002;181–182:577–80.

4. Mueller CM, Caporaso N, Greene MH. Familial and genetic risk of transitional cell carcinoma of the urinary tract. Urol Oncol. 2008;26(5):451–64.
5. Grignon DJ, Shum DT, Bruckschwaiger O. Transitional cell carcinoma in the Muir-Torre syndrome. J Urol. 1987;138(2):406–8.
6. Bapat B, Xia L, Madlensky L, et al. The genetic basis of Muir-Torre syndrome includes the hMLH1 locus. Am J Hum Genet. 1996;59(3):736–9.
7. Lynch HT, Smyrk T. An update on Lynch syndrome. Curr Opin Oncol. 1998;10(4):349–56.
8. Warthin AS. Heredity with reference to carcinoma. Arch Intern Med. 1913;12:546–55.
9. Modrich P. Strand-specific mismatch repair in mammalian cells. J Biol Chem. 1997;272(40): 24727–30.
10. Clark AB, Cook ME, Tran HT, Gordenin DA, Resnick MA, Kunkel TA. Functional analysis of human MutSalpha and MutSbeta complexes in yeast. Nucleic Acids Res. 1999;27(3): 736–42.
11. Harfe BD, Jinks-Robertson S. DNA mismatch repair and genetic instability. Annu Rev Genet. 2000;34:359–99.
12. Lipkin SM, Wang V, Jacoby R, et al. MLH3: a DNA mismatch repair gene associated with mammalian microsatellite instability. Nat Genet. 2000;24(1):27–35.
13. Catto JW, Azzouzi AR, Amira N, et al. Distinct patterns of microsatellite instability are seen in tumours of the urinary tract. Oncogene. 2003;22(54):8699–706.
14. Yates DR, Catto JW. Distinct patterns and behavior of urothelial carcinoma with respect to anatomical location: how molecular biomarkers can augment clinico-pathological predictors in upper urinary tract tumours. World J Urol. 2013;31(1):21–9.
15. Lynch HT, Watson P, Kriegler M, et al. Differential diagnosis of hereditary nonpolyposis colorectal cancer (Lynch syndrome I and Lynch syndrome II). Dis Colon Rectum. 1988;31(5): 372–7.
16. Lynch HT, Smyrk TC, Watson P, et al. Genetics, natural history, tumor spectrum, and pathology of hereditary nonpolyposis colorectal cancer: an updated review. Gastroenterology. 1993;104(5):1535–49.
17. Watson P, Lynch HT. Extracolonic cancer in hereditary nonpolyposis colorectal cancer. Cancer. 1993;71(3):677–85.
18. Vasen HF, Stormorken A, Menko FH, et al. MSH2 mutation carriers are at higher risk of cancer than MLH1 mutation carriers: a study of hereditary nonpolyposis colorectal cancer families. J Clin Oncol. 2001;19(20):4074–80.
19. Lynch HT, Ens JA, Lynch JF. The Lynch syndrome II and urological malignancies. J Urol. 1990;143(1):24–8.
20. Greenland JE, Weston PM, Wallace DM. Familial transitional cell carcinoma and the Lynch syndrome II. Br J Urol. 1993;72(2):177–80.
21. Orphali SL, Shols GW, Hagewood J, Tesluk H, Palmer JM. Familial transitional cell carcinoma of renal pelvis and upper ureter. Urology. 1986;27(5):394–6.
22. Vasen HF, Offerhaus GJ, den Hartog Jager FC, et al. The tumour spectrum in hereditary nonpolyposis colorectal cancer: a study of 24 kindreds in the Netherlands. Int J Cancer. 1990;46(1):31–4.
23. Sijmons RH, Kiemeney LALM, Witjes JA, Vasen HFA. Urinary tract cancer and hereditary nonpolyposis colorectal cancer: risks and screening options. J Urol. 1998;160:466–70.
24. Vasen HF, Wijnen JT, Menko FH, et al. Cancer risk in families with hereditary nonpolyposis colorectal cancer diagnosed by mutation analysis. Gastroenterology. 1996;110(4):1020–7.
25. Aarnio M, Mecklin JP, Aaltonen LA, Nystrom-Lahti M, Jarvinen HJ. Life-time risk of different cancers in hereditary non-polyposis colorectal cancer (HNPCC) syndrome. Int J Cancer. 1995;64(6):430–3.
26. Skeldon SC, Semotiuk K, Aronson M, et al. Patients with Lynch syndrome mismatch repair gene mutations are at higher risk for not only upper tract urothelial cancer but also bladder cancer. Eur Urol. 2013;63(2):379–85.
27. Audenet F, Yates DR, Cussenot O, Roupret M. The role of chemotherapy in the treatment of urothelial cell carcinoma of the upper urinary tract (UUT-UCC). Urol Oncol. 2013;31(4): 407–13.

28. Vasen HF, Mecklin JP, Khan PM, Lynch HT. The International Collaborative Group on Hereditary Non-Polyposis Colorectal Cancer (ICG-HNPCC). Dis Colon Rectum. 1991;34(5): 424–5.
29. Ladabaum U, Wang G, Terdiman J, et al. Strategies to identify the Lynch syndrome among patients with colorectal cancer: a cost-effectiveness analysis. Ann Intern Med. 2011;155(2): 69–79.
30. Lynch HT, Lynch JF, Lynch PM. Toward a consensus in molecular diagnosis of hereditary nonpolyposis colorectal cancer (Lynch syndrome). J Natl Cancer Inst. 2007;99(4):261–3.
31. Kwon JS, Scott JL, Gilks CB, Daniels MS, Sun CC, Lu KH. Testing women with endometrial cancer to detect Lynch syndrome. J Clin Oncol. 2011;29(16):2247–52.
32. Gryfe R, Kim H, Hsieh ET, et al. Tumor microsatellite instability and clinical outcome in young patients with colorectal cancer. N Engl J Med. 2000;342(2):69–77.
33. Roupret M, Fromont G, Azzouzi AR, et al. Microsatellite instability as predictor of survival in patients with invasive upper urinary tract transitional cell carcinoma. Urology. 2005;65(6): 1233–7.
34. Drummond JT, Anthoney A, Brown R, Modrich P. Cisplatin and adriamycin resistance are associated with MutLalpha and mismatch repair deficiency in an ovarian tumor cell line. J Biol Chem. 1996;271(33):19645–8.
35. Meyers M, Wagner MW, Hwang HS, Kinsella TJ, Boothman DA. Role of the hMLH1 DNA mismatch repair protein in fluoropyrimidine-mediated cell death and cell cycle responses. Cancer Res. 2001;61(13):5193–201.
36. Ribic CM, Sargent DJ, Moore MJ, et al. Tumor microsatellite-instability status as a predictor of benefit from fluorouracil-based adjuvant chemotherapy for colon cancer. N Engl J Med. 2003;349(3):247–57.
37. Mackay HJ, Cameron D, Rahilly M, et al. Reduced MLH1 expression in breast tumors after primary chemotherapy predicts disease-free survival. J Clin Oncol. 2000;18(1):87–93.
38. Jacob S, Aguado M, Fallik D, Praz F. The role of the DNA mismatch repair system in the cytotoxicity of the topoisomerase inhibitors camptothecin and etoposide to human colorectal cancer cells. Cancer Res. 2001;61(17):6555–62.
39. Catto JWF, Azzouzi AR, Rehman I, et al. Promoter hypermethylation is associated with tumor location, stage and subsequent progression in transitional cell carcinoma. J Clin Oncol. 2005;23:2903–10.
40. Catto JWF, Meuth M, Hamdy FC. Genomic instability in transitional cell carcinoma. BJU Int. 2004;93:19–24.
41. Jung I, Messing E. Molecular mechanisms and pathways in bladder cancer development and progression. Cancer Control. 2000;7(4):325–34.
42. Bringuier PP, McCredie M, Sauter G, et al. Carcinomas of the renal pelvis associated with smoking and phenacetin abuse: p53 mutations and polymorphism of carcinogen-metabolising enzymes. Int J Cancer. 1998;79(5):531–6.
43. Katoh T, Inatomi H, Nagaoka A, Sugita A. Cytochrome P4501A1 gene polymorphism and homozygous deletion of the glutathione S-transferase M1 gene in urothelial cancer patients. Carcinogenesis. 1995;16(3):655–7.
44. Katoh T, Inatomi H, Kim H, Yang M, Matsumoto T, Kawamoto T. Effects of glutathione S-transferase (GST) M1 and GSTT1 genotypes on urothelial cancer risk. Cancer Lett. 1998; 132(1–2):147–52.
45. Roupret M, Cancel-Tassin G, Comperat E, et al. Phenol sulfotransferase SULT1A1*2 allele and enhanced risk of upper urinary tract urothelial cell carcinoma. Cancer Epidemiol Biomarkers Prev. 2007;16(11):2500–3.
46. Rothman N, Garcia-Closas M, Chatterjee N, et al. A multi-stage genome-wide association study of bladder cancer identifies multiple susceptibility loci. Nat Genet. 2010;42(11): 978–84.
47. Roupret M, Drouin SJ, Cancel-Tassin G, Comperat E, Larre S, Cussenot O. Genetic variability in 8q24 confers susceptibility to urothelial carcinoma of the upper urinary tract and is linked with patterns of disease aggressiveness at diagnosis. J Urol. 2012;187(2):424–8.

48. Freedman ND, Silverman DT, Hollenbeck AR, Schatzkin A, Abnet CC. Association between smoking and risk of bladder cancer among men and women. JAMA. 2011;306(7):737–45.
49. Burger M, Catto JW, Dalbagni G, et al. Epidemiology and risk factors of urothelial bladder cancer. Eur Urol. 2013;63(2):234–41.
50. La Vecchia C, Boyle P, Franceschi S, et al. Smoking and cancer with emphasis on Europe. Eur J Cancer. 1991;27(1):94–104.
51. Pommer W, Bronder E, Klimpel A, Helmert U, Greiser E, Molzahn M. Urothelial cancer at different tumour sites: role of smoking and habitual intake of analgesics and laxatives. Results of the Berlin Urothelial Cancer Study. Nephrol Dial Transplant. 1999;14(12):2892–7.
52. McLaughlin JK, Silverman DT, Hsing AW, et al. Cigarette smoking and cancers of the renal pelvis and ureter. Cancer Res. 1992;52(2):254–7.
53. Colin P, Koenig P, Ouzzane A, et al. Environmental factors involved in carcinogenesis of urothelial cell carcinomas of the upper urinary tract. BJU Int. 2009;104(10):1436–40.
54. Doll R, Peto R. The causes of cancer: quantitative estimates of avoidable risks of cancer in the United States today. J Natl Cancer Inst. 1981;66(6):1191–308.
55. Rushton L, Bagga S, Bevan R, et al. Occupation and cancer in Britain. Br J Cancer. 2010;102(9):1428–37.
56. Wilson RT, Donahue M, Gridley G, Adami J, El Ghormli L, Dosemeci M. Shared occupational risks for transitional cell cancer of the bladder and renal pelvis among men and women in Sweden. Am J Ind Med. 2008;51(2):83–99.
57. McCredie M, Stewart JH. Risk factors for kidney cancer in New South Wales. IV. Occupation. Br J Ind Med. 1993;50(4):349–54.
58. Grollman AP, Scarborough J, Jelakovic B. Aristolochic acid nephropathy: an environmental and iatrogenic disease. In: Fishbein J, editor. Advances in molecular toxicology, vol. 3. Amsterdam: Elsevier; 2009.
59. Dawson W. Birthwort: a study of the progress of medical botany through twenty-two centuries. Pharm J Pharm. 1927;396–397:427–30.
60. Kumar V, Poonam, Prasad AK, Parmar VS. Naturally occurring aristolactams, aristolochic acids and dioxoaporphines and their biological activities. Nat Prod Rep. 2003;20(6):565–83.
61. Pohl J. Ueber das Aristolochin, einin giften Bestandtheil der Aristolochiaarten. Arch Exp Path Pharm. 1892;29:282–302.
62. Mengs U. Acute toxicity of aristolochic acid in rodents. Arch Toxicol. 1987;59(5):328–31.
63. Mengs U. Tumour induction in mice following exposure to aristolochic acid. Arch Toxicol. 1988;61(6):504–5.
64. Mengs U. On the histopathogenesis of rat forestomach carcinoma caused by aristolochic acid. Arch Toxicol. 1983;52(3):209–20.
65. Nortier JL, Martinez MC, Schmeiser HH, et al. Urothelial carcinoma associated with the use of a Chinese herb (Aristolochia fangchi). N Engl J Med. 2000;342(23):1686–92.
66. National TP. Aristolochic acids. Rep Carcinog. 2011;12:45–9.
67. IARC. Plants containing aristolochic acid. IARC Monogr Eval Carcinog Risk Chem Hum. 2012;100A:347–61.
68. Vanherweghem JL, Depierreux M, Tielemans C, et al. Rapidly progressive interstitial renal fibrosis in young women: association with slimming regimen including Chinese herbs. Lancet. 1993;341(8842):387–91.
69. Vanhaelen M, Vanhaelen-Fastre R, But P, Vanherweghem JL. Identification of aristolochic acid in Chinese herbs. Lancet. 1994;343(8890):174.
70. Schmeiser HH, Bieler CA, Wiessler M, van Ypersele de Strihou C, Cosyns JP. Detection of DNA adducts formed by aristolochic acid in renal tissue from patients with Chinese herbs nephropathy. Cancer Res. 1996;56(9):2025–8.
71. Gillerot G, Jadoul M, Arlt VM, et al. Aristolochic acid nephropathy in a Chinese patient: time to abandon the term "Chinese herbs nephropathy"? Am J Kidney Dis. 2001;38(5):E26.
72. Cosyns JP, Jadoul M, Squifflet JP, De Plaen JF, Ferluga D, van Ypersele de Strihou C. Chinese herbs nephropathy: a clue to Balkan endemic nephropathy? Kidney Int. 1994;45(6):1680–8.

73. Reginster F, Jadoul M, van Ypersele de Strihou C. Chinese herbs nephropathy presentation, natural history and fate after transplantation. Nephrol Dial Transplant. 1997;12(1):81–6.
74. Depierreux M, Van Damme B, Vanden Houte K, Vanherweghem JL. Pathologic aspects of a newly described nephropathy related to the prolonged use of Chinese herbs. Am J Kidney Dis. 1994;24(2):172–80.
75. Cosyns JP, Jadoul M, Squifflet JP, Van Cangh PJ, van Ypersele de Strihou C. Urothelial malignancy in nephropathy due to Chinese herbs. Lancet. 1994;344(8916):188.
76. Cosyns JP, Jadoul M, Squifflet JP, Wese FX, van Ypersele de Strihou C. Urothelial lesions in Chinese-herb nephropathy. Am J Kidney Dis. 1999;33(6):1011–7.
77. Zlotta AR, Roumeguere T, Kuk C, et al. Select screening in a specific high-risk population of patients suggests a stage migration toward detection of non-muscle-invasive bladder cancer. Eur Urol. 2011;59(6):1026–31.
78. Lemy A, Wissing KM, Rorive S, et al. Late onset of bladder urothelial carcinoma after kidney transplantation for end-stage aristolochic acid nephropathy: a case series with 15-year follow-up. Am J Kidney Dis. 2008;51(3):471–7.
79. Bamias G, Boletis J. Balkan nephropathy: evolution of our knowledge. Am J Kidney Dis. 2008;52(3):606–16.
80. Tatu CA, Orem WH, Finkelman RB, Feder GL. The etiology of Balkan endemic nephropathy: still more questions than answers. Environ Health Perspect. 1998;106(11):689–700.
81. Petkovic SD. Epidemiology and treatment of renal pelvic and ureteral tumors. J Urol. 1975;114(6):858–65.
82. Nikolić J. Uzrok endemske nefropatije I tumora gornjec urotela. Beograd: Srpsko Lekarsko Društvo; 2013.
83. Petronić V. Tumors of the upper urothelium and endemic nephropathy. In: Radovanović ZSM, Polenaković M, Dukanović L, Petronić V, editors. Endemic nephropathy. Beograd: Zavod za udzbenike i nastavna sredstva; 2000. p. 350–439.
84. Voice TC, Long DT, Radovanovic Z, et al. Critical evaluation of environmental exposure agents suspected in the etiology of Balkan endemic nephropathy. Int J Occup Environ Health. 2006;12(4):369–76.
85. Fink-Gremmels J. Ochratoxin A, in food: recent developments and significance. Food Addit Contam. 2005;22 Suppl 1:1–5.
86. Ivkovic V, Karanovic S, Fistrek Prlic M, et al. Is herbal tea consumption a factor in endemic nephropathy? Eur J Epidemiol. 2014. doi:10.1007/s10654-014-9886-3.
87. Ivić M. The problem of etiology of endemic nephropathy. Lij vjes. 1969;91:1273–81.
88. Hranjec T, Kovac A, Kos J, et al. Endemic nephropathy: the case for chronic poisoning by Aristolochia. Croat Med J. 2005;46(1):116–25.
89. Grollman AP, Shibutani S, Moriya M, et al. Aristolochic acid and the etiology of endemic (Balkan) nephropathy. Proc Natl Acad Sci USA. 2007;104(29):12129–34.
90. Jelakovic B, Karanovic S, Vukovic-Lela I, et al. Aristolactam-DNA adducts are a biomarker of environmental exposure to aristolochic acid. Kidney Int. 2012;81(6):559–67.
91. Dickman KG, Sweet DH, Bonala R, Ray T, Wu A. Physiological and molecular characterization of aristolochic acid transport by the kidney. J Pharmacol Exp Ther. 2011;338(2):588–97.
92. Sidorenko V, Attaluri S, Zaitseva I, et al. Bioactivation of the human carcinogen aristolochic acid. Carcinogenesis 2014;35(8):1814–22.
93. Sidorenko VS, Yeo JE, Bonala RR, Johnson F, Scharer OD, Grollman AP. Lack of recognition by global-genome nucleotide excision repair accounts for the high mutagenicity and persistence of aristolactam-DNA adducts. Nucleic Acids Res. 2012;40(6):2494–505.
94. Attaluri S, Bonala RR, Yang IY, et al. DNA adducts of aristolochic acid II: total synthesis and site-specific mutagenesis studies in mammalian cells. Nucleic Acids Res. 2010;38(1):339–52.
95. Petitjean A, Hainaut P, Caron de Fromentel C. TP63 gene in stress response and carcinogenesis: a broader role than expected. Bull Cancer. 2006;93(12):E126–135.

96. Moriya M, Slade N, Brdar B, et al. TP53 mutational signature for aristolochic acid: an environmental carcinogen. Int J Cancer. 2011;129(6):1532–6.
97. Hollstein M, Moriya M, Grollman AP, Olivier M. Analysis of TP53 mutation spectra reveals the fingerprint of the potent environmental carcinogen, aristolochic acid. Mutat Res. 2013;753(1):41–9.
98. De Broe ME. Chinese herbs nephropathy and Balkan endemic nephropathy: toward a single entity, aristolochic acid nephropathy. Kidney Int. 2012;81(6):513–5.
99. Zhu YP. Toxicity of the Chinese herb mu tong (Aristolochia manshuriensis). What history tells us. Adverse Drug React Toxicol Rev. 2002;21(4):171–7.
100. Lai MN, Wang SM, Chen PC, Chen YY, Wang JD. Population-based case–control study of Chinese herbal products containing aristolochic acid and urinary tract cancer risk. J Natl Cancer Inst. 2010;102(3):179–86.
101. Hsieh SC, Lin IH, Tseng WL, Lee CH, Wang JD. Prescription profile of potentially aristolochic acid containing Chinese herbal products: an analysis of National Health Insurance data in Taiwan between 1997 and 2003. Chin Med. 2008;3:13.
102. Chen CH, Dickman KG, Huang CY, et al. Aristolochic acid-induced upper tract urothelial carcinoma in Taiwan: clinical characteristics and outcomes. Int J Cancer. 2013;133(1):14–20.
103. Chen CH, Dickman KG, Moriya M, et al. Aristolochic acid-associated urothelial cancer in Taiwan. Proc Natl Acad Sci USA. 2012;109(21):8241–6.
104. Arlt VM, Stiborova M, Schmeiser HH. Aristolochic acid as a probable human cancer hazard in herbal remedies: a review. Mutagenesis. 2002;17(4):265–77.
105. Grollman AP. Aristolochic acid nephropathy: Harbinger of a global iatrogenic disease. Environ Mol Mutagen. 2013;54(1):1–7.
106. Debelle FD, Vanherweghem JL, Nortier JL. Aristolochic acid nephropathy: a worldwide problem. Kidney Int. 2008;74(2):158–69.
107. Heinrich M, Chan J, Wanke S, Neinhuis C, Simmonds MS. Local uses of Aristolochia species and content of nephrotoxic aristolochic acid 1 and 2–a global assessment based on bibliographic sources. J Ethnopharmacol. 2009;125(1):108–44.
108. Vaclavik L, Krynitsky AJ, Rader JI. Quantification of aristolochic acids I and II in herbal dietary supplements by ultra-high-performance liquid chromatography-multistage fragmentation mass spectrometry. Food Addit Contam Part A Chem Anal Control Expo Risk Assess. 2014;31(5):784–91.
109. Martena MJ, van der Wielen JC, van de Laak LF, Konings EJ, de Groot HN, Rietjens IM. Enforcement of the ban on aristolochic acids in Chinese traditional herbal preparations on the Dutch market. Anal Bioanal Chem. 2007;389(1):263–75.
110. Cheung TP, Xue C, Leung K, Chan K, Li CG. Aristolochic acids detected in some raw Chinese medicinal herbs and manufactured herbal products–a consequence of inappropriate nomenclature and imprecise labelling? Clin Toxicol (Phila). 2006;44(4):371–8.
111. Li HZ, Xia M, Han Y, Xu XG, Zhang YS. De novo urothelial carcinoma in kidney transplantation patients with end-stage aristolochic acid nephropathy in China. Urol Int. 2009;83(2): 200–5
112. Wu F, Wang T. Risk assessment of upper tract urothelial carcinoma related to aristolochic acid. Cancer Epidemiol Biomarkers Prev. 2013;22(5):812–20.
113. Gokmen MR, Cosyns JP, Arlt VM, et al. The epidemiology, diagnosis, and management of aristolochic acid nephropathy: a narrative review. Ann Intern Med. 2013;158(6):469–77.
114. Li XB, Xing NZ, Wang Y, Hu XP, Yin H, Zhang XD. Transitional cell carcinoma in renal transplant recipients: a single center experience. Int J Urol. 2008;15(1):53–7.
115. Zhou L, Cao YL, Li WG, et al. Transitional cell carcinoma associated with aristolochic acid nephropathy: most common cancer in chronic hemodialysis patients in China. Chin Med J (Engl). 2012;125(24):4460–5.
116. Fang D, Zhang L, Li X, et al. Risk factors and treatment outcomes of new contralateral upper urinary urothelial carcinoma after nephroureterectomy: the experiences of a large Chinese center. J Cancer Res Clin Oncol. 2014;140(3):477–85.
117. Spuhler O, Zollinger HU. [Chronic interstitial nephritis]. Z Klin Med. 1953;151(1):1–50.

118. Nanra RS. Renal effects of antipyretic analgesics. Am J Med. 1983;75(5A):70–81.
119. Prescott LF. Analgesic nephropathy: a reassessment of the role of phenacetin and other analgesics. Drugs. 1982;23(1–2):75–149.
120. Hultengren N, Lagergren C, Ljungqvist A. Carcinoma of the renal pelvis in renal papillary necrosis. Acta Chir Scand. 1965;130(4):314–20.
121. McCredie M, Coates MS, Ford JM, Disney AP, Auld JJ, Stewart JH. Geographical distribution of cancers of the kidney and urinary tract and analgesic nephropathy in Australia and New Zealand. Aust NZ J Med. 1990;20(5):684–8.
122. De Broe M. Urinary tract malignancy and atherosclerotic disease in patients with chronic analgesic abuse. Up-to-Date. 2014; http://www.uptodate.com.
123. IARC. Phenacetin. IARC Monogr Eval Carcinog Risk Chem Hum. 2012;100A:377–98.
124. McCredie M, Stewart JH, Mathew TH, Disney AP, Ford JM. The effect of withdrawal of phenacetin-containing analgesics on the incidence of kidney and urothelial cancer and renal failure. Clin Nephrol. 1989;31(1):35–9.
125. McCredie M, Stewart J, Smith D, Supramaniam R, Williams S. Observations on the effect of abolishing analgesic abuse and reducing smoking on cancers of the kidney and bladder in New South Wales, Australia, 1972–1995. Cancer Causes Control. 1999;10(4):303–11.
126. Mihatsch MJ, Khanlari B, Brunner FP. Obituary to analgesic nephropathy–an autopsy study. Nephrol Dial Transplant. 2006;21(11):3139–45.
127. Hinson JA. Reactive metabolites of phenacetin and acetaminophen: a review. Environ Health Perspect. 1983;49:71–9.
128. Stewart JH, Hobbs JB, McCredie MR. Morphologic evidence that analgesic-induced kidney pathology contributes to the progression of tumors of the renal pelvis. Cancer. 1999;86(8):1576–82.
129. Novara G, De Marco V, Dalpiaz O, et al. Independent predictors of contralateral metachronous upper urinary tract transitional cell carcinoma after nephroureterectomy: multi-institutional dataset from three European centers. Int J Urol. 2009;16(2):187–91.
130. Wright JL, Hotaling J, Porter MP. Predictors of upper tract urothelial cell carcinoma after primary bladder cancer: a population based analysis. J Urol. 2009;181(3):1035–9. discussion 1039.
131. Giannarini G, Kessler TM, Thoeny HC, Nguyen DP, Meissner C, Studer UE. Do patients benefit from routine follow-up to detect recurrences after radical cystectomy and ileal orthotopic bladder substitution? Eur Urol. 2010;58(4):486–94.
132. Picozzi S, Ricci C, Gaeta M, et al. Upper urinary tract recurrence following radical cystectomy for bladder cancer: a meta-analysis on 13,185 patients. J Urol. 2012;188(6):2046–54.
133. Huguet-Pérez J, Palou J, Millán-Rodríguez F, Salvador-Bayarri J, Villavicencio-Mavrich H, Vicente-Rodríguez J. Upper tract transitional cell carcinoma following cystectomy for bladder cancer. Eur Urol. 2001;40(3):318–23.
134. Millán-Rodríguez F, Chéchile-Toniolo G, Salvador-Bayarri J, Huguet-Pérez J, Vicente-Rodríguez J. Upper urinary tract tumors after primary superficial bladder tumors: prognostic factors and risk groups. J Urol. 2000;164(4):1183–7.
135. Solsona E, Iborra I, Rubio J, Casanova J, Dumont R, Monrós JL. Late oncological occurrences following radical cystectomy in patients with bladder cancer. Eur Urol. 2003;43(5):489–94.
136. Tran W, Serio AM, Raj GV, et al. Longitudinal risk of upper tract recurrence following radical cystectomy for urothelial cancer and the potential implications for long-term surveillance. J Urol. 2008;179(1):96–100.
137. Akkad T, Gozzi C, Deibl M, et al. Tumor recurrence in the remnant urothelium of females undergoing radical cystectomy for transitional cell carcinoma of the bladder: long-term results from a single center. J Urol. 2006;175(4):1268–71. discussion 1271.
138. Meissner C, Giannarini G, Schumacher MC, Thoeny H, Studer UE, Burkhard FC. The efficiency of excretory urography to detect upper urinary tract tumors after cystectomy for urothelial cancer. J Urol. 2007;178(6):2287–90.

139. Stein JP, Lieskovsky G, Cote R, et al. Radical cystectomy in the treatment of invasive bladder cancer: long-term results in 1,054 patients. J Clin Oncol. 2001;19(3):666–75.
140. Hurle R, Losa A, Manzetti A, Lembo A. Intravesical bacille Calmette-Guérin in Stage T1 grade 3 bladder cancer therapy: a 7-year follow-up. Urology. 1999;54(2):258–63.
141. Volkmer BG, Schnoeller T, Kuefer R, Gust K, Finter F, Hautmann RE. Upper urinary tract recurrence after radical cystectomy for bladder cancer–who is at risk? J Urol. 2009;182(6): 2632–7.
142. Solsona E, Iborra I, Ricós JV, Dumont R, Casanova JL, Calabuig C. Upper urinary tract involvement in patients with bladder carcinoma in situ (Tis): its impact on management. Urology. 1997;49(3):347–52.
143. Sved PD, Gomez P, Nieder AM, Manoharan M, Kim SS, Soloway MS. Upper tract tumour after radical cystectomy for transitional cell carcinoma of the bladder: incidence and risk factors. BJU Int. 2004;94(6):785–9.
144. Gakis G, Schilling D, Perner S, Schwentner C, Sievert K-D, Stenzl A. Sequential resection of malignant ureteral margins at radical cystectomy: a critical assessment of the value of frozen section analysis. World J Urol. 2011;29(4):451–6.
145. Osman Y, El-Tabey N, Abdel-Latif M, Mosbah A, Moustafa N, Shaaban A. The value of frozen-section analysis of ureteric margins on surgical decision-making in patients undergoing radical cystectomy for bladder cancer. BJU Int. 2007;99(1):81–4.
146. Schumacher MC, Scholz M, Weise ES, Fleischmann A, Thalmann GN, Studer UE. Is there an indication for frozen section examination of the ureteral margins during cystectomy for transitional cell carcinoma of the bladder? J Urol. 2006;176(6 Pt 1):2409–13. discussion 2413.
147. Raj GV, Tal R, Vickers A, et al. Significance of intraoperative ureteral evaluation at radical cystectomy for urothelial cancer. Cancer. 2006;107(9):2167–72.
148. Sanderson KM, Cai J, Miranda G, Skinner DG, Stein JP. Upper tract urothelial recurrence following radical cystectomy for transitional cell carcinoma of the bladder: an analysis of 1,069 patients with 10-year followup. J Urol. 2007;177(6):2088–94.
149. Gakis G, Efstathiou J, Lerner SP, et al. ICUD-EAU International Consultation on Bladder Cancer 2012: Radical cystectomy and bladder preservation for muscle-invasive urothelial carcinoma of the bladder. Eur Urol. 2013;63(1):45–57.
150. Burger M, Oosterlinck W, Konety B, et al. ICUD-EAU International Consultation on Bladder Cancer 2012: Non-muscle-invasive urothelial carcinoma of the bladder. Eur Urol. 2013; 63(1):36–44.
151. Messer J, Shariat SF, Brien JC, et al. Urinary cytology has a poor performance for predicting invasive or high-grade upper-tract urothelial carcinoma. BJU Int. 2011;108(5):701–5.
152. Wang L-J, Wong Y-C, Huang C-C, Wu C-H, Hung S-C, Chen H-W. Multidetector computerized tomography urography is more accurate than excretory urography for diagnosing transitional cell carcinoma of the upper urinary tract in adults with hematuria. J Urol. 2010; 183(1):48–55.

Chapter 2
Diagnosis and Evaluation of Upper Tract Urothelial Carcinoma (UTUC)

Pierre Colin, Wassim Kassouf, Badrinath R. Konety, Yair Lotan, and Morgan Rouprêt

Abstract Upper tract urothelial carcinomas (UTUC) are scarce and account for only 5–10 % of urothelial carcinomas. The estimated annual incidence of UTUC in Western countries is about 1–2 new cases per 100,000 inhabitants. Pyelocaliceal tumors are about twice as common as ureteral tumors. The diagnosis of a UTUC may be fortuitous or related to the exploration of symptoms. The symptoms are generally restricted. The most common symptom of UTUC is gross or microscopic haematuria (70–80 %). Flank pain occurs in 20–40 % of cases, and a lumbar mass is present in 10–20 %. In case of UTUC, a cystoscopy is mandatory to rule out a concomitant bladder tumor. Positive urine cytology is highly suggestive of UTUC when bladder cystoscopy is normal and if CIS of the bladder or prostatic urethra has been largely excluded (e.g., by biopsies of any suspicious lesion, possibly guided

P. Colin, MD, PhD
Department of Urology, Hôpital privé de la Louvière,
Générale de santé, 69, rue de la Louvière, Lille, France
e-mail: docpierrecolin@gmail.com

W. Kassouf, MD, CM, FRCS(C)
Department of Surgery (Urology), McGill University Health Center,
1650 Cedar Ave, L8-315, Montreal, QC H4R 3H1, Canada
e-mail: wassim.kassouf@muhc.mcgill.ca

B.R. Konety, MD, MBA
Department of Urology, Dougherty Family Chair in Prostate Cancer,
Institute for Prostate and Urologic Cancers, University of Minnesota,
420 Delaware St. SE, RM B535 Mayo, MMC 394, Minneapolis, MN 55455, USA
e-mail: brkonety@umn.edu

Y. Lotan, MD
Department of Urology, University of Texas Southwestern Medical Center,
5323 Harry Hines Blvd., Dallas, TX 75390-9110, USA
e-mail: yair.lotan@utsouthwestern.edu

M. Rouprêt, MD, PhD (✉)
Department of Urology, Pitié-Salpétrière Hospital (Assistance Publique - Hôpitaux de Paris),
83, Boulevard de l'Hopital Batiment Gaston Cordier, 75013 Université Paris 6, Paris, France
e-mail: morgan.roupret@psl.aphp.fr

© Springer Science+Business Media New York 2015
S.F. Shariat, E. Xylinas (eds.), *Upper Tract Urothelial Carcinoma*,
DOI 10.1007/978-1-4939-1501-9_2

by photodynamic diagnosis). Cytology is less sensitive for UTUC than for bladder tumors, even for high-grade lesions, and it should ideally be performed in situ (i.e., in the renal cavities). Retrograde ureteropyelography (through a ureteral catheter or during ureteroscopy) remains an option for the exclusion of a tumor in the upper urinary tract. Computed tomography (CT) urography is the imaging technique with the highest diagnostic accuracy for UTUC and has replaced intravenous excretory urography and ultrasonography as the first-line imaging test for investigating high-risk patients. In addition, the possible advantages of ureteroscopy should be discussed in the preoperative assessment of any UTUC patient. Flexible ureteroscopy is used to visualize and biopsy the ureter, renal pelvis, and collecting system with a technical success approaching 95 %. Such ureteroscopic biopsies can determine tumor grade in 90 % of cases with a low false-negative rate regardless of the size of the sample. Ureteroscopy also facilitates selective ureteral sampling for cytology in situ. Flexible ureteroscopy is especially useful when there is diagnostic uncertainty, in patients with a solitary kidney, or when conservative treatment is being considered.

Keywords Renal pelvis • Ureter • Urothelial carcinoma • Ureteroscopy • Computed tomography • Urinary cytology

Introduction

Because of their low incidence, upper tract urothelial carcinomas (UTUC) are often discovered during a symptomatic episode or during surveillance of bladder cancers. Over the past 10 years, technical advances in both imaging and endoscopy have improved the evaluation of these tumors preoperatively. We are entering a new era of preoperative assessment for both clinical imaging and endoscopy. This multimodal predictive assessment should lead, in the near future, to a more conservative treatment when possible or to a more intensive and multimodal adapted radical treatment (extended lymphadenectomy, neoadjuvant or adjuvant therapy).

Elements of Diagnosis

Clinical Revelation

Hematuria

Hematuria is the most common symptom found in the diagnosis of UTUC (75–82 % of cases) [1, 2]. However, among patients with isolated hematuria, the diagnosis of UTUC is rare involving only 0.32 % of cases. Hematuria may be gross or microscopic, often total, and sometimes terminal when a tumor of the lower ureter is prolapsed at the meatus. Its abundance is variable, as is its frequency (intermittent, recurrent, and permanent). This typically painless disorder can sometimes be responsible for pain (renal colic) in cases of clotting or tumor-related obstruction in the upper tract.

Pain

Flank and lumbar pain is the second most frequent symptom of UTUC (20–30 % of cases). The most common disease etiology is ureteral obstruction by either intraluminal clotting or due to a bulky tumor. Progressive upper tract obstruction by the tumor is responsible for lumbar pain due to the dilatation of the proximal ureter and kidney [3]. Locoregional tumor extension is an infrequent cause of constant and poorly localized pain. Metastatic tumor dissemination to regions including the bone can also be responsible for pain.

Other Clinical Signs

Other clinical signs are present in approximately 10 % of cases. A palpable mass is correlated with very advanced tumors of the renal pelvis or the caliceal system or a hydronephrotic kidney. Due to the rising rates of obesity and location of the kidney behind the rib cage, a palpable mass is rarely noted.

Irritative or infectious symptoms may also be present at UTUC diagnosis. Urinary frequency can be caused by tumors in the lower ureter that are located in the intramural ureter or prolapsed at the meatus or due to concomitant bladder cancer (especially Carcinoma In Situ). Pyelonephritis may complicate the hydronephrosis caused by the tumor obstruction.

The deterioration of patients' general condition and development of constitutional symptoms (e.g., weight loss, anorexia) is possible but rare. When present, this deterioration often indicates advanced or metastatic tumors [3].

Asymptomatic Patients

In several recent series, the rate of asymptomatic tumors varies from 10 to 15 % of cases. However, these diagnoses are fortuitous because they are revealed following image analysis (including abdominopelvic CT) performed for other reasons.

Another circumstance of UTUC diagnosis in asymptomatic patients occurs after examination for non-muscle invasive bladder cancer (NMIBC). While upper tract tumor recurrence is a rare event (less than 5 %) for patients with NMIBC, a previous history of NMIBC was found in 10–30 % of UTUC cases.

Upper tract recurrence is a lifelong risk in patients with bladder cancer. A recent publication has described the practicality of routine surveillance by CT urography in this population to detect recurrence in the upper tract [4]. However, in case of previous NMIBC, systematic routine upper tract imaging appears to have a low profitability and is not currently recommended (i.e., overall efficacy of less than 0.5 %) [5].

Conversely, after cystectomy for muscle invasive bladder urothelial carcinoma (MIBC), regular follow-ups with CT urography combine the advantage to explore the urinary tract functionally and oncologically [6]. While these recurrences are rare (0.75–6.4 %), routine follow-up investigations detect them in only 38 %. However, the use of CT urography was recommended to improve detection especially in high-risk patients after cystectomy (high-grade tumor, carcinoma in situ, multifocal disease, history of multiple urothelial recurrences, the presence of ureteral tumors/CIS, positive ureteral margins, positive urethral margins, urethral involvement, or history of upper urinary tract urothelial carcinoma) who undergo CT urography might more efficiently detect recurrence.

Imaging

CT Urography

The opacification of the urinary tract has been the most commonly used diagnostic tool for the diagnosis of UTUC. Urinary excretion of contrast or retrograde opacification of the urinary tract can usually locate the lesion in the urinary tract, given its size and endo-luminal characteristics, and help to objectify other lesions. Intravenous urography (IVU) has been the radiological standard for UTUC characterization. The opacification is achieved by the intravenous injection of a hypo-osmolar iodinated contrast agent and by simple radiographs of the abdomen. However, it is currently no longer recommended as a first-line procedure.

The development of CT urography using thin slices (<2 mm), various protocols to visualize the entire urinary tract (hyperhydration, diuretic injection), and excretory acquisition time (6–8 min after injection) now offers improved accuracy over IVU. Indeed, Wang et al. reported the sensitivity of IVU is 75 % vs. 95.8 % for CT urography and the specificity of IVU is 86 % vs. 100 % for CT urography [7].

Chlapoutakis et al. compiled the results of five studies in a meta-analysis and found that the sensitivity of CT urography for the diagnosis of UTUC was 96 % (88–100 %) and the specificity was 99 % (98–99 %) [8].

However, the cutoff for lesion detection by CT urography is 2–3 mm in terms of spatial resolution. For lesions <3 mm, the detection sensitivity drops to 40 %.

Moreover, CT urography facilitates a more comprehensive assessment of the lesion through MPR (multiplanar reformatted imaging) type reconstructions and the evaluation of its extension on the nodes and metastasis. Unfortunately, it is impossible to accurately determine the depth of tumor invasion (cT stage: cTa to cT2) due to insufficient spatial resolution.

Radiological appearance of intraluminal lesions is identical on IVU and CT urography:

- Within pelvicaliceal cavities, the CT images of these tumors depend on their growth (papillary or non-papillary invasive). Papillary tumors are seen as intraluminal masses with tissue density [40–50 hounsefield units (HU)]. These mass lesions are sometimes heterogeneous but rarely calcified (<3 %). Their enhancement after injection of contrast is often discrete (50–60 HU), whereas during the excretory time, UTUCs appear as gaps with a sessile or pedunculated base. Infiltrative forms correspond to a nonspecific thickening of the wall that is more or less circumferential and/or irregular [9]. In case of hydronephrosis, it is sometimes possible to distinguish the UTUC due to higher density than the non-opaque urine.
- Within the ureter, UTUC can take the appearance of wall thickening or a filling defect. The radiographic images allow the detection of Bergman's sign (widening of the ureter below the lesion), which is not present with obstructions due to ureteral stones. In case of poor opacification of a dilated ureter, the suspicion of tumor presence is high, especially if there is an enhancement of the ureter wall at this level. It is then necessary to repeat the exam after placing the patient in the prone position [9].

The disadvantages of this technique include a relatively large radiation dose (16–35 mSv), the potential side effects associated with the injected iodinated contrast agent (anaphylaxis, acute tubular necrosis), and the high cost (approximately 3 times higher than the IVU).

Today, CT urography remains the gold standard for the diagnosis of UTUC (grade A recommendation) [2].

MR Urography

Magnetic Resonance Urography is the modality of choice in cases where CT urography is not recommended because of an allergy to iodinated contrast agents or moderate renal impairment. However, gadolinium contrast used for MRI is contraindicated in patients with severe chronic renal impairment with creatinine clearance <30 mL/min, due to the risk of nephrogenic systemic fibrosis. In those cases, retrograde pyelogram is preferred.

The radiological findings are identical to those described for CT urography. Usually, the lesions appear iso-attenuating on T1 and hyper-attenuating on T2 compared to the muscle. Enhancement of the lesion after the injection of gadolinium can distinguish a suspected lesion from a calculus (Fig. 2.1).

Several different sequences are needed to improve performance. Thus, it is possible to obtain reconstructions of urinary tracts comparable to IVU sequences with TSE (turbo spin-echo), HASTE (T2-weighted apnea), and MIP (3D T1-weighted gadolinium and furosemide). The MR urography has a lower spatial resolution and

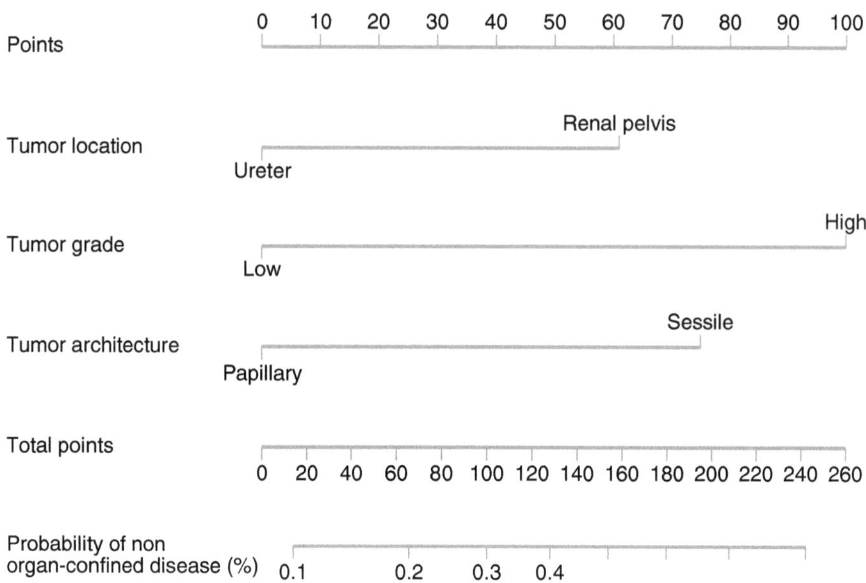

Fig. 2.1 Preoperative nomogram for prediction of organ-confined stage of the UTUC (adapted from Margulis V, et al.: Preoperative multivariable prognostic model for prediction of nonorgan confined urothelial carcinoma of the upper urinary tract. J Urol. 184: 453-8, 2010)

more artifacts by hematuria or the presence of a ureteral catheter than CT urography. Although only a few results have been published on this subject, the detection of UTUCs with MR urography has been demonstrated with a sensitivity of 70–80 % and specificity close to 100 % [10].

More recently, DWI (diffusion-weighted images) with calculation of apparent diffusion coefficient (ADC) was evaluated in the diagnosis of UTUC [11]. This technique, which does not require injection of gadolinium, is based on the diffusion of water molecules in tissue. This allows the calculation of the ADC for the renal parenchyma, dilated urinary system, and tumor. Several studies agree that the ADC of the pelvicaliceal cavities UTUC is significantly lower that of the adjacent tissue, making this sequence of interest for diagnosis in addition to conventional sequences [12]. The value of ADC in tumor staging is currently limited with conflicting data in the literature but appears to be associated with the tumor grade and proliferation markers [12, 13].

As with CT urography, MR urography has limited accuracy in staging cTa-cT2 grade tumors [14].

Endoscopy

Retrograde Ureteropyelography

Retrograde ureteropyelography (RUP) is usually performed during cystoscopy and/or flexible ureteroscopy under general anesthesia and is therefore not a diagnostic modality in its own right. This procedure consists of retrograde opacification by prior catheterization of the upper urinary tract with a ureteral catheter.

Using this approach, the delineation of the upper urinary tract following opacification demonstrates performance comparable to CT urography in terms of diagnostic sensitivity and specificity (96 % and 97 %, respectively) [15]. However, there is a bias since many patients already have a suspected lesion prior to going to the operating room for a RUP. This examination is recommended by several guidelines including that of the EAU (grade C) [2] and AUA.

Flexible Ureteroscopy and In Situ Biopsies

Technological advances have made ureteroscopy a valuable diagnostic tool for the evaluation of suspicious lesions in the upper urinary tract. Indeed, the use of flexible devices enables the complete examination of the upper tract, including the lower pole renal calices.

Ureteroscopy is particularly useful in cases of uncertain diagnoses, in cases of patients with a solitary kidney, or when conservative treatment is considered. Ureteroscopic examination is now recommended by the guidelines for the first-line screening of UTUC (recommendation of grade C) [2].

Flexible ureteroscopy allows a visual diagnosis in 95 % of cases [2]. Advances in image resolution with digital ureteroscopes reinforce the quality of this examination. The detection sensitivity could be improved by photodiagnosis using 5-aminolevulinic acid (5-ALA), especially for small lesions and carcinoma in situ, or Narrow Band Imaging (NBI) [16, 17]. The NBI system uses only a part of the visible spectra (between 415 and 540 nm), which enhances the contrast of the tumor neovascularization and thus the detection of the small lesion. The preliminary results are promising, with 22.7 % more lesions detected using this technique than with white light [17]. Further studies are warranted to evaluate whether tangential viewing within the ureter poses a limitation towards the use of these new technologies within the upper tract.

Morel et al. showed the limited applicability of rigid ureteroscopy in this context due to inability to explore the pyelocaliceal cavities [18].

However, the macroscopic visual diagnosis does not allow the infiltrating nature of the tumor to be determined. According to El-Hakim et al., the endoscopic appearance of tumors leads to errors of staging in at least 30 % of cases [19].

During the procedure, the surgeon can perform selective cytology and biopsy of a visualized suspicious lesion in addition to the visual macroscopic diagnosis. This pathologic biopsy can confirm the diagnosis with a sensitivity of 89–95 % and obtain a prognostic tumor grade and stage [20]. The reliability of biopsies for tumor staging is poor, with 45 % of tumors classified as Ta, but these are actually more invasive tumors. However, the biopsy grade is adequately correlated with the final histopathological grade in 69–91 % of cases and the final tumor stage. Often the grade of the tumor gives information about the likely stage. In fact, the detection of a grade 1 tumor on biopsy corresponds to a noninvasive tumor (≤pT1) in 68–100 % and the detection of a grade 3 tumor on biopsy corresponds to an invasive tumor (≥pT2) in 62–100 % cases [21–24]. Upper tract ureteroscopy may not identify any tumor up to 50 % of the time even in patients with positive urine cytology.

However, obtaining biopsies is not always possible. Indeed, the introduction of biopsy forceps through the working channel of the ureteroscope may limit deflection and therefore the accessibility of the lower calyx.

The assessment of UTUC depth invasion remains a challenging task in ureteroscopy. The use of endoscopic ultrasonography has been described for this task but has not been routinely used in daily practice [25]. New imaging techniques such as optical coherence tomography (OCT) or endoscopic confocal microscopy are now in development and could eventually be used for this specific evaluation and as a complement to lesion biopsies [26, 27].

The hypothesis of the possible "seeding" of cancer cells during the procedure (by hyperpressure of the cavities or trauma to the wall) is not currently discussed [28]. The delay attributable to the performance of a diagnostic ureteroscopy with biopsy does not significantly affect the long-term prognosis of the disease [29].

Although rare, complications associated with diagnostic ureteroscopy are possible (0.5–5 % of cases). These consist of perforations, stripping of the ureter, stenosis, or parenchymal infections.

Cystoscopy

This simple test is recommended (grade A) as a first-line screening to rule out any synchronous bladder tumors.

Urine Cytology

Urine cytology is based on the analysis of cells exfoliated in urine and remains recommended for the diagnosis of UTUC (grade A) [2].

The cells can be obtained following urination or samples taken by bladder wash during cystoscopy or in situ during ureteroscopy. Although easy and noninvasive, voided urinary cytology is limited by its variable sensitivity (35–65 %) according to the large interindividual variability in the interpretation and the increased level of false positives in cases of trauma of urothelium or inflammation. The specificity of this technique is also excellent (>90 %).

In cases of positive urine cytology with normal cystoscopy, the likelihood of UTUC is very high. However, urine cytology is poor at predicting final tumor stage and grade. Messer et al. reported that positive urine cytology predicts a high-grade tumor with a sensitivity of 56 % and an invasive tumor with a sensitivity of 62 % [30]. Additionally, a positive preoperative urine cytology appears to be a risk factor for intravesical recurrence [31].

This cytology examination can be optimized with the detection of chromosomal abnormalities by FISH (fluorescence in situ hybridization) [32, 33], but the results using this approach are still preliminary and the cost of this technique is high.

Predictive Tools

Currently, treatment decisions regarding UTUC are based on the clinician's ability to predict the risk of progression based on the individual pathology of each patient.

Therefore, predictive and prognostic statistical tools have been developed to assist the clinician in predicting the progression risk of the disease.

The combination of the various elements previously described should increase the prediction performance of such tools.

Margulis et al. developed a nomogram based on clinical criteria (biopsy grade, tumor architecture, and location) to estimate the probability of locally advanced disease [34]. Their tool showed an accuracy of 76.7 %.

Similarly, Favaretto et al. developed a tool to predict the invasiveness or locally advanced nature of UTUC based on the criteria of imaging data and ureteroscopy, which includes biopsy grade [35]. This tool predicts the infiltrating character with 71 % accuracy and the locally advanced nature with 70 % accuracy.

Currently, no molecular parameter has yet been incorporated into these nomograms, unlike with other pathologies such as colon cancer (K-ras status) and breast cancer (HER2 status).

These tools could be helpful for selected patients who require radical treatment and/or extensive lymphadenectomy and/or neoadjuvant chemotherapy; however, independent validation of these tools is required today as they are not currently used in clinical practice, external validation is not yet available, and these tools are not yet used in clinical practice.

We now propose the flowchart in Fig. 2.2 to summarize this chapter.

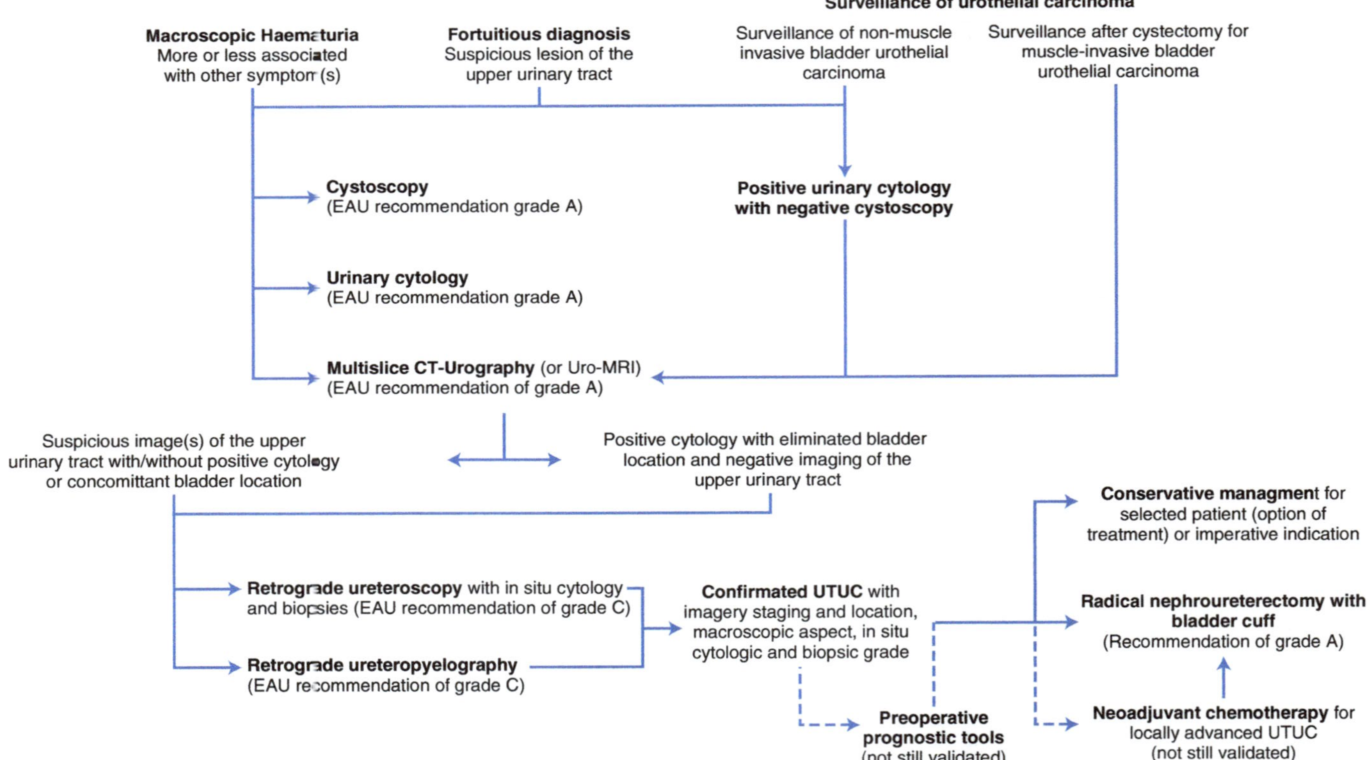

Fig. 2.2 Flowchart summarizing the diagnosis and evaluation of UTUC

Conclusion

Due to recent advances in imaging and endoscopy, the diagnostic management of UTUC has evolved in recent years. CT urography is now the tool for the detection of UTUC. Flexible ureteroscopy is often needed for the pretreatment patient evaluation. Future developments are expected to further refine the preoperative staging of these tumors.

Executive Summary

- The most common symptom of UTUC is gross hematuria (75–80 %).
- Systemic symptoms (i.e., weight loss, malaise, fever) associated with UTUC should prompt consideration of a rigorous metastatic evaluation.
- UTUC are diagnosed using imaging, cystoscopy, urinary cytology, and diagnostic ureteroscopy. The benefits of ureteroscopy in preoperative assessment should also be discussed with the patient.
- The diagnosis of UTUC may be fortuitous or related to the explorations of symptoms.
- Computed tomography (CT) urography is the imaging technique with the highest accuracy for UTUC.
- Magnetic resonance (MR) urography is indicated in patients who cannot undergo CT urography (i.e., radiation or iodinated contrast media are contraindicated).
- Retrograde ureteropyelography through a ureteral catheter is an option for the exclusion of a UTUC.
- Positive urine cytology is highly suggestive of UTUC when bladder cystoscopy is normal and if CIS of the bladder has been ruled out.
- Flexible ureteroscopy is used to visualize and biopsy lesions in the ureter, which can be helpful to determine tumor grade in 90 % of cases.
- Ureteroscopy facilitates selective ureteral sampling for cytology in situ.

References

1. Sudakoff GS, Dunn DP, Guralnick ML, Hellman RS, Eastwood D, See WA. Multidetector computerized tomography urography as the primary imaging modality for detecting urinary tract neoplasms in patients with asymptomatic hematuria. J Urol. 2008;179:862–7.
2. Roupret M, Babjuk M, Comperat E, Zigeuner R, Sylvester R, Burger M, Cowan N, Bohle A, Van Rhijn BW, Kaasinen E, et al. European guidelines on upper tract urothelial carcinomas: 2013 update. Eur Urol. 2013;63:1059–71.
3. Raman JD, Shariat SF, Karakiewicz PI, Lotan Y, Sagalowsky AI, Roscigno M, Montorsi F, Bolenz C, Weizer AZ, Wheat JC, et al. Does preoperative symptom classification impact prognosis in patients with clinically localized upper-tract urothelial carcinoma managed by radical nephroureterectomy? Urol Oncol. 2011;29:716–23.

4. Xu AD, Ng CS, Kamat A, Grossman HB, Dinney C, Sandler CM. Significance of upper urinary tract urothelial thickening and filling defect seen on MDCT urography in patients with a history of urothelial neoplasms. AJR Am J Roentgenol. 2010;195:959–65.
5. Sternberg IA, Keren Paz GE, Chen LY, Herr HW, Donat SM, Bochner BH, Dalbagni G. Upper tract surveillance is not effective in diagnosing upper tract recurrences in patients followed for non-muscle-invasive bladder cancer. J Urol. 2013. doi:10.1016/j.juro.2013.05.020.
6. Picozzi S, Ricci C, Gaeta M, Ratti D, Macchi A, Casellato S, Bozzini G, Carmignani L. Upper urinary tract recurrence following radical cystectomy for bladder cancer: a meta-analysis on 13,185 patients. J Urol. 2012;188:2046–54.
7. Wang LJ, Wong YC, Huang CC, Wu CH, Hung SC, Chen HW. Multidetector computerized tomography urography is more accurate than excretory urography for diagnosing transitional cell carcinoma of the upper urinary tract in adults with hematuria. J Urol. 2010;183:48–55.
8. Chlapoutakis K, Theocharopoulos N, Yarmenitis S, Damilakis J. Performance of computed tomographic urography in diagnosis of upper urinary tract urothelial carcinoma, in patients presenting with hematuria: systematic review and meta-analysis. Eur J Radiol. 2008;73:334–8.
9. Anderson EM, Murphy R, Rennie AT, Cowan NC. Multidetector computed tomography urography (MDCTU) for diagnosing urothelial malignancy. Clin Radiol. 2007;62:324–32.
10. Takahashi N, Glockner JF, Hartman RP, King BF, Leibovich BC, Stanley DW, Fitz-Gibbon PD, Kawashima A. Gadolinium enhanced magnetic resonance urography for upper urinary tract malignancy. J Urol. 2010;183:1330–65.
11. Akita H, Jinzaki M, Kikuchi E, Sugiura H, Akita A, Mikami S, Kuribayashi S. Preoperative T categorization and prediction of histopathologic grading of urothelial carcinoma in renal pelvis using diffusion-weighted MRI. AJR Am J Roentgenol. 2011;197:1130–6.
12. Sufana Iancu A, Colin P, Puech P, Villers A, Ouzzane A, Fantoni JC, Leroy X, Lemaitre L. Significance of ADC value for detection and characterization of urothelial carcinoma of upper urinary tract using diffusion-weighted MRI. World J Urol. 2012;31:13–9.
13. Yoshida S, Kobayashi S, Koga F, Ishioka J, Ishii C, Tanaka H, Nakanishi Y, Matsuoka Y, Numao N, Saito K, et al. Apparent diffusion coefficient as a prognostic biomarker of upper urinary tract cancer: a preliminary report. Eur Radiol. 2013;23(8):2206–14.
14. Obuchi M, Ishigami K, Takahashi K, Honda M, Mitsuya T, Kuehn DM, Stolpen AH, Brown BP, Nishie A. Gadolinium-enhanced fat-suppressed T1-weighted imaging for staging ureteral carcinoma: correlation with histopathology. AJR Am J Roentgenol. 2007;188:W256–61.
15. Cowan NC, Turney BW, Taylor NJ, McCarthy CL, Crew JP. Multidetector computed tomography urography for diagnosing upper urinary tract urothelial tumour. BJU Int. 2007;99:1363–70.
16. Audenet F, Traxer O, Yates DR, Cussenot O, Roupret M. Potential role of photodynamic techniques combined with new generation flexible ureterorenoscopes and molecular markers for the management of urothelial carcinoma of the upper urinary tract. BJU Int. 2012;109:608–13; discussion 613–4.
17. Traxer O, Geavlete B, de Medina SG, Sibony M, Al-Qahtani SM. Narrow-band imaging digital flexible ureteroscopy in detection of upper urinary tract transitional-cell carcinoma: initial experience. J Endourol. 2011;25:19–23.
18. Morel Journel N, Manel A, Chaffanges P, Champetier D, Devonec M, Perrin P. [Rigid ureteroscopy in the case of suspected tumor of the upper urinary tract: report of 63 cases]. Prog Urol. 2002;12:15–20.
19. El-Hakim A, Weiss GH, Lee BR, Smith AD. Correlation of ureteroscopic appearance with histologic grade of upper tract transitional cell carcinoma. Urology. 2004;63:647–50.
20. Lam JS, Gupta M. Ureteroscopic management of upper tract transitional cell carcinoma. Urol Clin North Am. 2004;31:115–28.
21. Cutress ML, Stewart GD, Zakikhani P, Phipps S, Thomas BG, Tolley DA. Ureteroscopic and percutaneous management of upper tract urothelial carcinoma (UTUC): systematic review. BJU Int. 2012;110:614–28.
22. Keeley FX, Kulp DA, Bibbo M, McCue PA, Bagley DH. Diagnostic accuracy of ureteroscopic biopsy in upper tract transitional cell carcinoma. J Urol. 1997;157:33–7.

23. Brown GA, Matin SF, Busby JE, Dinney CP, Grossman HB, Pettaway CA, Munsell MF, Kamat AM. Ability of clinical grade to predict final pathologic stage in upper urinary tract transitional cell carcinoma: implications for therapy. Urology. 2007;70:252–6.
24. Brien JC, Shariat SF, Herman MP, Ng CK, Scherr DS, Scoll B, Uzzo RG, Wille M, Eggener SE, Terrell JD, et al. Preoperative hydronephrosis, ureteroscopic biopsy grade and urinary cytology can improve prediction of advanced upper tract urothelial carcinoma. J Urol. 2010; 184:69–73.
25. Ingram MD, Sooriakumaran P, Palfrey E, Montgomery B, Massouh H. Evaluation of the upper urinary tract using transureteric ultrasound – a review of the technique and typical imaging appearances. Clin Radiol. 2008;63:1026–34.
26. Bui D, Jen-Jane Liu JJ, Chang T, Hsiao S, Mohan R, Mach K, Liao J. Optical biopsy of upper tract urotheial carcinoma with confocal laser endomicroscopy: AUA Annual Meeting 2013. San Diego, USA, 2013, Abstract number 892.
27. Mueller-Lisse UL, Bader M, Bauer M, Engelram E, Hocaoglu Y, Püls M, Meissner OA, Babaryka G, Sroka R, Stiefa CG, et al. Optical coherence tomography of the upper urinary tract: review of initial experience ex vivo and in vivo. Med Laser Appl. 2010;25:44–52.
28. Ishikawa S, Abe T, Shinohara N, Harabayashi T, Sazawa A, Maruyama S, Kubota K, Matsuno Y, Osawa T, Shinno Y, et al. Impact of diagnostic ureteroscopy on intravesical recurrence and survival in patients with urothelial carcinoma of the upper urinary tract. J Urol. 2010;184: 883–7.
29. Nison L, Roupret M, Bozzini G, Ouzzane A, Audenet F, Pignot G, Ruffion A, Cornu JN, Hurel S, Valeri A, et al. The oncologic impact of a delay between diagnosis and radical nephroureterectomy due to diagnostic ureteroscopy in upper urinary tract urothelial carcinomas: results from a large collaborative database. World J Urol. 2012;31:69–76.
30. Messer J, Shariat SF, Brien JC, Herman MP, Ng CK, Scherr DS, Scoll B, Uzzo RG, Wille M, Eggener SE, et al. Urinary cytology has a poor performance for predicting invasive or high-grade upper-tract urothelial carcinoma. BJU Int. 2011;108:701–5.
31. Kobayashi Y, Saika T, Miyaji Y, Saegusa M, Arata R, Akebi N, Takenaka T, Manabe D, Nasu Y, Kumon H. Preoperative positive urine cytology is a risk factor for subsequent development of bladder cancer after nephroureterectomy in patients with upper urinary tract urothelial carcinoma. World J Urol. 2012;30:271–5.
32. Xu C, Zeng Q, Hou J, Gao L, Zhang Z, Xu W, Yang B, Sun Y. Utility of a modality combining FISH and cytology in upper tract urothelial carcinoma detection in voided urine samples of Chinese patients. Urology. 2011;77:636–41.
33. Mian C, Mazzoleni G, Vikoler S, Martini T, Knuchel-Clark R, Zaak D, Lazica A, Roth S, Mian M, Pycha A. Fluorescence in situ hybridisation in the diagnosis of upper urinary tract tumours. Eur Urol. 2010;58:288–92.
34. Margulis V, Youssef RF, Karakiewicz PI, Lotan Y, Wood CG, Zigeuner R, Kikuchi E, Weizer A, Raman JD, Remzi M, et al. Preoperative multivariable prognostic model for prediction of nonorgan confined urothelial carcinoma of the upper urinary tract. J Urol. 2010;184:453–8.
35. Favaretto RL, Shariat SF, Savage C, Godoy G, Chade DC, Kaag M, Bochner BH, Coleman J, Dalbagni G. Combining imaging and ureteroscopy variables in a preoperative multivariable model for prediction of muscle-invasive and non-organ confined disease in patients with upper tract urothelial carcinoma. BJU Int. 2012;109:77–82.

Chapter 3
Upper Urinary Tract Urothelial Carcinoma Pathology

Kiril Trpkov, Steven Christopher Smith, Premal Patel, and Mahul B. Amin

Abstract Urothelial carcinomas of the upper tract are malignant neoplasms arising from the pelvicalyceal and ureteral mucosal lining and sharing the same pathologic spectrum and overall classification as urothelial neoplasms of the urinary bladder. However, upper tract urothelial carcinomas are more frequently high grade and high stage and show frequent variant differentiation. The histologic differential diagnosis of upper tract urothelial carcinoma, when it involves the kidney, includes collecting duct carcinoma, high-grade renal cell carcinoma, and metastasis, for which contemporary immunohistochemical panels may complement integration of gross, histomorphological, clinical, and radiographic assessment. Grossly, these lesions appear as papillary, polypoid, ulcerative, or infiltrative masses, with thickening of the ureteral or the renal pelvic wall. Careful gross examination and comprehensive sampling of the tumor in this region are essential to reliably distinguish a noninvasive from an invasive tumor, as well as to assign appropriate stage to invasive cases, given the paramount importance of pathologic stage to prognosis. Recently, a growing body of data implicates similar molecular pathways in the genesis of upper tract urothelial carcinoma to those in the genesis of urothelial carcinomas of the lower tract. Evaluation of these markers as diagnostic, predictive, and prognostic biomarkers is ongoing.

K. Trpkov, MD, FRCPC (✉)
Department of Pathology and Laboratory Medicine,
University of Calgary, Calgary Laboratory Services, Rockyview General Hospital,
7007 14 street, Calgary, AB, Canada, T2V 1P9
e-mail: kiril.trpkov@cls.ab.ca

S.C. Smith, MD, PhD • M.B. Amin, MD
Department of Pathology and Laboratory Medicine,
Cedars-Sinai Medical Center, Los Angeles, CA, USA
e-mail: Steven.smith@cshs.org; mahul.amin@cshs.org

P. Patel, MD
Department of Pathology and Laboratory Medicine,
University of Calgary and Calgary Laboratory Services, Calgary, AB, Canada
e-mail: premalpatel8@gmail.com

© Springer Science+Business Media New York 2015

S.F. Shariat, E. Xylinas (eds.), *Upper Tract Urothelial Carcinoma*,
DOI 10.1007/978-1-4939-1501-9_3

Keywords Urothelial carcinoma • Upper tract • Papilloma • Papillary urothelial neoplasm of low malignant potential • Stage • Grade • Biopsy • Resection • Collecting duct carcinoma • Renal cell carcinoma • Immunohistochemistry • Biomarkers • Morphology

Introduction

Upper tract urothelial carcinoma is a malignant neoplasm that involves the segment of the urinary tract that extends from the renal calyces to the ureteral orifices at the bladder. These neoplasms share the same pathologic spectrum and the same classification with the urothelial neoplasia of the bladder. However, they also exhibit significant differences, resulting from the different anatomy of the ureter and the renal pelvis. Because these sites are characterized by a relatively thin lamina propria and smooth muscle layer (muscularis propria), these tumors demonstrate higher incidence of muscle invasion and present at more advanced tumor stage [1, 2]. Upper tract urothelial carcinomas are also more difficult to access clinically than lower tract (bladder/urethral) urothelial carcinomas, because they are less directly accessible endoscopically and they are biopsied only in selected cases. Most patients with upper tract urothelial carcinoma present with microscopic or gross painless hematuria or flank pain. Ureteral tumors may also present with episodic colicky pain. On imaging, there is usually a filling defect or an obstruction caused by a tumoral mass, resulting in hydronephrosis or hydroureter. Additionally, these cases are often associated with nephrolithiasis.

Anatomic Distribution, Epidemiology, and Risk Factors

Upper tract urothelial carcinomas are less common neoplasms and account for about 7–8 % of all urothelial tumors and 5–10 % of all renal tumors [3–6]. Upper tract urothelial carcinomas more commonly affect the renal pelvis, and only about 25–30 % of cases involve the ureters [7, 8]. They occur with equal frequency in both kidneys, with approximately 2–4 % of cases showing bilateral involvement. In certain high-risk groups, bilateral neoplasms have been documented in up to 10 % of patients [6, 9]. Some cases demonstrate contiguous involvement of the renal pelvicalyceal system and the ureter. Furthermore, multifocality is relatively common, and between 6 and 38 % of patients demonstrate synchronous neoplasms in both the renal pelvis and the ureter [6–8, 10–12]. Involvement of the bladder is frequent and is seen in up to 50 % of patients. The bladder involvement may either precede or follow the upper tract urothelial carcinoma, and less commonly it occurs synchronously with the upper tract lesion [6].

The incidence of upper tract urothelial carcinoma ranges from 0.7 to 1.1 per 100,000 individuals, with an increasing trend over the past 30 years [4, 13]. Similar

Table 3.1 Risk factors for upper urinary tract carcinoma

Risk factors
Tobacco smoking
Increased lifetime risk with increased consumption and intensity of smoking
Analgesic abuse
Long-term use of analgesics, especially phenacetin
Balkan nephropathy
Papillary necrosis
Occupation carcinogen exposure
α/β-Naphthylamine, benzidine, aniline dye, petrochemicals, plastic materials, coal,
asphalt, tar, and thorium-containing contrast media (Thorotrast)
Previous urinary bladder carcinoma
>2/3 of patients have prior, concurrent, or subsequent bladder carcinomas
Chronic irritation
Urinary stones
Infection
Cyclophosphamide therapy
Hereditary non-polyposis colon carcinoma

to bladder cancers, upper tract cases are more common in older patients, between the sixth and eight decade, with a mean age of 70 years [4]. There is a male predominance with a male to female ratio of 1.7–1, but the incidence in females has been increasing in recent years [4]. Various risk factors have been associated with upper tract urothelial carcinoma, including environmental, occupational, or chemotherapeutic exposures; additional factors include previous history of urinary bladder carcinoma and genetic predisposition. The risk factors are summarized in Table 3.1.

Histologic Classification of Upper Tract Urothelial Carcinoma

Multiple series confirm that the predominant type of carcinoma arising in the mucosa of the upper urinary tract is urothelial carcinoma, which is diagnosed in >90 % of cases [1–6]. A histologic classification of the different types of carcinomas of the urothelial tract is shown in Table 3.2. Upper tract carcinomas are noted for showing a wide spectrum of variant morphologies. Recent reviews identify that aberrant squamous and glandular differentiation and the micropapillary variant are most frequent at these sites [14]. Additional morphologies include lymphoepithelioma-like, sarcomatoid, clear cell, rhabdoid, small cell neuroendocrine, signet-ring, small and large nested, and plasmacytoid urothelial carcinomas [15]. In fact, these variants may be more prevalent in the upper urothelial tract than in the bladder [2].

Table 3.2 Classification of neoplasms of the ureter and renal pelvis[a]

Urothelial neoplasms
Benign
Urothelial papilloma
Inverted papilloma
Papillary urothelial neoplasm of low malignant potential
Malignant
Papillary
Typical, noninvasive
Typical, with invasion
Variant (with squamous or glandular differentiation)
Micropapillary
Non-papillary (flat)
Carcinoma in situ
Invasive carcinoma, including the variants below:
Variants containing or exhibiting deceptively benign features
Nested pattern (resembling von Brunn's nests)
Large nested pattern
Small nested pattern
Small tubular pattern
Microcystic pattern
Inverted pattern
Squamous differentiation
Glandular differentiation
Undifferentiated carcinoma
Small cell carcinoma/high-grade neuroendocrine carcinoma
Large cell neuroendocrine carcinoma
Micropapillary
Giant Cell Carcinoma
Lymphoepithelioma-like carcinoma
Sarcomatoid foci ("sarcomatoid carcinoma")
Urothelial carcinoma with unusual cytoplasmic features
Clear cell
Plasmacytoid
Rhabdoid
Urothelial carcinoma with syncytiotrophoblasts
With unusual stromal reactions
Pseudosarcomatous stroma
Stromal osseous or cartilaginous metaplasia
Osteoclast-type giant cells
With prominent lymphoid infiltrate
Myxoid stroma/chordoid differentiation
Squamous Cell Carcinoma
Typical
Variant histology, including verrucous carcinoma and basaloid squamous cell carcinoma

(continued)

Table 3.2 (continued)

Adenocarcinoma
Histologic variants
Typical (Enteric type)
Mucinous (including colloid)
Signet-ring cell
Clear cell
Hepatoid
Mixed Adenocarcinoma, not otherwise specified (NOS)
Undifferentiated Carcinoma (pure/no synchronous or history of urothelial carcinoma)
Small cell carcinoma (pure/no synchronous or history of urothelial carcinoma)
Large cell neuroendocrine carcinoma (pure/no synchronous or history of urothelial carcinoma)
Lymphoepithelioma-like carcinoma (pure/no synchronous or history of urothelial carcinoma)
Giant cell carcinoma (pure/no synchronous or history of urothelial carcinoma)
Metastatic Carcinoma

[a]Compiled from the WHO Classification of Pathology and Genetics of Tumours of the Urinary System and Male Genital Organs [126], CAP Protocol for the examination of specimens from patients with carcinoma of the ureter and renal pelvis [34], Consensus Statements of the International Society of Urological Pathology [30, 93], and AJCC Staging Manual [33]

The morphologic variation present in these tumors can present diagnostic challenges: while a conventional papillary or flat urothelial carcinoma is quite familiar to the surgical pathologist, the remarkable variety of variants is not, with some studies suggesting that variant differentiation may be under-recognized by surgical pathologists [16, 17]. Additionally, cases of urothelial carcinoma with extensive variant differentiation underscore one of the limitations of interpretation of small biopsies and the importance of appropriate sampling of resection specimens; a carcinoma showing an extensive pattern of squamous differentiation may only be recognized as a urothelial carcinoma with squamous differentiation if an unequivocal urothelial carcinoma component (whether in situ, invasive, or papillary in architecture) is identified, at least focally [15].

Gross Features

Grossly, urothelial carcinomas of the upper tract may appear as papillary, polypoid, ulcerative, or infiltrative masses, with thickening of the renal pelvic or ureteral wall (Fig. 3.1a–d). Tumors with papillary or polypoid features are more likely

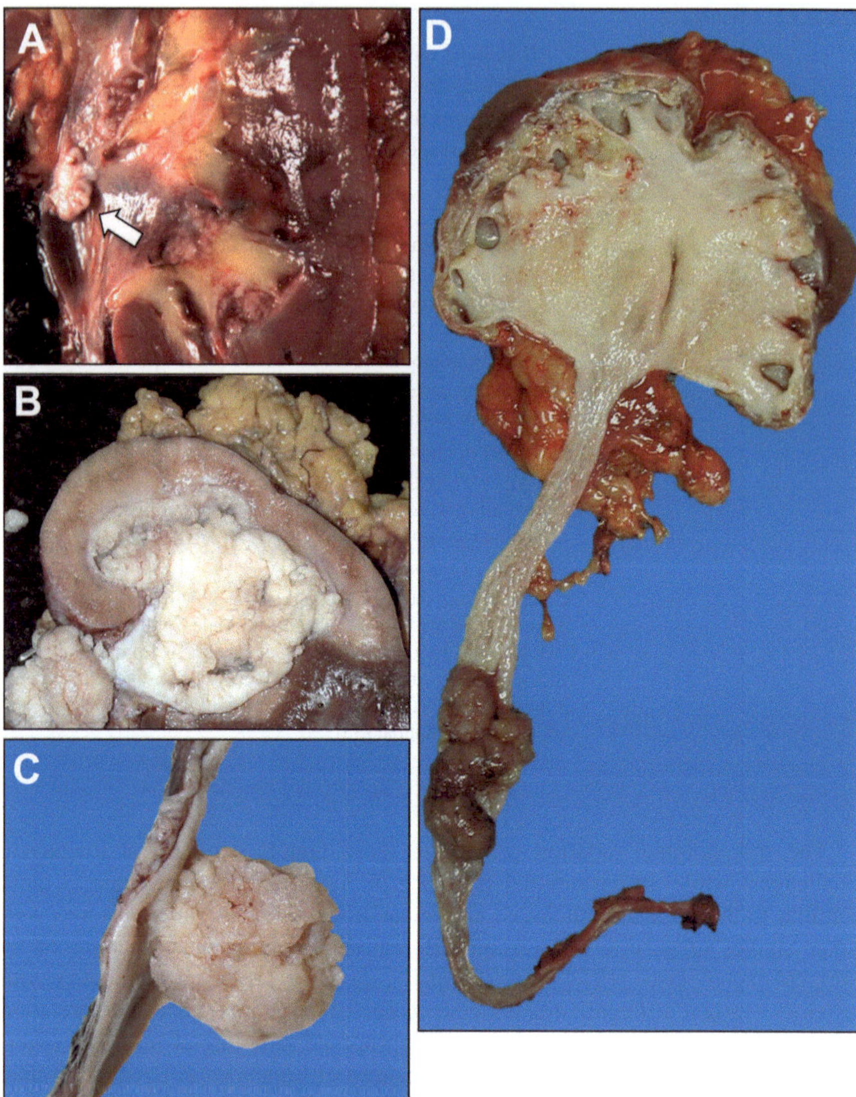

Fig. 3.1 Gross appearance of urothelial neoplasms of upper urinary tract. (**a**) A small noninvasive papillary urothelial carcinoma of the renal pelvis (*arrow*). (**b**) Urothelial carcinoma extensively involving the renal pelvis, minor calyces, and proximal ureter. (**c**) Urothelial carcinoma of the ureter showing papillary and polypoid appearance. (**d**) Urothelial carcinoma of the ureter causing complete obstruction, resulting in hydronephrosis

noninvasive; such cases may grow significantly and completely fill the lumen of the ureter and the pelvicalyceal system. An expansion into the lumen of the distal ureter, the most common tumor location, can cause an obstruction, resulting in hydronephrosis [13]. Carcinomas that invade the renal parenchyma may grossly mimic a high-grade primary renal carcinoma, from which it may be difficult to distinguish, especially in core biopsies or limited samples [18–21].

Intraoperative assessment by frozen section may complement the imaging findings to determine whether a tumor originates from the urothelial lining or the renal parenchyma, a distinction which may direct the surgical or chemotherapeutic management. Invasive carcinomas of urothelial origin typically require a radical nephroureterectomy, whereas primary renal cortical tumors may be managed by radical or "nephron-sparing" partial nephrectomy. Another important aspect of the gross evaluation of the tumor is to assess for multifocality, because the pathologic stage may vary for different tumors [13].

Urothelial carcinomas of the renal pelvis may present either as large papillary/polypoid tumors expanding the pelvicalyceal system or as broadly infiltrative cancers of the renal parenchyma. These tumors are often centered on the renal pelvis and medulla, but in some instances this may not be apparent grossly. Careful dissection is necessary to preserve the relationship of infiltrative tumors within the renal medulla to the pelvicalyceal mucosa and the renal parenchyma. Thus, multiple histologic sections are often necessary to demonstrate the anatomic relationships and clarify the differential diagnosis and the pathologic stage. Infiltrative carcinomas, particularly if arising in or centered on the minor calyces, may also grossly mimic renal cortical neoplasms. Ulcerative or infiltrative lesions may cause mucosal defect or thickening of the ureteral or the pelvic wall, which sometimes may be more difficult to appreciate grossly [13], underscoring the importance of a careful gross evaluation and sectioning.

Histopathology and Differential Diagnoses

The histopathology of upper urinary tract tumors is analogous to the histopathology of the urothelial neoplasia of the urinary bladder, as illustrated in Table 3.2, and demonstrates the same histopathologic diversity seen in bladder tumors [2, 4, 6, 10, 13, 22]. The basic histopathology of upper urinary tract tumors includes papillary noninvasive tumors (papilloma, papillary urothelial neoplasm of low malignant potential "PUNLMP," low-grade papillary carcinoma, or high-grade papillary carcinoma), carcinoma in situ, and invasive carcinoma. PUNLMP appears to be extremely rare in the upper urinary tract, and low-grade carcinoma is also less common compared to lesions in the bladder. High-grade carcinomas are the most common upper urinary tract tumors, and they are often invasive at presentation. About 70 % of all tumors in the renal pelvis are high-grade urothelial carcinomas [2, 6]. Although the broad histologic spectrum seen in the bladder can also be seen in the upper urinary tract, several divergent carcinoma morphologies occur more frequently in the pelvicalyceal system. These patterns include micropapillary, lymphoepithelioma-like, sarcomatoid, squamous or glandular differentiation, rhabdoid, signet-ring, small cell, or plasmacytoid, as well as a variety of lesions with giant cells, even with trophoblastic differentiation [2]. Some of these are illustrated in Fig. 3.2a, b. Table 3.3

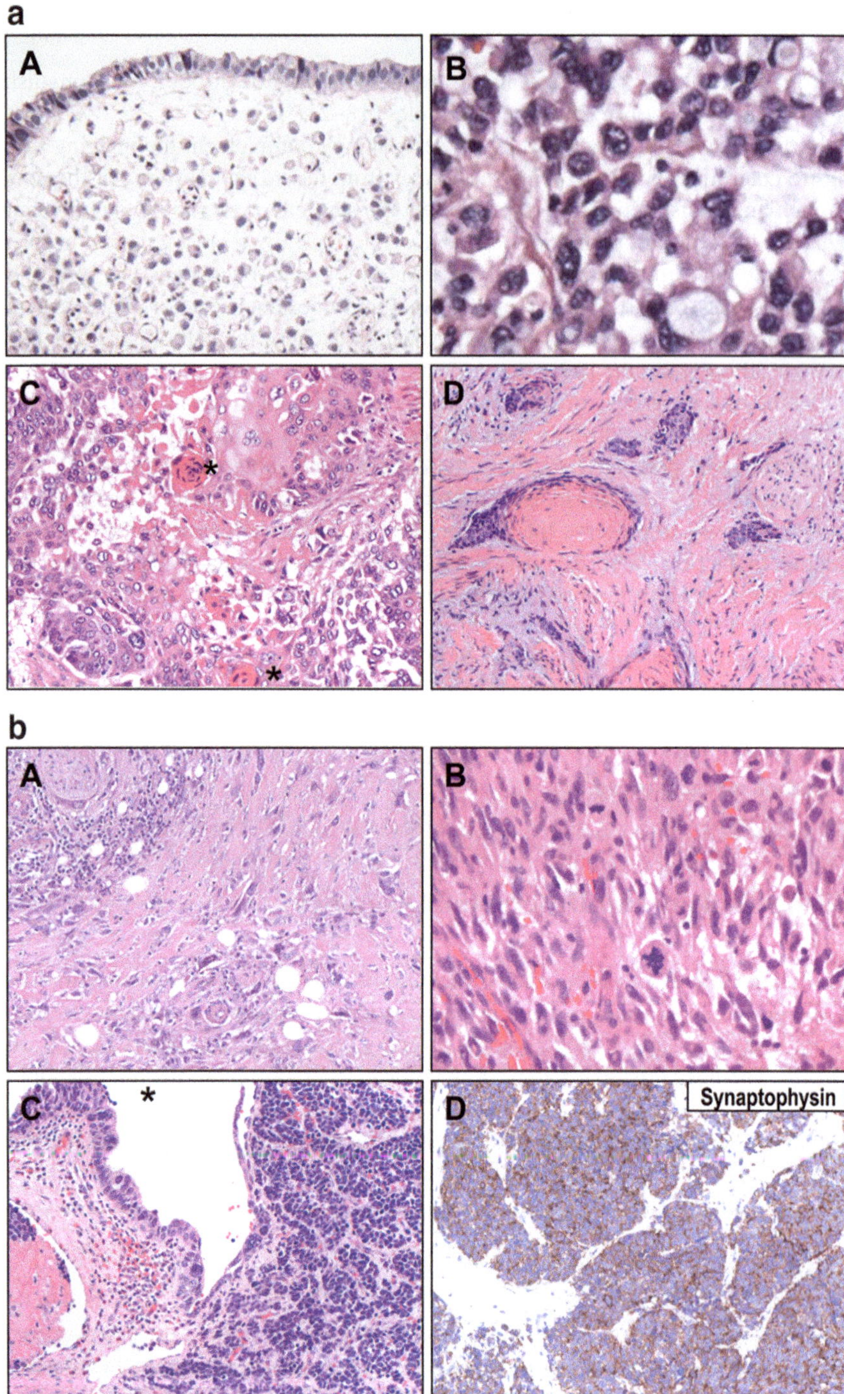

Fig. 3.2 (**a**) Urothelial carcinomas of upper tract demonstrate divergent morphologies. A. Plasmacytoid variant of urothelial carcinoma is characterized by single-cell discohesive appearance. B. Plasmacytoid urothelial carcinomas frequently demonstrate areas of signet ring cell morphology. C. Squamous differentiation is often seen in urothelial carcinoma of the upper tract.

Table 3.3 Most frequent patterns of variant differentiation in upper tract urothelial carcinoma

Variant	Differential diagnosis	Significance
Squamous	Primary squamous cell carcinoma; keratinizing and non-keratinizing squamous metaplasia; condyloma acuminatum with extension into the bladder	Poor prognosis overall; possible inferior response to chemoradiation
Glandular	Primary adenocarcinoma, including clear cell and enteric variants; intestinal metaplasia; villous adenoma; urachal adenocarcinoma; metastatic adenocarcinomas	Poor prognosis overall; limited data on treatment implications
Sarcomatoid	Primary sarcomas of the bladder, including leiomyosarcoma, undifferentiated pleomorphic sarcoma, malignant peripheral nerve sheath tumors, and rhabdomyosarcoma; urothelial carcinomas with pseudosarcomatous stromal changes; pseudosarcomatous myofibroblastic proliferations/inflammatory myofibroblastic tumors	Remarkably poor prognosis, including median survival of 1 year; consideration of sarcoma-directed chemotherapy
Micropapillary	Adenocarcinomas with micropapillary morphology of other sites, including breast and papillary serous adenocarcinomas of the gynecologic tract	High stage disease at presentation, including vascular invasion and nodal metastasis; poor prognostic histology; may be associated with Her2/neu molecular alterations
Small Cell	Primary small cell carcinoma (not arising from a urothelial carcinoma), metastatic small cell carcinoma from lung or by direct extension from prostate; small round blue cell tumors (rhabdomyosarcoma); lymphoma	High stage disease with poor prognosis, wide metastatic dissemination, and possible paraneoplastic syndromes; chemotherapy used for pulmonary counterparts often offered

Fig. 3.2 (continued) A morphologic hallmark of squamous differentiation is keratinization and formation of keratin pearls (adjacent to *asterisks*) in this low power micrograph. D. Urothelial carcinoma with prominent squamous differentiation. In a case with extensive squamous (or other variant) differentiation, urothelial vs. primary squamous carcinoma requires careful sampling and inspection for a conventional urothelial component. This distinction may guide therapy selection. (**b**) Urothelial carcinomas of upper tract demonstrate divergent morphologies. A. Sarcomatoid differentiation may also occur with urothelial carcinomas of the upper tract, characterized by markedly atypical, spindled cell growth. B. Higher power view of a sarcomatoid urothelial carcinoma shows pleomorphic spindled cells with atypical mitoses, reminiscent of a pleomorphic sarcoma. C. Small cell carcinoma can also be seen in the upper tract. Urothelial carcinoma in situ (*asterisk*) is shown, a variant of high-grade neuroendocrine (small cell) differentiation. A primary small cell carcinoma or a metastasis from another site, such as lung, needs to be ruled out clinically in these cases. D. Neuroendocrine differentiation may be confirmed immunohistochemically by appropriate immunostains, such as synaptophysin (illustrated), chromogranin, or CD56

outlines the five most common forms of variant differentiation as recently reported in a large multi-institutional cohort [14], including pathologic lesions in the differential diagnosis and clinicopathological significance.

In one large study, these variant morphologic features were present in 40 % of renal pelvis tumors [2]. To add to the morphologic diversity of these lesions, recent reports have identified three additional variants of urothelial carcinoma, urothelial carcinoma with myxoid stroma (so-called "chordoid" differentiation), which may simulate mucinous adenocarcinoma, myxoid sarcomas, or myoepithelial neoplasms [23], large nested urothelial carcinoma, which is low-grade appearing and a mimic of benign processes [24], and large cell undifferentiated carcinoma, which engenders a wide differential, including metastatic carcinomas of other sites, sarcomas, and even melanoma [25]. In most studies, variant differentiation has been associated with advanced stage and poor outcomes [15]; recent studies suggest that the association with poor outcome is related to advanced stage at presentation or at surgery rather than as an independent prognostic or predictive factor [14].

The microscopic diagnosis of urothelial carcinoma of the upper urinary tract may be either straightforward, or it may mimic collecting duct carcinoma, high-grade undifferentiated renal cell carcinoma (RCC), or a metastasis. Urothelial carcinomas and carcinomas of the collecting ducts of Bellini (collecting duct carcinomas) or high-grade undifferentiated RCC may demonstrate similar features, such as an infiltrative pattern and a desmoplastic response in the renal medullary region [13]. A predominantly nested, solid, or trabecular invasive architecture with a variable squamous or glandular component favors urothelial carcinoma. Additional features in favor of urothelial carcinoma include history of urothelial cancer, coexisting papillary urothelial neoplasia involving the pelvicalyceal system, or presence of carcinoma in situ. In contrast, collecting duct carcinoma is essentially a high-grade adenocarcinoma with recognizable glandular architecture. Dysplastic features may often be present in the adjacent renal tubules, and urothelial carcinoma in situ should be absent. Figure 3.3 illustrates key points in the differential diagnosis of urothelial carcinoma versus collecting duct carcinoma.

Importantly, as collecting duct carcinomas are rare and represent a diagnosis of exclusion, metastatic adenocarcinoma must be ruled out before establishing such a diagnosis. Metastatic carcinoma can be favored when the histology does not conform to any of the known subtypes of urothelial carcinoma or RCC, and when multifocality is documented, clinically, grossly, or microscopically. Metastatic carcinomas are often associated with extensive lymphovascular invasion and interstitial growth [13]. Metastases to the upper urinary tract generally involve the ureters and may originate from primary breast, kidney, stomach, colon, and hematologic malignancies [26–28]. A careful microscopic and gross examination with appropriate clinicopathological correlation will help resolve the differential diagnosis in most cases. Renal medullary carcinoma is another differential diagnostic consideration; however, this aggressive type of renal carcinoma is uncommon and usually occurs in younger African-American patients with sickle cell disease or trait [29]. In some instances, however, immunohistochemistry may play an important ancillary role in resolving the differential diagnosis [18–21].

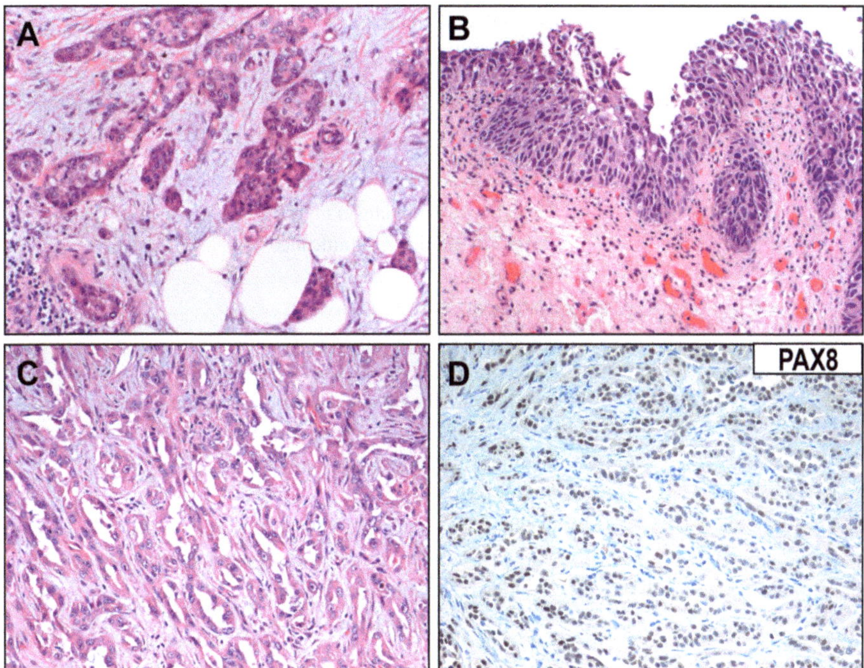

Fig. 3.3 Differentiating urothelial carcinoma from collecting duct carcinoma can be challenging. (**a**) An invasive upper tract urothelial carcinoma showing small, infiltrative nests simulating the malignant glandular morphology of collecting duct carcinoma. (**b**) Identification of an in situ urothelial carcinoma may be helpful in establishing urothelial origin for the neoplasm. (**c**) A representative field showing collecting duct carcinoma morphology, composed of invading cords and trabeculae in a desmoplastic stroma. (**d**) Reactivity for immunohistochemical marker PAX8 (illustrated) can be helpful in establishing a diagnosis of collecting duct carcinoma (rather than urothelial carcinoma with glandular differentiation)

Histopathologic Grading

The grading scheme of urothelial tumors of the upper urinary tract is identical to that used for bladder neoplasms. Consistent with mounting evidence that flat and papillary lesions proceed from significantly different molecular pathways, papillary and flat lesions are graded separately, though the cytologic criteria used for grading are similar. The basis of classification of urothelial neoplasms of the urinary bladder was a consensus report, published in 1998, which standardized both classification and the grading system [30]. This system was provided as a consensus approach by the World Health Organization and International Society of Urologic Pathology was adopted in the WHO 2004 “Blue Book” [4]; this approach has become the international standard. Importantly, though this system was developed and implemented as a consensus approach to lower tract urothelial neoplasms, it is applied to upper tract urothelial lesions as well. Table 3.4 summarizes this classification system.

Table 3.4 Consensus for classification and grading of urothelial lesions[a]

Normal urothelium
Hyperplasia
Flat
Papillary
Mixed
Flat Lesions with Atypia
Reactive (inflammatory) atypia
Atypia of unknown significance
Dysplasia
Carcinoma in situ
Exophytic Papillary Neoplasms
Papilloma
Papillary urothelial neoplasm of low malignant potential
Papillary carcinoma, low-grade
Papillary carcinoma, high-grade
Inverted Papilloma
Papilloma
Papillary urothelial neoplasm of low malignant potential
Papillary carcinoma, low-grade
Papillary carcinoma, high-grade
Mixed Exophytic and Endophytic
Papilloma
Papillary urothelial neoplasm of low malignant potential
Papillary carcinoma, low-grade
Papillary carcinoma, high-grade
Invasive Neoplasms
Lamina propria invasion
Muscularis propria invasion

[a]Compiled from the WHO Classification of Pathology and Genetics of Tumours of the Urinary System and Male Genital Organs [126], CAP Protocol for the examination of specimens from patients with carcinoma of the ureter and renal pelvis [34], Consensus Statements of the International Society of Urological Pathology [30, 93], and AJCC Staging Manual [33]

Among papillary neoplasms, broadly there are four groups of lesions. The first group includes benign neoplasms, which include papillomas and inverted papillomas (see below section on "benign tumors"), which are not graded because they are benign. Among papillary lesions with malignant potential, there are three types of lesions: papillary urothelial neoplasms with low malignant potential (PUNLMP), low-grade papillary urothelial carcinomas, and high-grade papillary urothelial carcinomas. Among flat neoplasms, two groups are identified: urothelial dysplasia and urothelial carcinoma in situ. Grading of urothelial carcinoma is based on architectural and cytologic features. These include lack of differentiation from the base to the surface, loss of polarity and cell orientation, and the nuclear features such as nuclear atypia, chromatin texture, hyperchromasia, macronucleoli, and mitotic activity (Fig. 3.4).

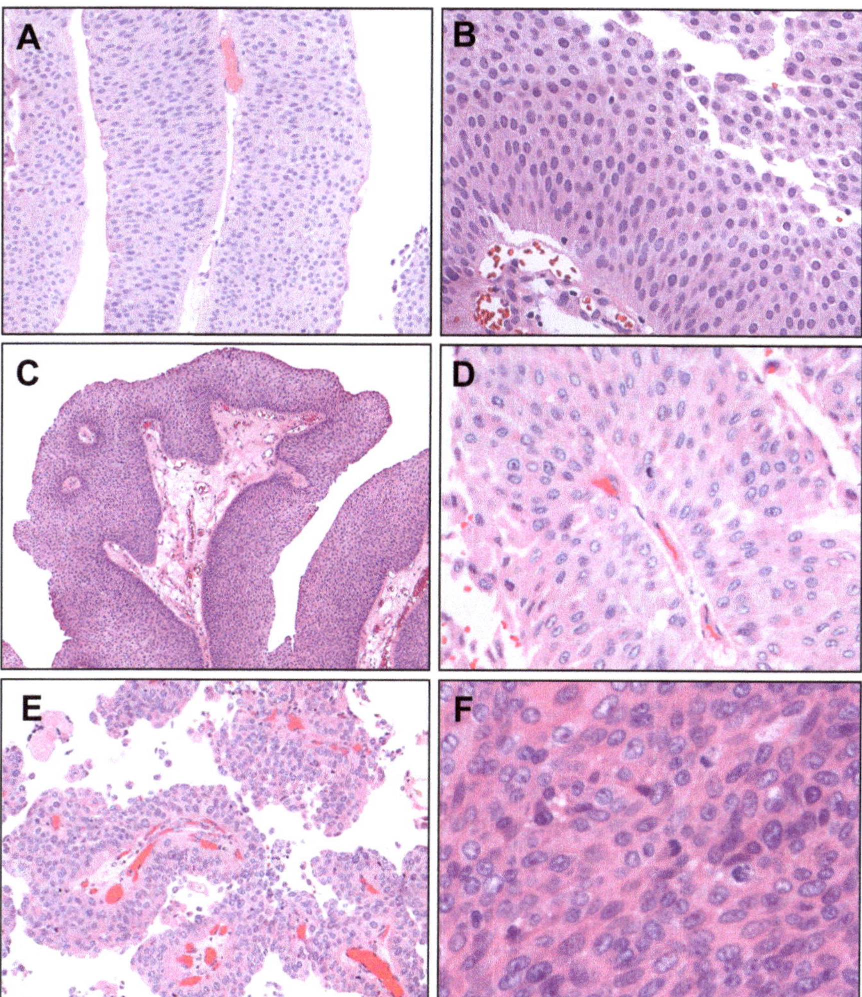

Fig. 3.4 Grading of papillary urothelial neoplasm. (**a**) Papillary urothelial neoplasm of low malignant potential (PUNLMP) demonstrates papillary growth with thickened epithelium exhibiting minimal architectural and cytologic atypia. (**b**) On higher power, it is apparent that urothelial cells in PUNLMP show mild atypia; mitotic figures are absent, or if present, they have a basal location. (**c**) Low-grade urothelial carcinoma exhibits greater architectural complexity of the papillae, with branching and fusion. (**d**) On higher power, there is more prominent cytologic atypia with variation in nuclear size, presence of small nucleoli, irregularities of nuclear membranes, and coarser chromatin. Importantly, the polarization of the epithelium is maintained. (**e**) High-grade papillary urothelial carcinoma exhibits complex architecture and the epithelium is markedly atypical, with variably sized rounded nuclei and loss of polarity. (**f**) On higher power, the degree of cell atypia is apparent. There is disordered architecture, cell crowding, frequent mitotic features, hyperchromasia and macronucleoli, markedly coarser chromatin, and marked nuclear irregularity

Generally speaking, the degree of cytologic atypia present is comparable between flat and papillary lesions of similar grades; for example, the cytologic atypia present in a low-grade papillary urothelial carcinoma is essentially equivalent to the degree of atypia present in urothelial dysplasia, though the latter flat lesion is much less prevalent. Similarly, the degree of atypia present in a high-grade papillary urothelial carcinoma is equivalent to a flat urothelial carcinoma in situ. The grade that is assigned is based on the worst area present for evaluation, and combinations of lesions may be present in a given individual (i.e., a low-grade papillary urothelial carcinoma with simultaneous adjacent flat urothelial carcinoma in situ or carcinoma in situ in a separate biopsy).

Invasive lesions are generally regarded as high-grade definitionally, with rare examples of invasive variants with a low-grade appearance, like the small and large nested variants of urothelial carcinoma [24, 31, 32]. For this reason, grade is generally only prognostic amongst noninvasive papillary tumors; most pT2 and higher stage tumors tend to be non-papillary and of higher grade [4]. Olgac et al. noted that although WHO/ISUP 2004 system stratifies renal pelvic tumors into distinct prognostic groups, the grade is not a significant prognostic factor on multivariate analysis [6]. Overall, and most pertinent to urothelial carcinomas of the upper tract, pelvicalyceal and ureteral urothelial carcinomas show a higher prevalence of high-grade lesions compared to bladder lesions [6].

Pathologic Stage

Pathologic staging of urothelial carcinoma of the upper tract is as outlined by the American Joint Committee on Cancer [33] and is summarized in Table 3.5. As is the case in other organ systems, lesions of the upper urothelial tract are staged by a "TNM"-based system, though given the differing anatomy and histology of pelvicalyceal lesions versus ureteral lesions, the staging of invasive lesions differs somewhat. In this system, the "T" refers to the primary tumor mass, and the letter or number associated refers to the depth of invasion. Noninvasive lesions are staged as Ta or Tis, indicative of papillary noninvasive Ta and flat noninvasive carcinoma in situ, respectively. Invasive lesions are staged as T1, T2, T3, or T4, each of which indicates varying depths of invasion. Similarly, the "N" refers to nodal status, which varies from N1-3 based on the number of involved regional lymph nodes and size of the metastasis. The "M" designation refers to distant metastasis, which may be either to a visceral site (e.g., liver) or to a lymph node that is beyond the regional lymph nodes specified by the AJCC for lesions of the renal pelvis or of the ureter (e.g., a supraclavicular lymph node). Also, similar to TNM-based systems, a lower case "p" assigned to the pT stage is indicative of pathologic staging, while a lower case "c" indicates clinical stage, as may be assigned based on examination and imaging findings before resection with pathologic staging, or in cases where pathologic staging is not possible. The TNM

Table 3.5 Pathologic staging of urothelial carcinoma of the upper tract (pTNM)[a]

Primary tumor (pT)
pTX: Cannot be assessed
pT0: No evidence of primary tumor
pTa: Papillary carcinoma without invasion
pTis: Flat carcinoma in situ without invasion
pT1: Carcinoma invades subepithelial connective tissue/stroma (lamina propria)
pT2: Carcinoma invades the muscularis propria of the ureter or pelvicalyceal mucosa
pT3: Pelvicalyceal-based carcinoma invades through muscularis of pelvis into peripelvic fat or into the renal parenchyma
Or
Ureter-based carcinoma invades beyond muscularis propria into periureteric fat
pT4: Pelvicalyceal carcinoma invades through the kidney into perinephric fat
Or
Ureteric carcinoma invades into adjacent organs, or through the kidney into the perinephric fat
Regional Lymph Nodes (pN)
pN0: No regional lymph node metastasis
pN1: Metastasis in a single regional lymph node, 2 cm or less in greatest dimension
pN2: Metastasis in a single regional lymph node, more than 2 cm but not more than 5 cm in greatest dimension, or multiple lymph nodes, none more than 5 cm in greatest dimension
pN3: Metastasis in a regional lymph node more than 5 cm in greatest dimension
Distant metastasis (pM)
Not applicable
pM1: Distant metastasis
TNM Descriptors (required only if applicable) (select all that apply)
m (multiple)
r (recurrent)
y (posttreatment)

[a]Compiled from the WHO Classification of Pathology and Genetics of Tumours of the Urinary System and Male Genital Organs [126], CAP Protocol for the examination of specimens from patients with carcinoma of the ureter and renal pelvis [34], Consensus Statements of the International Society of Urological Pathology [30, 93], and AJCC Staging Manual [33]

combination of each case may then be assigned to prognostic groupings, which vary from Stages I to IV and are of particular use for therapeutic decision-making and consideration of treatment guidelines.

In both lesions of the renal pelvis and the ureter, noninvasive lesions are staged as pTa (if papillary) or pTis (if flat carcinoma in situ), while flat or papillary lesions that invade the basement membrane and into the connective tissue of the lamina propria, whether beneath the lesion or within the stalk of papillary growths (infrequently occurring in papillary lesions), are staged as pT1. Unlike the urinary bladder, the mucosa of the ureter and renal pelvis generally does not exhibit a layer of fine, wispy muscle within the lamina propria, the so-called "muscularis mucosae," which can render staging interpretation difficult in bladder specimens. Instead, beyond the connective tissue of the lamina propria, in both the renal pelvis (including most of its major calyces) and the ureter, is the muscularis propria or definitive muscular layer of the organ, which if invaded is staged as pT2. In the ureter, invasion through this muscularis propria and into periureteral soft (predominantly adipose tissue) is staged as pT3; invasion through muscle and soft tissue into adjacent organs is staged as pT4. In the renal pelvis, definitive invasion into the renal parenchyma is staged as pT3, while invasion through the renal parenchyma into perirenal adipose tissue is pT4.

Difficulties in Pathologic Staging of Upper Tract Urothelial Carcinomas

The staging system in its present form has the advantage of providing an internationally standardized framework so that lesions of similar extent may be classified and stratified into prognostically and therapeutically actionable groups. However, there are several areas of difficulty in the staging that require utmost attention from surgical pathologists. The first issue pertains to the remarkable degree of variability in the histology of the upper tract, in particular, in the renal pelvis. Because invasion of the muscularis propria (pT2) is an important intermediate stage between "superficial" invasion of the connective tissue of the lamina propria (pT1) and invasion of the renal parenchyma (pT3), two stages with dramatically different prognoses, the patchy to absent nature of the muscularis propria in the minor calyces provides an important conundrum in pathologic staging. Similarly, at the medullary pyramids, the urothelium essentially directly overlies the collecting system. At these sites, a carcinoma that invades the lamina propria may only have to traverse less than a millimeter or two of basement membrane before meeting diagnostic criteria for invasion of the renal parenchyma (which by definition includes the collecting ducts of Bellini); thus, extensive sampling of these tumors and a liberal use of deeper sections to evaluate the extent of invasion are critical.

For that matter, minor calyceal carcinomas may also spread into the distal renal collecting ducts in an intraepithelial or so-called "pagetoid" fashion, which may mimic the histologic appearance of renal parenchymal invasion without actually invading the basement membrane. At issue is whether definitive invasion of the basement membrane (pT1) or whether true, parenchymal invasion is present (pT3). Careful review of histologic sections is necessary to ascertain whether this pagetoid spread, which is considered pTa/pTis noninvasive disease, is present, as the prognostic and therapeutic difference between such noninvasive or superficially invasive disease and parenchymal invasion is very significant. In contrast, stage pT3 parenchymal invasion is generally destructive, multifocal to broad, and associated with stromal reaction (desmoplasia) and necrosis. Figure 3.5 provides examples of these important staging dilemmas.

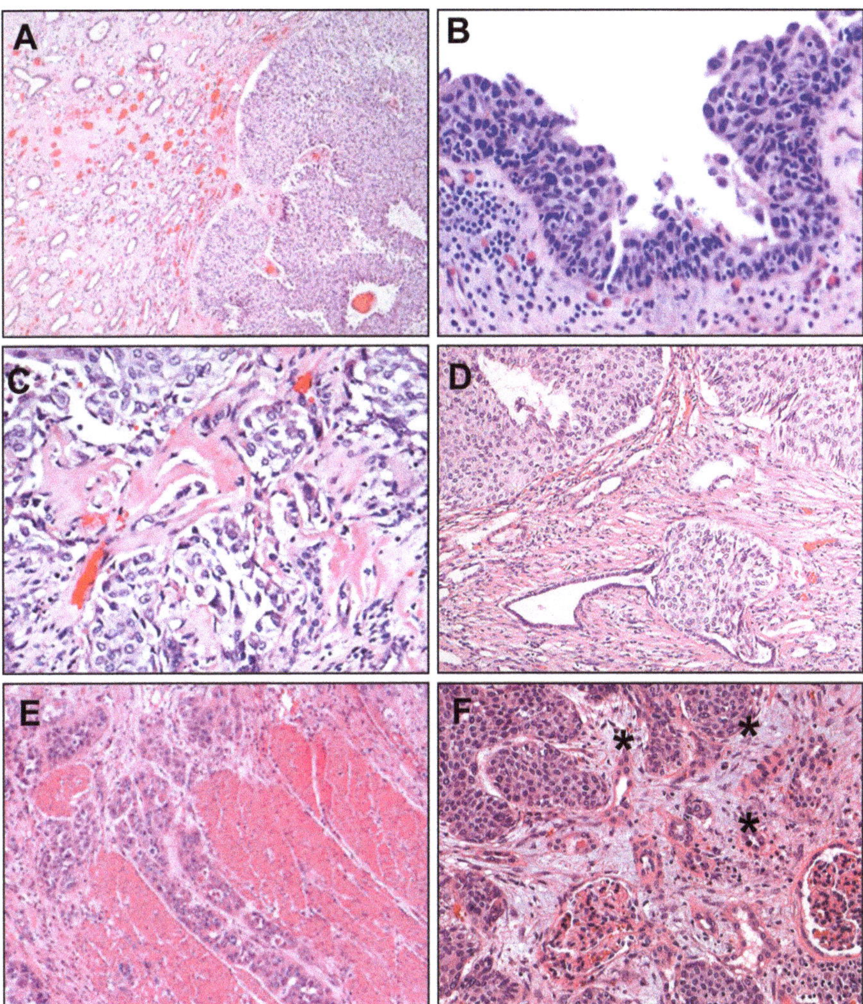

Fig. 3.5 Diagnostic challenges in pathologic staging of upper tract urothelial carcinoma (see also Table 3.4). (**a**) An upper tract urothelial carcinoma involving the minor calyces of the kidney presents a unique challenge, given the close apposition of the luminal tumor growth and the collecting system. In this example, a noninvasive tumor is present in a minor calyx, pushing and compressing the collecting ducts of Bellini. It is important to carefully sample and evaluate the tumor and the parenchymal interface, because an invasive tumor at this site may rapidly progress from early subepithelial stromal invasion (pT1) to renal parenchymal invasion (pT3) (**b**) In this example, flat urothelial carcinoma in situ shows significant cellular atypia, with nuclear hyperchromasia, nucleoli, and variability in nuclear size. Despite the associated inflammatory infiltrate in the lamina propria, this represents in situ disease (pTis). (**c**) A high power field demonstrating features of early stromal invasion, with small, irregular nests and single cells, accompanied by stromal desmoplasia and retraction artifact. This tumor is stage pT1. (**d**) An intraductal extension of low-grade papillary urothelial carcinoma is present into the collecting ducts, which does not represent true invasion, but an in situ disease (pTa or pTis, if flat lesion). A preserved layer of the tubular lining cells is apparent adjacent to the lesional cells. (**e**) Upper tract urothelial carcinoma invades well-formed smooth muscle bundles of ureteral muscularis propria (stage pT2). (**f**) Parenchymal invasion in the kidney parenchyma, illustrated at high power by individual malignant cells (*asterisks*) invading around a glomerulus, represents stage pT3

Upper Tract Urothelial Carcinoma Specimens: Processing, Sampling, and Reporting

Modern practices in urologic surgical oncology may result in a diversity of specimens being sent to surgical pathology. These range from tiny endoscopic biopsies from ureteroscopy to scant needle core biopsy fragments from image-guided biopsy protocols from interventional radiology to larger segmental ureterectomy, nephrectomy, and nephroureterectomy specimens undertaken by open, laparoscopic, and robot-assisted approaches. Fortunately, the College of American Pathologists provides evidence-based guidances in this regard, which may be referenced as a guide to establishing institutional procedures for laboratory processing of these specimens, as well as providing an outline of the reporting elements by specimen type and anatomical site [34].

Briefly, the tiny biopsies from ureteroscopic examination of upper tract lesions must be submitted entirely, with particular care in gross and histologic handling. One approach is to process such scant biopsies as cytologic specimens, using "cell block" preparations such as are used to process aspirates and other scant specimens. Other labs employ special protocols for tiny biopsy material to avoid unnecessary trim and waste of tissue when slides are being prepared. Needle core biopsies are also submitted entirely; given the shape and geometry of such specimens, multiple levels are often necessary for tissue interpretation; multiple precut levels may be made to preserve tissue should additional ancillary histochemical or immunohistochemical stains be necessary.

For larger specimens such as a segmental "partial" ureterectomy, such as may be performed for limited resection of lesions in the proximal or mid ureter, careful gross exam is important. First, the outer aspect of the specimen should be inked. The length and diameter of the specimen should be documented in the gross description, and the proximal and distal margins should be sampled en face. Then, the ureter may be opened longitudinally, with careful inspection and palpation for lesions that are not grossly apparent; carcinoma in situ, prior biopsy sites, and diminutive papillary lesions may appear as subtle mucosal abnormalities. A grossly apparent lesion should be measured, documenting its extent of surface involvement, depth of invasion, and relationship to the margins. Given the small size of these specimens, it may be advantageous to entirely submit the involved area if feasible in a reasonable number of sections. Overnight fixation in 10 % formalin is recommended to ensure appropriate sectioning of friable lesions. If gross lesions are absent, extensive sampling of the urothelium is necessary to look for in situ lesions.

Larger nephrectomy or nephroureterectomy with bladder cuff specimens also require careful gross examination, fixation, and documentation of anatomical relationships and extent of disease. Similarly, specimens should be inked on the exterior and mucosal margins (distal ureteral) and vascular (renal artery and vein) margins sampled. Sectioning should focus on demonstrating anatomical relationships most relevant to pathologic stage (relationship of tumor to lamina propria, muscular walls, renal parenchyma, perirenal or periureteral soft tissue). Additional sections of grossly uninvolved renal parenchyma and pelvicalyceal and ureteral mucosa should be taken to evaluate for glomerular disease and in situ lesions, respectively.

Definitive resection specimens such as nephroureterectomies may or may not include a lymphadenectomy as an attached or separate specimen. As in all cancer resection specimens, the perirenal and periureteral adipose tissue should be carefully examined to identify any associated lymph nodes, which should be submitted for evaluation of metastatic disease. Whether attached or separately submitted, any lymph nodes appearing grossly to be involved by metastatic disease should be measured and a representative section submitted. Any grossly negative lymph nodes should be submitted entirely, as identification of even microscopic nodal metastasis impacts the therapeutic approach. While lymph node metastasis is only identified in ~10 % of cases, in cases where lymph nodes are dissected at resection, the rate of lymph node involvement approaches one in four cases, underscoring the aggressiveness of this disease.

One harbinger of metastatic disease that may be apparent even in cases that do not show lymph node involvement is invasion of the lymphovascular space, also known as vascular invasion, lymphovascular invasion, or angiolymphatic invasion. This finding, defined as the identification outside the main tumor mass of tumor cells adherent to or floating within lymphatics and small veins, is a relatively frequent finding in urothelial carcinomas at any site. Though friable tumor cells and necrotic debris may be seen floating in vascular spaces as an artifact of sampling and histologic preparation, identification of true vascular invasion often shows the features of adherent, "vessel-shaped" balls of carcinoma, often covered with a layer of endothelial cells or adherent to the muscular wall of a vessel. In any case of suspicious but not definitive for vascular invasion, liberal use of deeper sections and even immunohistochemical stains to confirm that the lumen is indeed vascular (i.e., CD31, CD34, Erg, or other vascular markers) may be undertaken.

For that matter, a nephroureterectomy with bladder cuff is a complex specimen that includes mucosal, vascular, and radial soft tissue margins. These should be sampled with care, which, as always, requires communication with the surgical team to ensure appropriate evaluation of margin status. For margins sampled by frozen section at the time of intraoperative consultation, frozen-permanent section correlation should be undertaken as a routine quality assurance measure.

Finally, guidelines from the College of American Pathologists for evaluation of renal resection margins call for submission of tissue sections of grossly uninvolved tumor tissue for evaluation of medical renal kidney disease. Large series of renal resections find that arterionephrosclerosis, hypertensive nephropathy, or diabetic nephropathy may be present in a substantial minority of cases [35]. Such changes have been associated with a decline in renal function post-nephrectomy [36]. Histochemical stains such as PAS and Jones silver stains may be necessary to appropriately evaluate for glomerular disease. Consultation with a medical renal pathologist may be undertaken in equivocal or worrisome cases.

Pathologic Diagnostic Issues in Evaluating Ureteroscopic Biopsies and Other Upper Urinary Tract Specimens

The management of upper tract urothelial carcinoma has significantly changed with the introduction of modern imaging techniques and endoscopic visualization of all levels of the urinary tract. The development of better imaging techniques, including computed tomography urogram and magnetic resonance urogram and the use of novel endoscopic instruments, including flexible and digital ureteroscopes, has greatly improved the ability to identify and characterize these cases. These technical advances have led to increased frequency of performing ureteroscopic biopsies of the upper urinary tract. The relatively low frequency of these tumors, however, has been an impediment to conducting randomized trials that would allow definitive conclusions about staging, grading, and treatment impact on patient prognosis.

From a diagnostic standpoint, suspected upper tract urothelial carcinomas are usually evaluated by retrograde ureteropyelography, upper urinary tract cytology, and cystoureteroscopy with biopsy. Ureteroscopic biopsy is crucial for the diagnosis, follow-up, and management of the upper ureter and renal pelvis lesions and is the current gold standard for diagnosis. Ureteroscopy and pyeloscopy allow visualization of the suspected lesion and an ability to perform a targeted biopsy. The biopsy can potentially provide accurate histologic type and grade, and in some instances, such approaches may even be able to stage an upper tract urothelial carcinoma, providing parameters crucial for selection of the appropriate treatment.

Ureteroscopic biopsies are generally smaller than cystoscopic biopsies due to the size of the instrument, which results in less accurate visualization of the lesion. Therefore, the specimens from the upper urinary tract are often challenging for pathologists with regard to accurate tumor diagnosis, grading, and staging. In a great majority of cases, the evaluation is based on limited and scant amounts of tissue, often consisting of a few minute fragments of urothelium with loss of tissue orientation. Ureteroscopic biopsy provides grading accuracy of 71 % for low-grade and 80 % for high-grade urothelial neoplasms when compared to definitive assessment at resection [37, 38]. These biopsies have been reported to yield a sensitivity of 85 % for the ureter, 78 % for the renal pelvis, and 100 % for the ureteropelvic junction tumors [39]. Endoscopic biopsies have been recently reported to have a specificity of 100 % for all upper urinary tract locations and a diagnostic accuracy of 98 % [39]. Though highly specific, endoscopic biopsies result in a significant false-negative rate, owing to both sampling and diagnostic errors in the assessment of possible upper tract urothelial carcinoma. Vashistha et al. found that 87 % of tumors diagnosed on biopsy had concordant grade and 60 % had concordant pT stage, when correlated with the follow-up surgical resections and biopsies [39]. The biopsy samples with concordant tumor grades were larger (mean size 0.6 cm) than the biopsy samples with discordant grades (mean size 0.3 cm) ($p=0.04$) [39], suggesting that appropriate sampling is the key in evaluating these biopsies. The grade concordance was relatively high between ureteroscopic biopsies and definitive surgical resections, particularly for larger biopsy samples. This was in contrast to the staging of the tumor, which was inaccurate, regardless of the tissue size.

Pathologists and urologists should accept negative biopsy results with caution, particularly for limited or scant biopsy specimens. In almost 1 in 4 renal pelvis/ureteral biopsies, a definitive diagnosis cannot be made because of inadequate or suboptimal biopsy or the limited size of the obtained tissue [40]. On microscopy, in cases where a definitive diagnosis could not be established, it was mainly because of the absence of recognizable papillary fronds, crush artifact, and distorted tissue architecture [40]. Major diagnostic discrepancies on expert review by a genitourinary pathologist included an overdiagnosis of a neoplastic tissue by the initial pathologist when normal tissue was examined, containing either strips of urothelium without well-developed fibrovascular cores, or polypoid ureteritis/pyelitis, or reactive urothelium [40]. Thus, caution is necessary when evaluating limited biopsy specimens obtained by ureteroscopy, especially in the absence of a clinically suspected or visualized neoplasm. The sensitivity of the cytology is related to the degree of tumor differentiation, and overall it is poor in low-grade tumors, but significantly higher in high-grade tumors [41, 42]. Fluorescence in situ hybridization (FISH) analysis of abnormalities on chromosomes 3, 7, 9, and 17 provides greater sensitivity than cytology for the detection of urothelial carcinoma while providing a similar specificity [43].

Radical nephroureterectomy with ipsilateral bladder cuff resection, increasingly performed laparoscopically, is the most common surgical treatment for urothelial carcinoma of the upper tract [44]. Some of these lesions, however, may be overtreated by radical surgery, which necessitates an increasing role for accurate diagnostics and less invasive endoscopic management of these tumors. For example, patients with compromised renal function or small, low-grade neoplasms might be able to enjoy a significant degree of disease control by endoscopic ablation alone [45–47]. A diagnosis of high-grade and high-volume carcinoma may be an indication for neoadjuvant chemotherapy [48]. Despite the advances in endourology, nephroureterectomy remains the gold standard in the definitive treatment of urothelial carcinoma of the upper tract, mainly because of the high recurrence rate of urothelial carcinoma in unresected cases.

The presence of lesions in the upper tract progressively increases the risk of bladder carcinoma from 15 to 75 % over a 5-year period, thus mandating routine bladder surveillance and additional biopsies in these patients [38, 49, 50]. The tumors of the upper urinary tract are also characterized by multicentricity and frequent recurrences [50–54], which often necessitate removal of the entire ureter with a urinary bladder during nephroureterectomy [50–54].

Prognostic Factors

The most important prognostic factor for urothelial carcinoma of the upper tract is the tumor stage, as assigned by the TNM system of the AJCC. In particular, nodal metastatic disease and distant metastasis are harbingers of a dismal prognosis. Patient survival varies widely by stage, given that the survival of patients with noninvasive papillary (pTa) or flat in situ (pTis) carcinomas is essentially 100 %, while invasion of the muscularis (pT2), if not associated with lymphatic metastasis, is as much as 75 % [4]. Survival is quite poor for patients with pT3+ disease, especially with aforementioned nodal involvement, positive margins, or residual disease following definitive therapy. Other parameters that have been identified in univariate and multivariate analyses of patient series with upper tract urothelial carcinoma include tumor necrosis, lesional size, number of foci of carcinoma, presence and severity of concurrent in situ lesions and other neoplasia, as well as traditional clinical parameters, including age, sex, race, and treatment modality [2, 4, 6, 11, 51].

One key issue where controversy remains in the literature is whether the prognosis of an upper tract urothelial carcinoma varies by anatomic site in the upper tract. Some single-institutional series demonstrated that ureteric urothelial carcinoma had a worse prognosis than carcinomas of the renal pelvis [55, 56], although this has not been confirmed by others, particularly in higher stage disease [8]. Some investigators particularly noted that high stage tumors with renal parenchymal invasion (pT3) have actually done better than tumors invading peripelvic or periureteral adipose tissue (also pT3 by definition) [56–58], which could provide an explanation for the discordance of some of the aforementioned studies. In contrast, other studies have shown that tumors of the renal pelvis and proximal ureter demonstrate a worse 5-year cancer-specific survival [59], which might be explained by the relatively attenuated muscularis of the renal pelvis and proximal ureter. A large multicenter study and a separate population-based study found that renal pelvic tumors present with more advanced pathologic stage than ureteral urothelial carcinoma [60, 61]. Both studies however failed to demonstrate that the tumor location had an effect on disease recurrence and cancer-specific mortality, after adjusting for the effects of the pathological stage, grade, and nodal disease [60, 61]. A single-institution study of 253 patients also failed to show an association between the tumor location and either disease recurrence or cancer-specific survival [7]. In a large multi-institutional international study, ureteral tumor location, particularly when associated with renal pelvis disease, was found to be an independent predictor for both higher disease recurrence and cancer-specific survival [12]. Another large multicenter French study demonstrated that ureteral and multifocal tumors had a worse prognosis than renal pelvic tumors [11]. In a large multicenter Canadian study, Williamson et al. found no correlation between the tumor location and the survival, but they confirmed that synchronous multifocal tumors that involved both the ureter and the renal pelvis were associated with decreased disease-free and an overall patient survival [62]. In summary, it seems that patients with more extensive multifocal disease involving both the renal pelvis and the ureter may be candidates for adjuvant chemotherapy and may require closer surveillance, though greater experience and meta-analyses may be necessary to make formal recommendations.

Another prognostic question pertains to the depth/extent of invasion in stage pT3 upper tract carcinomas. pT3 tumors are defined as invasion beyond muscularis propria into the peripelvic or periureteral fat or into the renal parenchyma. Some studies demonstrated that "superficial invasion" (less than 5 mm in depth) have better prognosis and better disease-free and recurrence-free survival than patients with extensive parenchymal invasion or invasion into peripelvic or periureteral fat [8, 63]. Yoshimura et al. suggested dividing the cancers with renal parenchymal invasion into two prognostic subtypes: superficial and deep [63]. The superficial subtype would represent parenchymal invasion to a depth of less than 5 mm from the basement membrane, whereas the deep subtype was defined as extensive parenchymal invasion, which can be readily recognizable on gross evaluation [63].

Immunohistochemistry

The immunohistochemical profile of upper tract urothelial carcinoma recapitulates the one seen in urothelial carcinomas of the urinary bladder. In most cases, however, immunohistochemistry (IHC) is unnecessary, and a careful gross, microscopic, and clinicopathological correlation will be sufficient to reach a correct diagnosis. IHC may play an ancillary role, and in some instances even a crucial one in differentiating renal pelvis or ureteral tumors from renal collecting duct carcinoma (CDC), primary RCC, or metastatic carcinoma. A frequent and useful property of a number of lesions in the differential for a urothelial carcinoma of the upper tract is that the immunohistochemical properties of the cancer often match that of the primary tumor and are different from the immunoprofile of a urothelial carcinoma. In addition, IHC may also play a role in differentiating reactive atypia from urothelial carcinoma in situ or urothelial intraepithelial neoplasm.

Urothelial Carcinoma IHC

Several antibodies have been reported to confirm urothelial differentiation in a primary cancer with unusual morphology. These include GATA3, Thrombomodulin, Cytokeratin 7 and 20, p63, CK5/6, and high molecular weight cytokeratin. The reported sensitivity of these markers for urothelial carcinoma and its variants ranges from 20 to 100 %. Additionally, none of these antibodies are 100 % specific for urothelial differentiation, and a number of other cancers have demonstrated varying positivity for these markers. A currently recommended panel by the International Society of Urologic Pathology (ISUP) to confirm urothelial differentiation includes GATA3, S100P, Cytokeratin 20, p63, and high molecular weight cytokeratin [64]. Additionally, recent studies have confirmed the specificity of a family of proteins called uroplakins, which are constituents of the plaque-like lining of the luminal surface of the urothelium. Uroplakin III has shown a high degree of specificity as a urothelial marker in several studies and may be useful in the appropriate setting, though its sensitivity appears quite low [65–67]. Other members of the uroplakin family, especially uroplakin II, might prove to be more sensitive as urothelial markers; validation studies are under way in this regard. Figure 3.6 demonstrates examples of the use of key IHC markers of urothelial carcinoma.

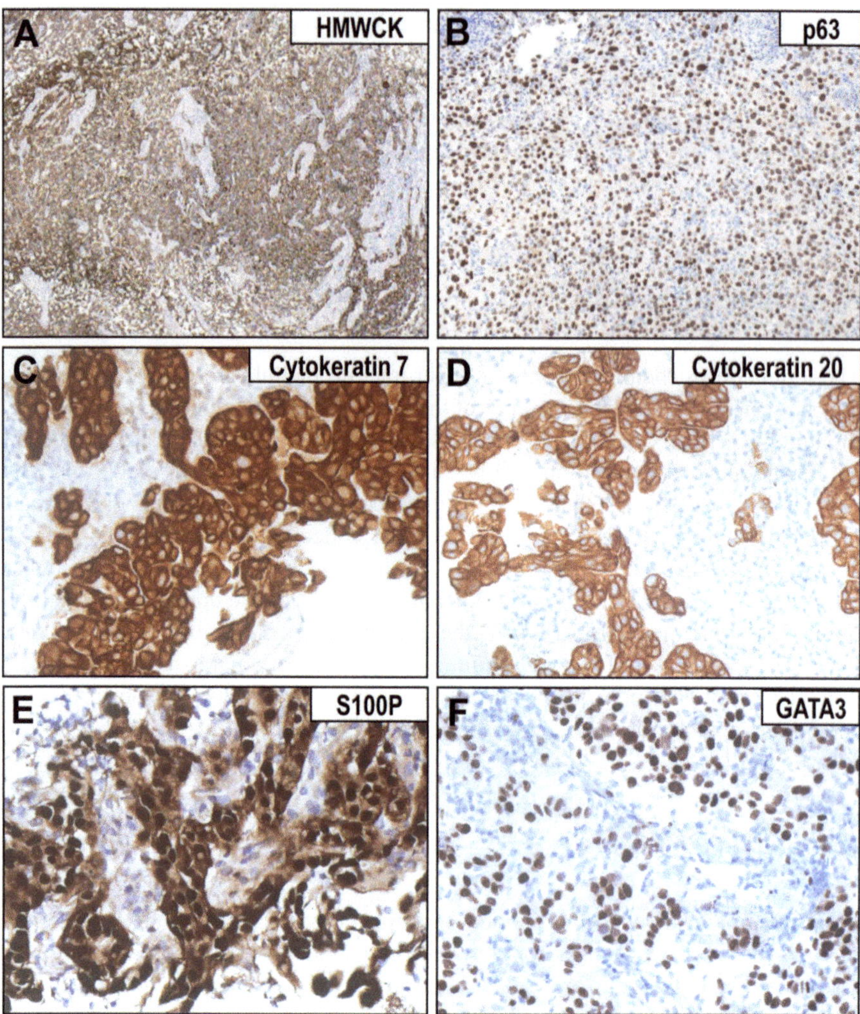

Fig. 3.6 Immunohistochemical biomarkers for urothelial carcinoma. (**a**–**b**) Traditional immunohistochemical markers for urothelial carcinoma include high molecular weight cytokeratin (HMWCK/CK903/34BE12), which demonstrates diffuse cytoplasmic positivity (*A*). Another useful marker is p63 (*B*), which demonstrates nuclear reactivity. Although both HMWCK and p63 can support a diagnosis of urothelial neoplasm in the appropriate setting, they can be also positive in a many squamous carcinomas of the urothelial tract or other organs. (**c**-**d**) Both cytokeratin 7 (*C*) and cytokeratin 20 (*D*) are diffuse cytoplasmic stains which are often positive in urothelial carcinoma. While more urothelial carcinomas show positivity for CK7 (70–100 %) than CK20 (40–70 %), positive staining for both CK7 and CK20, in the appropriate setting, favors urothelial carcinoma over carcinomas derived from breast and lung (both CK7+/CK20-) or gastrointestinal tract primaries (CK7-/CK20+). (**e**–**f**) Newer immunohistochemical markers, such as S100P (*E*), exhibiting cytoplasmic and nuclear stain, and GATA3 (*F*), a nuclear stain, demonstrate greater specificity for urothelial carcinoma as compared to other neoplasms

Collecting Duct Carcinoma IHC

CDC is a highly infiltrative neoplasm that may extensively involve the renal parenchyma and may mimic either undifferentiated urothelial carcinoma of the renal pelvis or primary RCC. Although IHC may not be discriminatory in separating urothelial carcinoma and CDC, potentially useful positive markers for CDC include EMA, p63, Cytokeratin 7, high molecular weight cytokeratin, PAX2, and PAX8. PAX 8 is more sensitive than PAX2; it is also reported to be positive only in minority (about 10–20 %) of upper tract urothelial carcinomas [18, 19, 21, 68]. Thus, recent reports suggest use of immunohistochemical panels to resolve the differential diagnosis in this setting [19, 69].

Renal Cell Carcinoma IHC

Morphology remains the key in distinguishing primary RCC, including the common types, such as clear cell and papillary RCC, from urothelial carcinoma arising in the renal pelvis. Useful IHC markers for clear cell RCC include PAX2 and PAX8, CD10, Vimentin, and CAIX; clear cell RCC is typically negative for Cytokeratin 7, Cytokeratin 20, high molecular weight cytokeratin and p63. Papillary RCC is typically positive for PAX2 and PAX8, CD10, Vimentin, Cytokeratin 7, and AMACR; negative markers include Cytokeratin 20, high molecular weight cytokeratin, and p63 [70–72].

Reactive Atypia Versus Carcinoma In Situ IHC

Cytokeratin 20 is a cytokeratin normally expressed in the umbrella cells, and it is restricted to the terminally differentiated cells in the normal urothelium in reactive atypia (or rarely may be expressed in the upper 1/3 of the urothelium). In contrast, Cytokeratin 20 demonstrates full thickness (>2/3) reactivity in carcinoma in situ [73–75]. *TP53* mutations are associated with high-grade tumors including carcinoma in situ; antibodies used in IHC detect both wild-type and mutant p53 protein, though mutant p53 often shows increased protein stability and nuclear accumulation. Negative to weak and patchy, or rarely, moderate nuclear reactivity is present in the normal urothelium and in reactive atypia. In contrast, strong nuclear positivity is frequently noted in the atypical cells of carcinoma in situ, reflecting the aforementioned phenomenon of accumulation of mutant protein, frequently involving all urothelial cell layers. Additionally, CD44 (standard isoform) is an adhesion molecule with membranous reactivity limited to the basal cells of the normal urothelium. It exhibits increased reactivity in reactive urothelial atypia (often full thickness), while it is typically absent in carcinoma in situ, although patchy and focal reactivity may be present in the residual basal cells. Recent reports have employed a three antibody "cocktail" using these markers for evaluation of problematic lesions of the urothelium, with some success [73–75]. In summary, although Cytokeratin 20, p53, and CD44 may play a potential role in

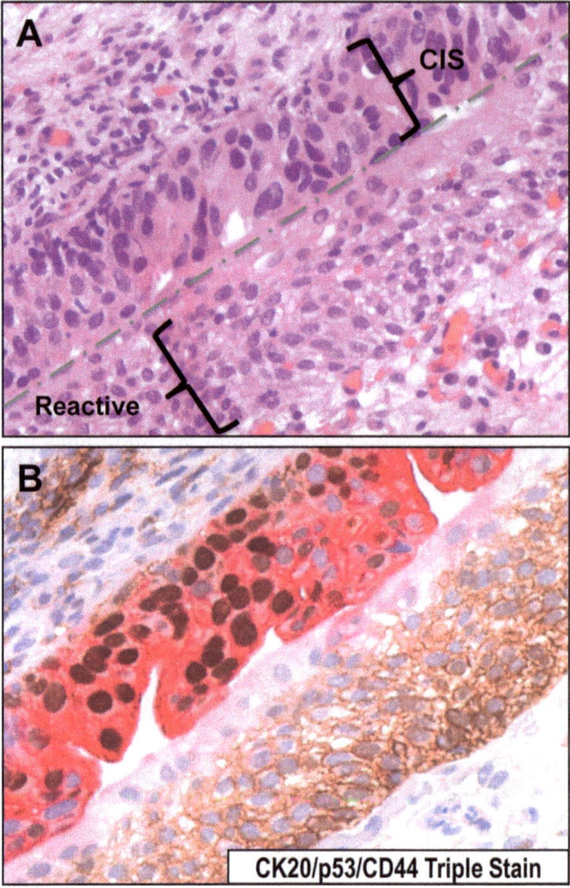

Fig. 3.7 Immunohistochemical markers for distinguishing reactive urothelium from carcinoma in situ. (**a**) Reactive urothelium (*lower* and *right* half of the field) is contrasted against urothelial carcinoma in situ (*upper* and *left* half of field), along the dashed diagonal line. (**b**) Triple immunostain for p53 (nuclear, *brown* chromogen), CD44 (membranous, with basolateral accentuation, *brown* chromogen), and cytokertain 20 (cytoplasmic, *red* chromogen) shows characteristic pattern in these lesions. CIS shows overexpression of p53 and full thickness expression of cytokeratin 20, the pattern of CIS (CD44 is negative) (*upper* and *left* half of field). In contrast, reactive urothelium shows membranous reactivity for CD44, weak nuclear p53, and focal expression of cytokeratin 20, restricted to the uppermost umbrella cell layer (*lower* and *right* half of the field)

differentiating reactive atypia and carcinoma in situ, these IHC markers must be interpreted in strict correlation with the histomorphology. Figure 3.7 shows representative examples of these immunostains used in a combination "cocktail" with dual color chromogens so that they may be evaluated on the same tissue section.

Genetics and Molecular Pathology

Urothelial carcinomas of the renal pelvis, the ureter, and the urinary bladder share similar genetic alterations. Deletions of genetic loci on chromosome 9p and 9q occur in 50–75 % of all patients and frequent deletions of 17p, in addition to p53 mutations, are seen in advanced high-grade tumors [4]. The association of upper tract lesions with non-polyposis colorectal cancer syndrome or Lynch syndrome II is well documented [76]. Urothelial carcinomas that demonstrate microsatellite instability are associated with non-polyposis colorectal cancer syndrome [77]. Microsatellite instability and mismatch repair proteins MSH2, MLH1, or MSH6 are present in 4–30 % of all upper tract cases [77, 78]. Mutations in genes with repetitive sequences, which are present in up to a third of cases with microsatellite instability, suggest a molecular carcinogenesis pathway similar to some mismatch repair-deficient colorectal cancers. These tumors have significantly different clinical and histopathologic features, including low grade and stage, and frequently exhibit inverted (endophytic) growth and higher prevalence in female patients [79]. Formal guidelines for consideration of testing are not published for upper tract urothelial carcinoma, though the Bethesda Guidelines and Amsterdam Criteria have been reported for colorectal carcinomas [80].

FGFR3 and *TP53* mutations have been recognized as key genetic pathways in the carcinogenesis of urothelial carcinoma [81, 82]. In general, non-muscle-invasive cancers are characterized by alterations in the tyrosine kinase receptor gene *FGFR3* and the oncogene *HRAS*, which lead to disruption of the *PI3K–AKT* pathway. The mutations in *FGFR3* seem to be mutually exclusive to *HRAS* mutations [83]. *FGFR3* appears to be the most frequently mutated oncogene in urothelial carcinoma. Its mutation is strongly associated with favorable disease parameters including low tumor grade, early stage, and low recurrence rate, which confer a better overall prognosis. Although a number of studies have shown promising results, the prognostic value of *FGFR3* mutation and protein expression levels still remains controversial [84].

The main genetic alterations underlying the muscle invasive cancers involve tumor suppressor genes encoding proteins that regulate cell cycle, DNA repair, and apoptosis pathways, including primarily *TP53* [85], but also other cell cycle-related markers. *TP53* mutations are associated with higher tumor grade, more advanced stage, more frequent tumor recurrences, and worse prognosis. Mutations of p53 are very common (>50 %) in high-grade invasive tumors and in flat carcinoma in situ [81, 82]. Most, but not all, studies found that a p53 mutation or overexpression is associated with cancer progression.

In addition, proliferation marker Ki-67 has been widely confirmed as potentially relevant for urothelial, primarily bladder cancer prognostication. Ki-67 and MIB-1, markers of tumor proliferation index, have been consistently shown to have a prognostic role in bladder cancer. MIB-1 and *FGFR3* have been used in a combined prognosticator for non-muscle-invasive cancer, designated molecular grade (mG) [86–88]. Proliferating index assessment has also been confirmed in a large multicenter study to have prognostic and predictive role in muscle-invasive cancers [89].

Prognostic and Predictive Markers

Although traditional pathologic parameters such as stage, nodal status, and grade provide information regarding the biological potential and clinical behavior of urothelial cancer, there is an ongoing quest to identify additional biomarkers which may clarify important pathogenetic mechanisms, improve staging, and provide useful prognostic or treatment information. Unfortunately, so far, there is no single prognostic or predictive biomarker that has been clinically validated and can be recommended for use in routine practice. Emerging evidence indicates that a panel or a combination of prognostic and predictive clinicopathological and molecular biomarkers will eventually improve the ability for more accurate tumor grading and classification, but also for outcome prediction and clinical decision-making for individual patient treatment [90–94]. Table 3.6 summarizes a list of emerging markers found to be associated with tumor progression in non-muscle-invasive and muscle-invasive urothelial, primarily bladder cancers. These are also potentially applicable to upper tract lesions [90–94], though prospective validation will be necessary in the unique clinical milieu of the upper tract. These markers include cell cycle regulators, apoptosis modulators, angiogenesis regulators, signal transduction factors, cell proliferation promoters, hormone receptors, and cell adhesion modulators.

Table 3.6 Emerging prognostic markers in urothelial cancers

Biomarker	Normal function	Abnormality	Prognostic role in	
			Non-muscle-invasive cancer	Muscle-invasive cancer
Cell cycle				
p53[a]	Tumor suppressor	Inactivation/accumulation	Yes (multimarker)/No	Yes/No
p21	CDK inhibitor	Downregulated expression/loss	Yes (multimarker)/No	Yes
p27	CDK inhibitor	Downregulated expression	Yes (multimarker)/No	Yes/No
p16	CDK inhibitor	Altered expression	No	Yes/No
pRB	Tumor suppressor	Deletion/mutation	Yes (multimarker)/No	Yes/No
Ki-67[a]	Cell proliferation	Increased expression	Yes (multimarker, mG)	Yes
Cyclins				
D1, D3, E1	Phosphorylate Rb	Increased expression	Yes/No	No
Apoptosis				
Survivin	Inhibitor of apoptosis	Increased expression	Yes/No	Yes
Angiogenesis				
MVD	Marker of angiogenesis	Increased density	Yes/No	Yes/No
VEGF, HIF1A	Promote angiogenesis	Increased expression	Yes/No	Yes/No
Signaling proteins				
FGFR3[a]	Tyrosine kinase receptor	Mutation/overexpression	Yes	No
Hormone receptors				
HER2	Tyrosine kinase receptor	Amplification	No	Yes/No
AR	Nuclear receptor	Loss of expression	No	No
ER	Nuclear receptor	Downregulated expression	No	No
Cell adhesion				
E-cadherin	Cell adhesion	Loss	Yes	Yes/No

[a]p53, FGFR3, and Ki-67 (bolded) have the strongest evidence as prognostic markers in bladder cancer

CDK cyclin-dependent kinase, *MVD* microvessel density, *VEGF* vascular endothelial growth factor, *HIF1A* hypoxia-induced factor 1A, *FGFR* fibroblast growth factor receptor, *HER2* human epidermal growth receptor 2, *AR* androgen receptor, *ER* estrogen receptor, *mG* molecular grade

Other Neoplasms and Non-neoplastic Tumorous Lesions of the Renal Pelvis and Ureter

Benign Tumors

Urothelial Papilloma and Inverted Papilloma

Both tumors are uncommon but may be incidentally found in the upper urinary tract [4]. They are twice as common in the ureter as in the renal pelvis, most likely because they become symptomatic earlier when they involve the ureter. Inverted papilloma is composed of endophytic interconnected urothelial trabeculae and cords, invaginating from the flat urothelial surface into lamina propria. The nuclei often show palisading at the periphery. They are not accompanied by desmoplastic reaction and the tumor periphery is circumscribed. Renal pelvic mucosa has also a greater predilection to demonstrate von Brunn's nests than bladder mucosa [95]. Representative micrographs of examples of papilloma and inverted papilloma are illustrated in Fig. 3.8.

Villous Adenoma and Squamous Papilloma

These benign tumors are quite rare in the upper urinary tract. Villous adenoma in this location is similar to the villous adenomas of the colon. The diagnosis of villous adenoma can be extremely challenging in a biopsy specimen and it may be impossible to entirely exclude the possibility of adjacent adenocarcinoma. Thus, complete excision of the entire clinically apparent lesion is essential [4, 13].

Malignant Tumors

Squamous Cell Carcinoma

Squamous cell carcinoma is the second most common malignant tumor in this region, and it is more common in the renal pelvis than in the ureter (Fig. 3.9). In general, it is rare in both locations. These carcinomas occur on the background of local irritation due to nephrolithiasis and are often accompanied by squamous metaplasia and dysplasia. Ureteral squamous cell carcinomas show a significant predilection for the distal third of the ureter. Pure squamous carcinomas are usually high grade and high stage and frequently infiltrate the kidney. The prognosis is extremely poor, and 5-year survival is infrequent [4, 13, 96].

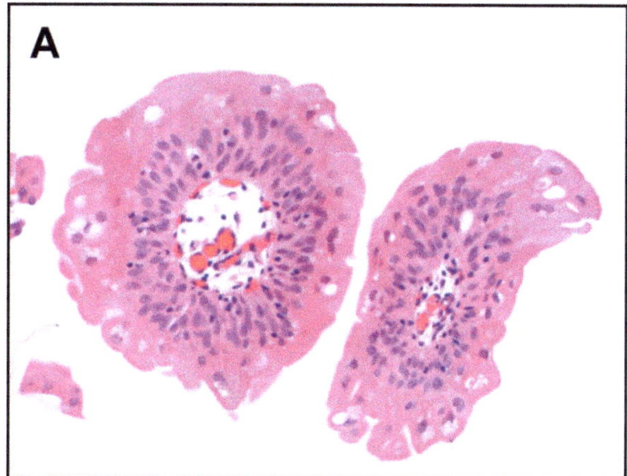

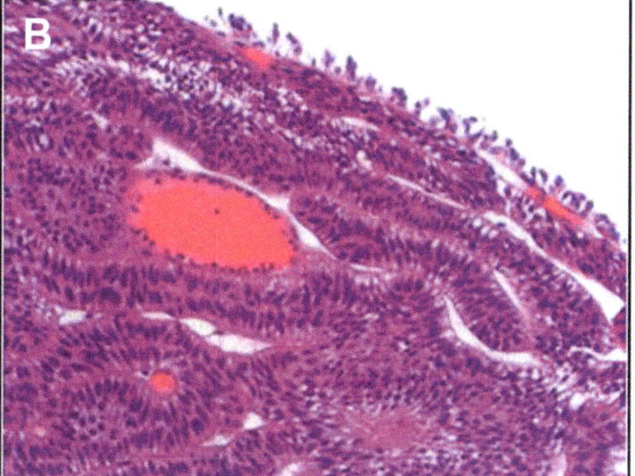

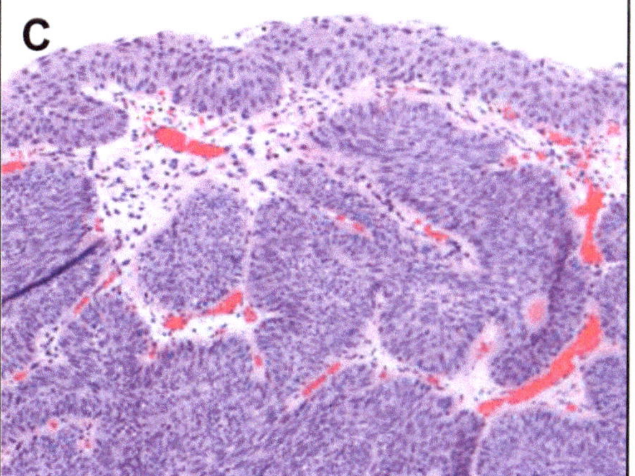

Fig. 3.8 Benign papillary lesions. (**a**) Urothelial papillomas are benign neoplasms characterized by normal thickness urothelium overlying delicate fibrovascular stalks. The urothelium is not thickened or hyperplastic (thus, not a PUNLMP) nor is it atypical. (**b**) Inverted papillomas are benign neoplasms that that show an endophytic growth pattern, "inverting" the architecture. Thus, the fibrovascular stromal tissue appears outside the ingrown epithelium. (**c**) A more spindled cellular morphology is often apparent in inverted papilloma, which may initially appear alarming on histologic review. Peripheral nuclear palisading is also evident

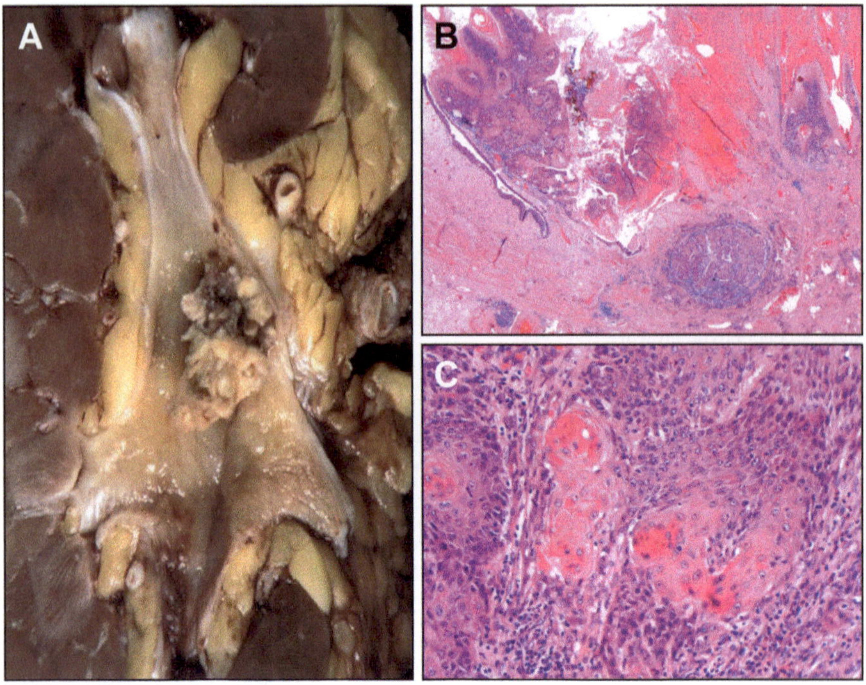

Fig. 3.9 Squamous cell carcinoma of the upper tract. (**a**) Pure squamous cell carcinomas (i.e., not urothelial carcinoma with squamous differentiation) are infrequent neoplasms of the upper tract. In this gross image, the neoplasm in the pelvis appears chalky white and plaque-like, compared to the often delicate papillary appearance of urothelial carcinoma. (**b**) At low power, the abundant keratinization of the neoplasm is apparent. (**c**) At higher power, the formation of typical keratin pearls is seen between the infiltrative nests and sheets composed of atypical squamous cells

Adenocarcinoma

Similarly, adenocarcinoma of the upper tract is rare and also occurs on a background of nephrolithiasis and repeated infections [4, 13]. Intestinal metaplasia is often seen in the non-neoplastic mucosa and is considered a potential precursor lesion. Adenocarcinomas of the upper tract frequently demonstrate concurrent enteric, mucinous, and signet-ring morphology [97, 98]. Most adenocarcinomas are high grade and broadly invasive at presentation, and they demonstrate clinically aggressive behavior. The differential diagnosis includes metastatic colonic carcinoma, lung adenocarcinoma, and other metastatic adenocarcinomas from pancreas, breast, or gynecologic primaries. Clinicopathological correlation and history are important in resolving this scenario. Careful dissection with extensive tissue sampling may be necessary to appreciate if such neoplasms are urothelium-based and if metaplastic and dysplastic precursor lesions are present, to rule out a possible collecting duct carcinoma. Metastatic disease should be considered particularly when multifocal lesions are present, mucosal disease is absent, and there is no history of chronic inciting factors (with hydronephrosis or stones) [13].

Miscellaneous Non-epithelial Tumors

A variety of benign and malignant non-epithelial neoplasms have been reported in the ureter and in the renal pelvis. These tumors do not differ from similar tumors documented at other body sites. They often arise in the perirenal and renal hilar soft tissue and secondarily involve the pelvicalyceal system and the renal parenchyma. Reported non-epithelial tumors in this region include hemangioma, angiomyoma, leiomyoma, neurofibroma, periureteric lipoma, leiomyosarcoma, rhabdomyosarcoma, fibrosarcoma, angiosarcoma, choriocarcinoma, malignant peripheral nerve sheath tumor, Ewing sarcoma/primitive neuroectodermal tumor, Wilms tumor, and solitary fibrous tumor [28, 99–113]. The most common mesenchymal primary malignancy of the upper urinary tract is leiomyosarcoma; however, its overall incidence is very low. It is important to recognize that these neoplasms on imaging may produce a filling defect or polypoid mass in the upper tract, simulating upper tract urothelial lesion. Figure 3.10 shows two examples of mesenchymal lesions, a primitive neuroectodermal tumor and a solitary fibrous tumor that each masqueraded as upper tract urothelial carcinoma during workup.

Proliferative Tumor-Like Lesions

Nephrogenic Adenoma/Metaplasia

Nephrogenic adenoma/metaplasia can also occur in the upper urinary tract, although the bladder remains the most common site. It may show a wide range of architectural patterns, such as papillary, tubular/glandular, single cell, and cysts. They are lined with cuboidal and single-layered, occasionally "hobnailed" epithelium; mixed patterns may also be present. The basement membrane underneath the epithelium is usually thick and hyalinized and frequently shows active chronic inflammation. Nephrogenic adenoma may be associated with a history of local irritation, infection, instrumentation, or stones. The histogenesis of this lesion is still a matter of debate, though recent findings suggest that it represents a neoplasm of renal tubular epithelial cells, which are shed in the urine [114]. A recently appreciated morphologic appearance of nephrogenic adenoma is its fibromyxoid variant, where the renal tubular cells exhibit a fine, gray-pink, myxoid stromal material [115]. Most important in the evaluation of nephrogenic adenoma/metaplasia is the recognition that these lesions may appear tumor-like and can demonstrate infiltrative growth,

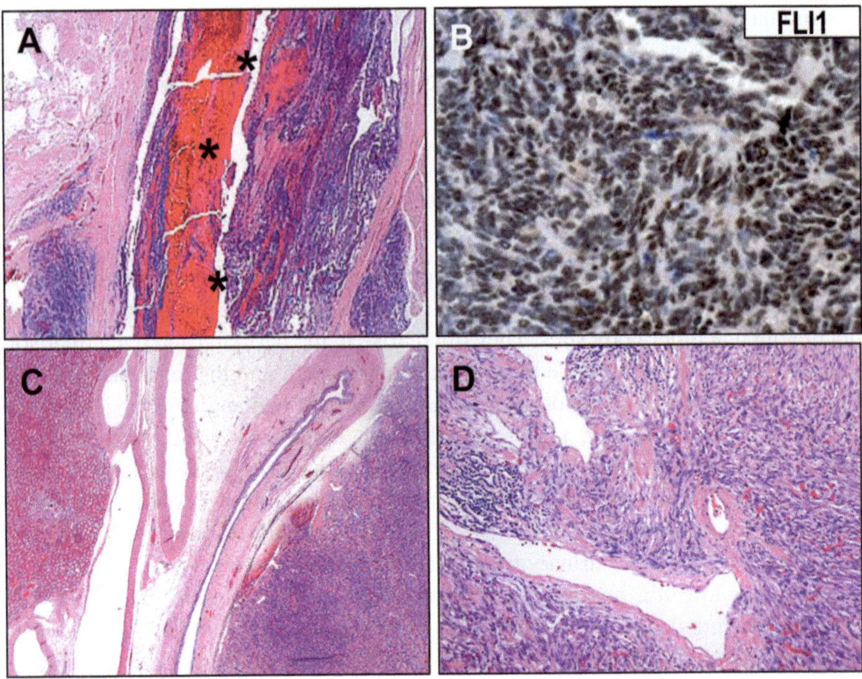

Fig. 3.10 Mesenchymal lesions may simulate upper tract urothelial carcinoma. (**a**) A low power field of a primitive neuroectodermal tumor (extraskeletal Ewing sarcoma) of the ureteral wall, showing a "small round blue cell morphology," erodes into this longitudinal section through the ureteral lumen (lumen denoted by *asterisks*). In this case, urothelial carcinoma with extensive high-grade neuroendocrine differentiation or a primary small cell carcinoma was considered during the case workup. (**b**) Immunostain for FLI1 was diffusely positive, indicative of t(11;22) translocation between the genes EWSR1 and FLI1, which may be confirmed by molecular testing. (**c**) In this low power view, a cellular spindle cell lesion (*lower right*) compresses the pelvic lumen and simulates a filling defect. On imaging, a polypoid lesion was noted to compress the renal pelvis, though cytology remained negative for atypial urothelial cells. (**d**) A higher power field shows a cellular spindle cell growth with so-called "patternless pattern" of haphazard spindle cells intimately admixed with ropy collagen, with hemangiopericytoma-like vessels, morphology classic for a solitary fibrous tumor

including rarely an extension into perirenal fat [116]. Figure 3.11 shows representative examples of nephrogenic adenoma simulating large and small papillary lesions which may appear worrisome on microscopy.

Fibroepithelial Polyp

Fibroepithelial polyps of the ureter and the renal pelvis are usually acquired rather than congenital [10, 117, 118]. Although they are more common in adults, they represent the most common benign polypoid ureteric tumors in children. Most polyps are hamartomatous growths that tend to occur in the proximal portion of the left ureter in

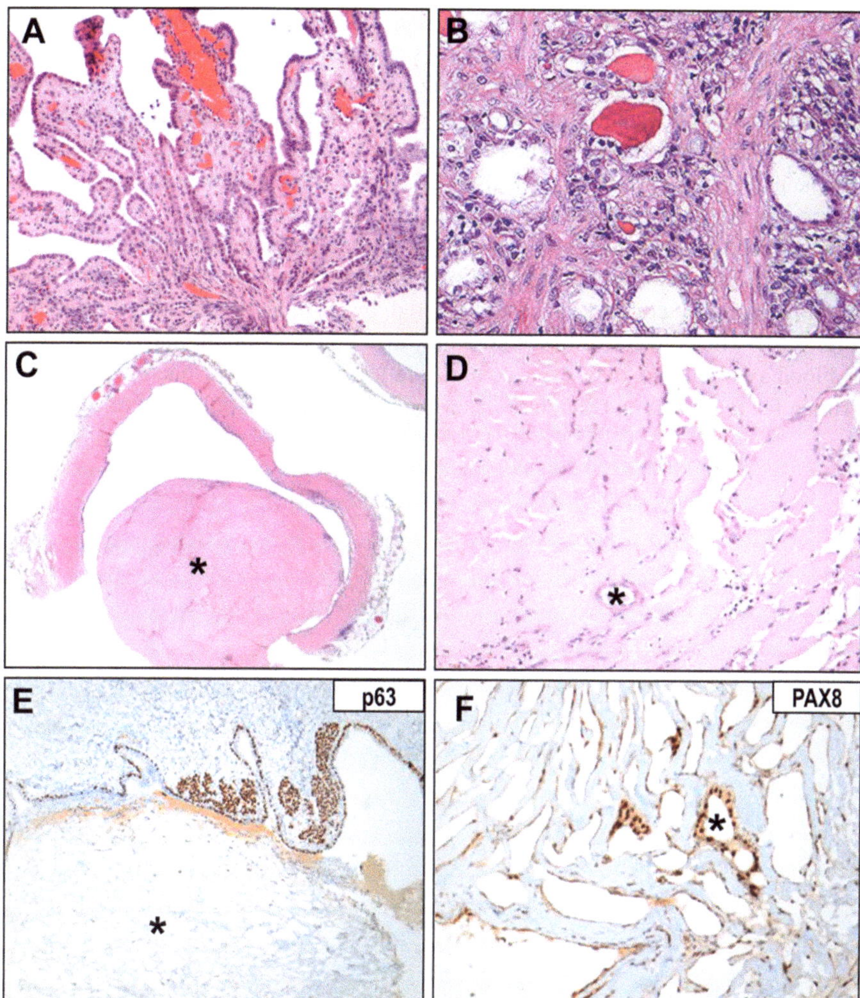

Fig. 3.11 Nephrogenic adenoma may simulate urothelial carcinoma. (**a**) The morphologic and clinical spectrum of nephrogenic adenoma (nephrogenic metaplasia) can be broad. Exuberant cases may show papillary pattern which may simulate a papillary urothelial neoplasm, as shown in this example. (**b**) At higher power, the reactive and inflammatory background of nephrogenic adenoma is more apparent, as is the classic cytologic appearance of cells with a hobnailed appearance, arranged in rudimentary tubules. Tangential sectioning can simulate invasion. (**c**) A recently described histologic variant of nephrogenic adenoma is the "fibromyxoid variant," where the cells are arrayed in a prominently myxoid matrix, which may simulate a mucinous carcinoma or urothelial carcinoma with myxoid stroma. In this case, the nephrogenic adenoma exhibited a tumor-like growth, as seen in the low power cross section of the opened ureter. On ureteroscopy, this was suspected to be a papillary urothelial carcinoma. (**d**) High power shows nephrogenic adenoma cells arranged both in tubules (*asterisk*) and as scattered spindled cells throughout the myxoid matrix. (**e**) Immunostain for p63 demonstrates that the cells in this lesion (*asterisk*) are negative (in contrast to the internal control urothelium and von Brunn's nests), which argues against urothelial carcinoma. (**f**) Nuclear immunoreactivity for PAX8 (*asterisk*) confirms the diagnosis of nephrogenic adenoma in the appropriate setting

males. Most often they are single tumors, but multiple and branching tumors have been documented. The clinical symptoms stem from the ureteral obstruction with flank pain and/or hematuria being the most common presenting symptoms. They can also be detected incidentally; urinary urgency or hesitancy has been reported as presenting symptoms in polyps of the lower urinary tract [118]. Fibroepithelial ureteral polyps may be resected endoscopically, which may allow avoiding an open surgical exploration with local excision or nephroureterectomy. Postoperative surveillance is recommended for potential early detection of ureteral stricture or recurrence [117].

These lesions grow as intraluminal masses and consist of a broad core of loose or more compact connective tissue covered by normal or denuded urothelium (Fig. 3.12). The connective tissue core may also contain smooth muscle, collagen, or blood vessels, and may even contain scattered lipid-laden macrophages [10]. Criteria for diagnosis and subclassification of fibroepithelial polyps were described

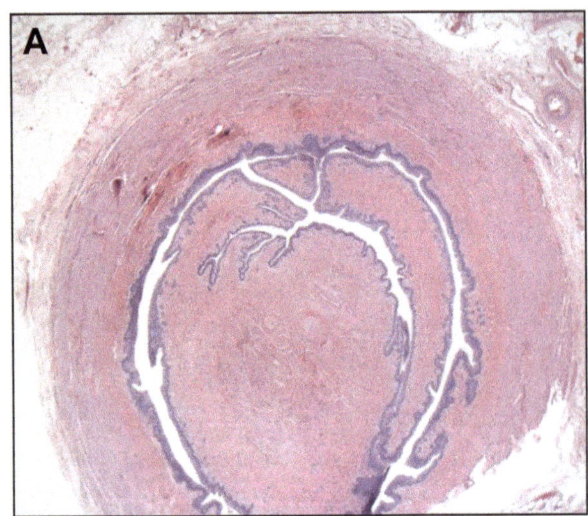

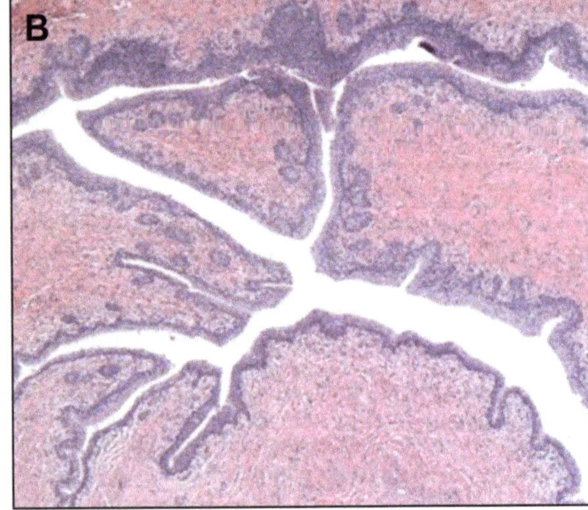

Fig. 3.12 Fibroepithelial polyp of ureter. (**a**) Fibroepithelial polyp of ureter may mimic upper tract urothelial carcinoma. This reactive lesion fills almost completely the ureteral lumen. It is lined by normal urothelium and is composed of broad papillary proliferations containing compact fibromuscular stroma—not the delicate fibrovascular stalks of urothelial neoplasms. (**b**) Higher magnification of the lesion

by Tsuzuki and Epstein [118]. Pattern 1 consists of fibroepithelial polyps with club-like projections resembling a cloverleaf with florid cystitis cystica and glandularis in the stalk. Pattern 2 fibroepithelial polyps are the most common in the ureter; they represent papillary tumors composed of numerous small, rounded fibrovascular cores containing dense fibrous tissue. Pattern 3 fibroepithelial polyps consist of polypoid lesions with secondary tall finger-like projections.

Idiopathic Retroperitoneal Fibrosis

Retroperitoneal fibrosis is an uncommon disease and it is characterized by development of fibrotic tissue and chronic inflammation in the retroperitoneum, which envelops the adjacent structures, such as the ureters and the abdominal aorta [119, 120]. The ureter is usually encased by firm fibrotic tissue, which mimics a neoplasm. Focally, there is a chronic inflammation with lymphocytes, plasma cells, and occasional lymphoid follicles. Stromal edema can also be present.

Idiopathic retroperitoneal fibrosis has been associated with IgG4-related autoimmune process [119, 121, 122]. This is a recently recognized entity that may manifest in many organs, including a mass forming tubulointerstitial nephritis in the kidney [122–124]. Approximately 50 % of patients with idiopathic retroperitoneal fibrosis are IgG4 positive and this entity should be included in the IgG4-related spectrum of sclerosing diseases [121].

Endometriosis

Endometriosis occurs most commonly in the bladder, but it may also occur in the upper urinary tract, most often in the ureter, usually affecting the lower third. The ureter may be compressed by endometriosis in an extrinsic fashion, thus mimicking a neoplasm (Fig. 3.13); intrinsic involvement, which is less common, may involve

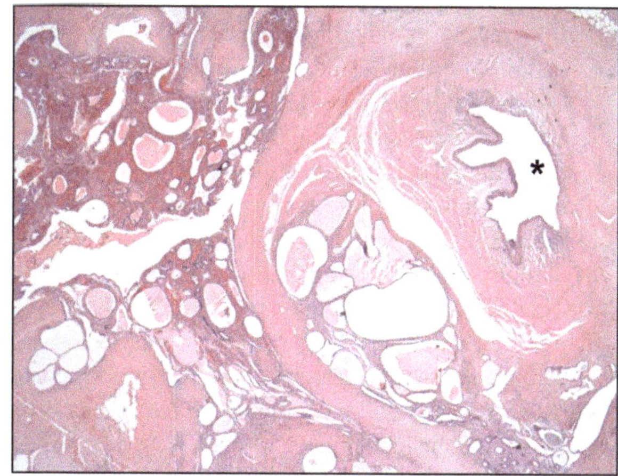

Fig. 3.13 Endometriosis of ureter. Ureteral lumen, which can be seen in the upper right, (*asterisk*) is compressed by extensive endometriosis at the periphery, which mimics a neoplasm. Ureteral wall involvement can also be seen involving the peripheral muscle propria

all the layers of the ureteral wall. It occurs typically in women of reproductive age or in postmenopausal women who are on estrogen replacement. Up to 50 % of patients demonstrate previous history of pelvic surgery. The symptoms, such as, flank pain, dysuria, and hematuria may have catamenial frequency. The lesion shares the same morphology as in other organs and consists of benign endometriotic glands and variable amount of stroma, with frequent presence of fresh or resorbed hemorrhage with hemosiderin pigment deposition [125].

Conclusions: Summary with Ten Most Important Points

1. Urothelial carcinomas represent the vast majority (>90 %) of carcinomas of the renal pelvis and ureter, and they share the same pathologic spectrum and the same classification with the urothelial neoplasms of the urinary bladder.
2. Urothelial cancers of the renal pelvis are more frequently high grade and high stage compared to the urinary bladder carcinomas.
3. Squamous cell carcinoma and adenocarcinoma also occur rarely in the upper tract, and typically arise on a background of nephrolithiasis and repeated infections. Both types are typically high grade, high stage, and broadly invasive at presentation.
4. Grossly, upper tract urothelial carcinomas may appear as papillary, polypoid, ulcerative, or infiltrative masses, with thickening of the ureteral or the renal pelvic wall. These lesions may grow significantly and completely fill the lumen of the ureter and the pelvicalyceal system. An expansion into the distal ureter can cause obstruction, resulting in hydronephrosis.
5. Careful gross examination and comprehensive sampling of the tumor in this region are essential to reliably distinguish a noninvasive from an invasive tumor. Regarding the normal histomorphology of the pelvicalyceal system, it is important to recognize that lamina propria is absent beneath the urothelium lining the renal papillae in the renal pelvis and the lamina propria is thin along the minor calyces. The muscularis propria within the renal sinus and minor calyces varies from absent to indistinguishable.
6. Pathologic stage is the single most important prognostic factor for urothelial carcinoma of the upper urinary tract.
7. Ureteroscopic biopsy is crucial for the diagnosis, follow-up, and management of urothelial carcinoma of the upper tract, and it is the current gold standard for the diagnosis of these tumors. Caution is however necessary when evaluating limited biopsy specimens obtained by ureteroscopy, especially in the absence of a clinically suspected neoplasm.
8. The main differential diagnosis of urothelial carcinoma includes renal collecting duct carcinoma, high-grade primary renal cell carcinoma, and metastatic carcinoma. In most cases, a thorough gross, microscopic, and clinicopathological correlation will be sufficient to reach the correct diagnosis, without the use of immunohistochemistry.

9. Immunohistochemical profile of upper tract urothelial carcinoma is identical to that of lower tract lesions. A currently recommended immunopanel to establish urothelial differentiation includes GATA3, Cytokeratin 20, p63, and high molecular weight cytokeratin (CK5/6). Upper tract urothelial carcinomas may rarely express PAX8.
10. Upper and lower tract urothelial carcinomas share similar genetic alterations, though the association between upper tract lesions with Lynch Syndrome (Hereditary Non-Polyposis Colorectal Carcinoma HNPCC) is stronger. Microsatellite instability and mismatch repair proteins are present in 5–30 % of all upper tract cases and are associated with low-grade and stage tumors, with inverted growth, occurring in females.

References

1. Stewart GD, Bariol SV, Grigor KM, Tolley DA, McNeill SA. A comparison of the pathology of transitional cell carcinoma of the bladder and upper urinary tract. BJU Int. 2005;95(6):791–3.
2. Perez-Montiel D, Wakely PE, Hes O, Michal M, Suster S. High-grade urothelial carcinoma of the renal pelvis: clinicopathologic study of 108 cases with emphasis on unusual morphologic variants. Mod Pathol. 2006;19(4):494–503.
3. Jemal A, Siegel R, Ward E, Murray T, Xu J, Smigal C, et al. Cancer statistics, 2006. CA Cancer J Clin. 2006;56(2):106–30.
4. Delahunt B, Amin MB, Hofstadter F. Tumors of the renal pelvis and the ureter. In: Eble JN, Sauter G, Epstein JI, editors. World Health Organisation classification of tumors: tumors of the urinary system and male genital organs. Lyon: IARC Press; 2004. p. 150–3.
5. Munoz JJ, Ellison LM. Upper tract urothelial neoplasms: incidence and survival during the last 2 decades. J Urol. 2000;164(5):1523–5.
6. Olgac S, Mazumdar M, Dalbagni G, Reuter VE. Urothelial carcinoma of the renal pelvis: a clinicopathologic study of 130 cases. Am J Surg Pathol. 2004;28(12):1545–52.
7. Favaretto RL, Shariat SF, Chade DC, Godoy G, Adamy A, Kaag M, et al. The effect of tumor location on prognosis in patients treated with radical nephroureterectomy at Memorial Sloan-Kettering Cancer Center. Eur Urol. 2010;58(4):574–80.
8. Wu CF, Pang ST, Chen CS, Chuang CK, Chen Y, Lin PY. The impact factors on prognosis of patients with pT3 upper urinary tract transitional cell carcinoma. J Urol. 2007;178(2):446–50. discussion 50.
9. Petkovic SD. Epidemiology and treatment of renal pelvic and ureteral tumors. J Urol. 1975;114(6):858–65.
10. Murphy WM, Grignon D, Perlman EJ. Tumors of the ureters and the renal pelvis. AFIP Atlas of tumor pathology: tumors of the kidney, bladder and related urinary structures. Washington, DC: American Registry of Pathology; 2004. p. 375–82.
11. Ouzzane A, Colin P, Xylinas E, Pignot G, Ariane MM, Saint F, et al. Ureteral and multifocal tumours have worse prognosis than renal pelvic tumours in urothelial carcinoma of the upper urinary tract treated by nephroureterectomy. Eur Urol. 2011;60(6):1258–65.
12. Yafi FA, Novara G, Shariat SF, Gupta A, Matsumoto K, Walton TJ, et al. Impact of tumour location versus multifocality in patients with upper tract urothelial carcinoma treated with nephroureterectomy and bladder cuff excision: a homogeneous series without perioperative chemotherapy. BJU Int. 2012;110(2 Pt 2):E7–13.
13. Gupta R, Paner GP, Amin MB. Neoplasms of the upper urinary tract: a review with focus on urothelial carcinoma of the pelvicalyceal system and aspects related to its diagnosis and reporting. Adv Anat Pathol. 2008;15(3):127–39.

14. Rink M, Robinson BD, Green DA, Cha EK, Hansen J, Comploj E, et al. Impact of histological variants on clinical outcomes of patients with upper urinary tract urothelial carcinoma. J Urol. 2012;188(2):398–404. Epub 2012/06/16.
15. Amin MB. Histological variants of urothelial carcinoma: diagnostic, therapeutic and prognostic implications. Mod Pathol. 2009;22 Suppl 2:S96–S118. Epub 2009/06/06.
16. Linder BJ, Boorjian SA, Cheville JC, Sukov WR, Thapa P, Tarrell RF, et al. The impact of histological reclassification during pathology re-review-evidence of a Will Rogers effect in bladder cancer? J Urol. 2013;190:1692–6.
17. Shah RB, Montgomery JS, Montie JE, Kunju LP. Variant (divergent) histologic differentiation in urothelial carcinoma is under-recognized in community practice: impact of mandatory central pathology review at a large referral hospital. Urol Oncol. 2013;31:1650–5.
18. Albadine R, Schultz L, Illei P, Ertoy D, Hicks J, Sharma R, et al. PAX8 (+)/p63 (-) immunostaining pattern in renal collecting duct carcinoma (CDC): a useful immunoprofile in the differential diagnosis of CDC versus urothelial carcinoma of upper urinary tract. Am J Surg Pathol. 2010;34(7):965–9.
19. Carvalho JC, Thomas DG, McHugh JB, Shah RB, Kunju LP. p63, CK7, PAX8 and INI-1: an optimal immunohistochemical panel to distinguish poorly differentiated urothelial cell carcinoma from high-grade tumours of the renal collecting system. Histopathology. 2012;60(4): 597–608.
20. Ozcan A, de la Roza G, Ro JY, Shen SS, Truong LD. PAX2 and PAX8 expression in primary and metastatic renal tumors: a comprehensive comparison. Arch Pathol Lab Med. 2012; 136(12):1541–51.
21. Young A, Kunju LP. High-grade carcinomas involving the renal sinus: report of a case and review of the differential diagnosis and immunohistochemical expression. Arch Pathol Lab Med. 2012;136(8):907–10.
22. Reuter VE. The urothelial tract: renal pelvis, ureter, urinary bladder, and urethra. In: Mills SE, Carter D, Greenson JK, Oberman HR, Reuter VE, Stoler MH, editors. Diagnostic surgical pathology. 4th ed. Philadelphia, PA: Lippincott Williams and Wilkins; 2004. p. 2035–81.
23. Cox RM, Schneider AG, Sangoi AR, Clingan WJ, Gokden N, McKenney JK. Invasive urothelial carcinoma with chordoid features: a report of 12 distinct cases characterized by prominent myxoid stroma and cordlike epithelial architecture. Am J Surg Pathol. 2009;33(8):1213–9.
24. Cox R, Epstein JI. Large nested variant of urothelial carcinoma: 23 cases mimicking von Brunn nests and inverted growth pattern of noninvasive papillary urothelial carcinoma. Am J Surg Pathol. 2011;35(9):1337–42.
25. Lopez-Beltran A, Cheng L, Comperat E, Roupret M, Blanca A, Menendez CL, et al. Large cell undifferentiated carcinoma of the urinary bladder. Pathology. 2010;42(4):364–8.
26. Cohen WM, Freed SZ, Hasson J. Metastatic cancer to the ureter: a review of the literature and case presentations. J Urol. 1974;112(2):188–9.
27. Hudolin T, Nola N, Milas I, Nola M, Juretic A. Ureteral metastasis of occult breast cancer. Breast. 2004;13(6):530–2.
28. Petersen RO, Sesterhenn IA, Davis CJ. Renal pelvis and ureter, Urologic pathology. 3rd ed. Philadelphia, PA: Lippincott Williams & Wilkins; 1986. p. 133–74.
29. Calderaro J, Moroch J, Pierron G, Pedeutour F, Grison C, Maille P, et al. SMARCB1/INI1 inactivation in renal medullary carcinoma. Histopathology. 2012;61(3):428–35.
30. Epstein JI, Amin MB, Reuter VR, Mostofi FK. The World Health Organization/International Society of Urological Pathology consensus classification of urothelial (transitional cell) neoplasms of the urinary bladder. Bladder Consensus Conference Committee. Am J Surg Pathol. 1998;22(12):1435–48.
31. Murphy WM, Deana DG. The nested variant of transitional cell carcinoma: a neoplasm resembling proliferation of Brunn's nests. Mod Pathol. 1992;5(3):240–3.
32. Wasco MJ, Daignault S, Bradley D, Shah RB. Nested variant of urothelial carcinoma: a clinicopathologic and immunohistochemical study of 30 pure and mixed cases. Hum Pathol. 2010;41(2):163–71. Epub 2009/10/06.

33. Edge SB, Byrd DR, Carducci MA, Compton CC. AJCC cancer staging manual. 7th ed. New York, NY: Springer; 2009.
34. Humphrey PA, Amin MB, Srigley JR, Chang A, Cohen AH, Delahunt B, et al. Protocol for the examination of specimens from patients with carcinoma of the ureter and renal pelvis. 7TH ed: Based on AJCC/UICC TNM 7th edition; 2011 February 1, 2011.
35. Henriksen KJ, Meehan SM, Chang A. Non-neoplastic renal diseases are often unrecognized in adult tumor nephrectomy specimens: a review of 246 cases. Am J Surg Pathol. 2007; 31(11):1703–8.
36. Bijol V, Mendez GP, Hurwitz S, Rennke HG, Nose V. Evaluation of the nonneoplastic pathology in tumor nephrectomy specimens: predicting the risk of progressive renal failure. Am J Surg Pathol. 2006;30(5):575–84.
37. El-Hakim A, Weiss GH, Lee BR, Smith AD. Correlation of ureteroscopic appearance with histologic grade of upper tract transitional cell carcinoma. Urology. 2004;63(4):647–50. discussion 50.
38. Hisataki T, Miyao N, Masumori N, Takahashi A, Sasai M, Yanase M, et al. Risk factors for the development of bladder cancer after upper tract urothelial cancer. Urology. 2000; 55(5):663–7.
39. Vashistha V, Shabsigh A, Zynger DL. Utility and diagnostic accuracy of ureteroscopic biopsy in upper tract urothelial carcinoma. Arch Pathol Lab Med. 2013;137(3):400–7.
40. Tavora F, Fajardo DA, Lee TK, Lotan T, Miller JS, Miyamoto H, et al. Small endoscopic biopsies of the ureter and renal pelvis: pathologic pitfalls. Am J Surg Pathol. 2009;33:1540–6.
41. Konety BR, Getzenberg RH. Urine based markers of urological malignancy. J Urol. 2001;165(2):600–11.
42. Lodde M, Mian C, Wiener H, Haitel A, Pycha A, Marberger M. Detection of upper urinary tract transitional cell carcinoma with ImmunoCyt: a preliminary report. Urology. 2001;58(3): 362–6.
43. Marin-Aguilera M, Mengual L, Ribal MJ, Musquera M, Ars E, Villavicencio H, et al. Utility of fluorescence in situ hybridization as a non-invasive technique in the diagnosis of upper urinary tract urothelial carcinoma. Eur Urol. 2007;51(2):409–15. discussion 15.
44. Hattori R, Yoshino Y, Gotoh M, Katoh M, Kamihira O, Ono Y. Laparoscopic nephroureterectomy for transitional cell carcinoma of renal pelvis and ureter: Nagoya experience. Urology. 2006;67(4):701–5.
45. Lam JS, Gupta M. Ureteroscopic management of upper tract transitional cell carcinoma. Urol Clin North Am. 2004;31(1):115–28.
46. Thompson RH, Krambeck AE, Lohse CM, Elliott DS, Patterson DE, Blute ML. Endoscopic management of upper tract transitional cell carcinoma in patients with normal contralateral kidneys. Urology. 2008;71(4):713–7.
47. Elliott DS, Segura JW, Lightner D, Patterson DE, Blute ML. Is nephroureterectomy necessary in all cases of upper tract transitional cell carcinoma? Long-term results of conservative endourologic management of upper tract transitional cell carcinoma in individuals with a normal contralateral kidney. Urology. 2001;58(2):174–8.
48. O'Donnell PH, Stadler WM. The role of chemotherapy in upper tract urothelial carcinoma. Adv Urol. 2009;2009:419028.
49. Miyake H, Hara I, Arakawa S, Kamidono S. A clinicopathological study of bladder cancer associated with upper urinary tract cancer. BJU Int. 2000;85(1):37–41.
50. Kang CH, Yu TJ, Hsieh HH, Yang JW, Shu K, Huang CC, et al. The development of bladder tumors and contralateral upper urinary tract tumors after primary transitional cell carcinoma of the upper urinary tract. Cancer. 2003;98(8):1620–6.
51. Sanderson KM, Roupret M. Upper urinary tract tumour after radical cystectomy for transitional cell carcinoma of the bladder: an update on the risk factors, surveillance regimens and treatments. BJU Int. 2007;100(1):11–6.
52. Kauffman EC, Raman JD. Bladder cancer following upper tract urothelial carcinoma. Expert Rev Anticancer Ther. 2008;8(1):75–85.

53. Sved PD, Gomez P, Nieder AM, Manoharan M, Kim SS, Soloway MS. Upper tract tumour after radical cystectomy for transitional cell carcinoma of the bladder: incidence and risk factors. BJU Int. 2004;94(6):785–9.
54. Tran W, Serio AM, Raj GV, Dalbagni G, Vickers AJ, Bochner BH, et al. Longitudinal risk of upper tract recurrence following radical cystectomy for urothelial cancer and the potential implications for long-term surveillance. J Urol. 2008;179(1):96–100.
55. Park S, Hong B, Kim CS, Ahn H. The impact of tumor location on prognosis of transitional cell carcinoma of the upper urinary tract. J Urol. 2004;171(2 Pt 1):621–5.
56. Park J, Ha SH, Min GE, Song C, Hong B, Hong JH, et al. The protective role of renal parenchyma as a barrier to local tumor spread of upper tract transitional cell carcinoma and its impact on patient survival. J Urol. 2009;182(3):894–9.
57. Guinan P, Vogelzang NJ, Randazzo R, Sener S, Chmiel J, Fremgen A, et al. Renal pelvic cancer: a review of 611 patients treated in Illinois 1975–1985. Cancer Incidence and End Results Committee. Urology. 1992;40(5):393–9.
58. Guinan P, Volgelzang NJ, Randazzo R, Fremgen A, Chmiel J, Sylvester J, et al. Renal pelvic transitional cell carcinoma. The role of the kidney in tumor-node-metastasis staging. Cancer. 1992;69(7):1773–5.
59. van der Poel HG, Antonini N, van Tinteren H, Horenblas S. Upper urinary tract cancer: location is correlated with prognosis. Eur Urol. 2005;48(3):438–44.
60. Raman JD, Ng CK, Scherr DS, Margulis V, Lotan Y, Bensalah K, et al. Impact of tumor location on prognosis for patients with upper tract urothelial carcinoma managed by radical nephroureterectomy. Eur Urol. 2010;57(6):1072–9.
61. Isbarn H, Jeldres C, Shariat SF, Liberman D, Sun M, Lughezzani G, et al. Location of the primary tumor is not an independent predictor of cancer specific mortality in patients with upper urinary tract urothelial carcinoma. J Urol. 2009;182(5):2177–81.
62. Williams AK, Kassouf W, Chin J, Rendon R, Jacobsen N, Fairey A, et al. Multifocality rather than tumor location is a prognostic factor in upper tract urothelial carcinoma. Urol Oncol. 2013;31:1161–5.
63. Yoshimura K, Arai Y, Fujimoto H, Nishiyama H, Ogura K, Okino T, et al. Prognostic impact of extensive parenchymal invasion pattern in pT3 renal pelvic transitional cell carcinoma. Cancer. 2002;94(12):3150–6.
64. Amin MB, Trpkov K, Lopez-Beltran A, Grignon D and Members of the ISUP Immunohistochemistry in Diagnostic Urologic Pathology Group. Best Practices Recommendations in the Application of Immunohistochemistry in the Bladder Lesions: Report from the International Society of Urologic Pathology Consensus Conference. Am J Surg Pathol. 2014;38:e20–e34.
65. Gruver AM, Amin MB, Luthringer DJ, Westfall D, Arora K, Farver CF, et al. Selective immunohistochemical markers to distinguish between metastatic high-grade urothelial carcinoma and primary poorly differentiated invasive squamous cell carcinoma of the lung. Arch Pathol Lab Med. 2012;136(11):1339–46.
66. Brown HM, Wilkinson EJ. Uroplakin-III to distinguish primary vulvar Paget disease from Paget disease secondary to urothelial carcinoma. Hum Pathol. 2002;33(5):545–8.
67. Shen SS, Truong LD, Scarpelli M, Lopez-Beltran A. Role of immunohistochemistry in diagnosing renal neoplasms: when is it really useful? Arch Pathol Lab Med. 2012;136(4):410–7.
68. Tong GX, Yu WM, Beaubier NT, Weeden EM, Hamele-Bena D, Mansukhani MM, et al. Expression of PAX8 in normal and neoplastic renal tissues: an immunohistochemical study. Mod Pathol. 2009;22(9):1218–27.
69. Chang A, Brimo F, Montgomery EA, Epstein JI. Use of PAX8 and GATA3 in diagnosing sarcomatoid renal cell carcinoma and sarcomatoid urothelial carcinoma. Hum Pathol. 2013;44(8):1563–8.
70. Memeo L, Jhang J, Assaad AM, McKiernan JM, Murty VV, Hibshoosh H, et al. Immunohistochemical analysis for cytokeratin 7, KIT, and PAX2: value in the differential diagnosis of chromophobe cell carcinoma. Am J Clin Pathol. 2007;127(2):225–9.

71. Carvalho JC, Wasco MJ, Kunju LP, Thomas DG, Shah RB. Cluster analysis of immunohistochemical profiles delineates CK7, vimentin, S100A1 and C-kit (CD117) as an optimal panel in the differential diagnosis of renal oncocytoma from its mimics. Histopathology. 2011;58(2):169–79.
72. Bing Z, Lal P, Lu S, Ziober A, Tomaszewski JE. Role of carbonic anhydrase IX, alpha-methylacyl coenzyme a racemase, cytokeratin 7, and galectin-3 in the evaluation of renal neoplasms: a tissue microarray immunohistochemical study. Ann Diagn Pathol. 2013;17(1):58–62.
73. McKenney JK, Desai S, Cohen C, Amin MB. Discriminatory immunohistochemical staining of urothelial carcinoma in situ and non-neoplastic urothelium: an analysis of cytokeratin 20, p53, and CD44 antigens. Am J Surg Pathol. 2001;25(8):1074–8.
74. Nese N, Gupta R, Bui MH, Amin MB. Carcinoma in situ of the urinary bladder: review of clinicopathologic characteristics with an emphasis on aspects related to molecular diagnostic techniques and prognosis. J Natl Compr Canc Netw. 2009;7(1):48–57.
75. Oliva E, Pinheiro NF, Heney NM, Kaufman DS, Shipley WU, Gurski C, et al. Immunohistochemistry as an adjunct in the differential diagnosis of radiation-induced atypia versus urothelial carcinoma in situ of the bladder: a study of 45 cases. Hum Pathol. 2013;44(5):860–6.
76. Lynch HT, Ens JA, Lynch JF. The Lynch syndrome II and urological malignancies. J Urol. 1990;143(1):24–8.
77. Blaszyk H, Wang L, Dietmaier W, Hofstadter F, Burgart LJ, Cheville JC, et al. Upper tract urothelial carcinoma: a clinicopathologic study including microsatellite instability analysis. Modern Pathol. 2002;15(8):790–7.
78. Roupret M, Yates DR, Comperat E, Cussenot O. Upper urinary tract urothelial cell carcinomas and other urological malignancies involved in the hereditary nonpolyposis colorectal cancer (lynch syndrome) tumor spectrum. Eur Urol. 2008;54(6):1226–36.
79. Hartmann A, Dietmaier W, Hofstadter F, Burgart LJ, Cheville JC, Blaszyk H. Urothelial carcinoma of the upper urinary tract: inverted growth pattern is predictive of microsatellite instability. Hum Pathol. 2003;34(3):222–7.
80. Rodriguez-Bigas MA, Boland CR, Hamilton SR, Henson DE, Jass JR, Khan PM, et al. A National Cancer Institute Workshop on Hereditary Nonpolyposis Colorectal Cancer Syndrome: meeting highlights and Bethesda guidelines. J Natl Cancer Inst. 1997;89(23):1758–62.
81. Wu XR. Urothelial tumorigenesis: a tale of divergent pathways. Nat Rev Cancer. 2005;5(9):713–25.
82. Mitra AP, Datar RH, Cote RJ. Molecular pathways in invasive bladder cancer: new insights into mechanisms, progression, and target identification. J Clin Oncol. 2006;24(35):5552–64.
83. Jebar AH, Hurst CD, Tomlinson DC, Johnston C, Taylor CF, Knowles MA. FGFR3 and Ras gene mutations are mutually exclusive genetic events in urothelial cell carcinoma. Oncogene. 2005;24(33):5218–25.
84. Hernandez S, Lopez-Knowles E, Lloreta J, Kogevinas M, Amoros A, Tardon A, et al. Prospective study of FGFR3 mutations as a prognostic factor in nonmuscle invasive urothelial bladder carcinomas. J Clin Oncol. 2006;24(22):3664–71.
85. Bakkar AA, Wallerand H, Radvanyi F, Lahaye JB, Pissard S, Lecerf L, et al. FGFR3 and TP53 gene mutations define two distinct pathways in urothelial cell carcinoma of the bladder. Cancer Res. 2003;63(23):8108–12.
86. van Rhijn BW. Combining molecular and pathologic data to prognosticate non-muscle-invasive bladder cancer. Urol Oncol. 2012;30(4):518–23.
87. van Rhijn BW, Vis AN, van der Kwast TH, Kirkels WJ, Radvanyi F, Ooms EC, et al. Molecular grading of urothelial cell carcinoma with fibroblast growth factor receptor 3 and MIB-1 is superior to pathologic grade for the prediction of clinical outcome. J Clin Oncol. 2003;21(10):1912–21.
88. van Rhijn BW, Zuiverloon TC, Vis AN, Radvanyi F, van Leenders GJ, Ooms BC, et al. Molecular grade (FGFR3/MIB-1) and EORTC risk scores are predictive in primary non-muscle-invasive bladder cancer. Eur Urol. 2010;58(3):433–41.

89. Margulis V, Lotan Y, Karakiewicz PI, Fradet Y, Ashfaq R, Capitanio U, et al. Multi-institutional validation of the predictive value of Ki-67 labeling index in patients with urinary bladder cancer. J Natl Cancer Inst. 2009;101(2):114–9.
90. Netto GJ. Molecular biomarkers in urothelial carcinoma of the bladder: are we there yet? Nat Rev Urol. 2012;9(1):41–51.
91. Mitra AP, Hansel DE, Cote RJ. Prognostic value of cell-cycle regulation biomarkers in bladder cancer. Semin Oncol. 2012;39(5):524–33.
92. Rink M, Cha EK, Green D, Hansen J, Robinson BD, Lotan Y, et al. Biomolecular predictors of urothelial cancer behavior and treatment outcomes. Curr Urol Rep. 2012;13(2):122–35.
93. Amin MB, McKenney JK, Paner GP, Hansel DE, Grignon DJ, Montironi R, et al. ICUD-EAU International Consultation on Bladder Cancer 2012: Pathology. Eur Urol. 2013;63(1):16–35.
94. Kamat AM, Hegarty PK, Gee JR, Clark PE, Svatek RS, Hegarty N, et al. ICUD-EAU international consultation on bladder cancer 2012: screening, diagnosis, and molecular markers. Eur Urol. 2013;63(1):4–15.
95. Volmar KE, Chan TY, De Marzo AM, Epstein JI. Florid von Brunn nests mimicking urothelial carcinoma: a morphologic and immunohistochemical comparison to the nested variant of urothelial carcinoma. Am J Surg Pathol. 2003;27(9):1243–52.
96. Blacher EJ, Johnson DE, Abdul-Karim FW, Ayala AG. Squamous cell carcinoma of renal pelvis. Urology. 1985;25(2):124–6.
97. Hes O, Curik R, Mainer K, Michal M. Urothelial signet-ring cell carcinoma of the renal pelvis with collagenous spherulosis: a case report. Int J Surg Pathol. 2005;13(4):375–8.
98. Takehara K, Nomata K, Eguchi J, Hisamatsu H, Maruta S, Hayashi T, et al. Mucinous adenocarcinoma of the renal pelvis associated with transitional cell carcinoma in the renal pelvis and the bladder. Int J Urol. 2004;11(11):1016–8.
99. Anderson JB, Lee JJ, Hancock RA, Black SR. Hemangioma of the kidney pelvis. J Urol. 1953;70(6):869–73.
100. Khater N, Khauli R, Shahait M, Degheili J, Khalifeh I, Aoun J. Solitary fibrous tumors of the kidneys: presentation, evaluation, and treatment. Urol Int. 2013;91:373–83.
101. Coup AJ. Angiosarcoma of the ureter. Br J Urol. 1988;62(3):275–6.
102. Kao VC, Graff PW, Rappaport H. Leiomyoma of the ureter. A histologically problematic rare tumor confirmed by immunohistochemical studies. Cancer. 1969;24(3):535–42.
103. Loomis RC. Primary leiomyosarcoma of the kidney: report of a case and review of the literature. J Urol. 1972;107(4):557–60.
104. Ogata S, Mizoguchi H, Arita M, Sakamoto S, Ogata J. A case of hemangiomyoma of the ureter in a child. Eur Urol. 1985;11(5):355–6.
105. Ravich A. Neurofibroma of the ureter: report of a case with operation and recovery. Arch Surg. 1935;30:442–8.
106. Rushton HG, Sens MA, Garvin AJ, Turner Jr WR. Primary leiomyosarcoma of the ureter: a case report with electron microscopy. J Urol. 1983;129(5):1045–6.
107. Uchida M, Watanabe H, Mishina T, Shimada N. Leiomyoma of the renal pelvis. J Urol. 1981;125(4):572–4.
108. Uhlir K. Hemangioma of the ureter. J Urol. 1973;110(6):647–9.
109. Vahlensieck Jr W, Riede U, Wimmer B, Ihling C. Beta-human chorionic gonadotropin-positive extragonadal germ cell neoplasia of the renal pelvis. Cancer. 1991;67(12):3146–9.
110. Weinberg AG, Currarino G, Hurt Jr GE. Botryoid Wilms' tumor of the renal pelvis. Arch Pathol Lab Med. 1984;108(2):147–8.
111. Smith EM, Resnick MI. Ureteropelvic junction obstruction secondary to periureteral lipoma. J Urol. 1994;151(1):150–1.
112. Charny CK, Glick RD, Genega EM, Meyers PA, Reuter VE, La Quaglia MP. Ewing's sarcoma/primitive neuroectodermal tumor of the ureter: a case report and review of the literature. J Pediatr Surg. 2000;35(9):1356–8.
113. Fein RL, Hamm FC. Malignant schwannoma of the renal pelvis: a review of the literature and a case report. J Urol. 1965;94(4):356–61.

114. Mazal PR, Schaufler R, Altenhuber-Muller R, Haitel A, Watschinger B, Kratzik C, et al. Derivation of nephrogenic adenomas from renal tubular cells in kidney-transplant recipients. N Engl J Med. 2002;347(9):653–9.
115. Hansel DE, Nadasdy T, Epstein JI. Fibromyxoid nephrogenic adenoma: a newly recognized variant mimicking mucinous adenocarcinoma. Am J Surg Pathol. 2007;31(8):1231–7.
116. Diolombi M, Ross HM, Mercalli F, Sharma R, Epstein JI. Nephrogenic adenoma: a report of 3 unusual cases infiltrating into perinephric adipose tissue. Am J Surg Pathol. 2013;37(4): 532–8.
117. Childs MA, Umbreit EC, Krambeck AE, Sebo TJ, Patterson DE, Gettman MT. Fibroepithelial polyps of the ureter: a single-institutional experience. J Endourol. 2009;23(9):1415–9.
118. Tsuzuki T, Epstein JI. Fibroepithelial polyp of the lower urinary tract in adults. Am J Surg Pathol. 2005;29(4):460–6.
119. Corradi D, Maestri R, Palmisano A, Bosio S, Greco P, Manenti L, et al. Idiopathic retroperitoneal fibrosis: clinicopathologic features and differential diagnosis. Kidney Int. 2007;72(6):742–53.
120. Vaglio A, Salvarani C, Buzio C. Retroperitoneal fibrosis. Lancet. 2006;367(9506):241–51.
121. Zen Y, Onodera M, Inoue D, Kitao A, Matsui O, Nohara T, et al. Retroperitoneal fibrosis: a clinicopathologic study with respect to immunoglobulin G4. Am J Surg Pathol. 2009;33(12): 1833–9.
122. Zen Y, Nakanuma Y. IgG4-related disease: a cross-sectional study of 114 cases. Am J Surg Pathol. 2010;34(12):1812–9.
123. Okazaki K, Uchida K, Fukui T. Recent advances in autoimmune pancreatitis: concept, diagnosis, and pathogenesis. J Gastroenterol. 2008;43(6):409–18.
124. Rudmik L, Trpkov K, Nash C, Kinnear S, Falck V, Dushinski J, et al. Autoimmune pancreatitis associated with renal lesions mimicking metastatic tumours. CMAJ. 2006;175(4):367–9.
125. Trpkov K, Guggisberg K, Yilmaz A. Arias-Stella reaction as a diagnostic pitfall in a bladder biopsy with endometriosis: case report and review of the pseudoneoplastic bladder lesions. Pathol Res Pract. 2009;205(9):653–6.
126. Eble JN, World Health Organization., International Agency for Research on Cancer. Pathology and genetics of tumours of the urinary system and male genital organs. Lyon, Oxford: IARC Press; 2004. p. 359. Oxford University Press (distributor).

Chapter 4
Prognostics Factors, Molecular Markers, and Predictive Tools in Upper Tract Urothelial Carcinoma

Evanguelos Xylinas, Giacomo Novara, Mesut Remzi, Pierre Karakiewicz, and Shahrokh F. Shariat

Abstract Upper urinary tract urothelial carcinoma (UTUC) is a rare disease. Thus, little evidence-based data are available to guide clinical decision-making. The aim of the study was to provide an overview of the currently available prognostic factors for UTUC.

A systematic literature search was conducted using the PubMed databases to identify original articles regarding prognostic factors in patients with UTUC.

We divided the prognostic factors for UTUC in four different categories: clinical factors, preoperative characteristics, intraoperative/surgical factors, and postoperative/pathologic factors. Prognostic factors described in order of importance are tumor stage and grade, lymph node involvement, a concomitant cis, age at the diagnostic, lymphovascular invasion, tumor architecture and necrosis, tumor location and

E. Xylinas, MD
Department of Urology, Weill Cornell Medical College, New York-Presbyterian Hospital, New York, NY, USA

Department of Urology, Cochin Hospital, APHP, Paris Descartes University, Paris, France
e-mail: evanguelosxylinas@hotmail.com

G. Novara, MD
Department of Surgical, Oncological and Gastroenterologic Sciences, Urology Clinic, University of Padua, Padua, Italy
e-mail: giacomo.novara@unipd.it

M. Remzi, MD
Department of Urology, Landeskrankenhaus Korneuburg, Korneuburg, Austria
e-mail: mRemzi@gmx.at

P. Karakiewicz, MD
Department of Urology, University of Montreal, Montreal, QC, Canada
e-mail: Pierre.karakiewicz@umontreal.ca

S.F. Shariat, MD (✉)
Department of Urology, Weill Cornell Medical College, New York-Presbyterian Hospital, New York, NY, USA

Department of Urology, Medical University of Vienna, Währinger Gürtel 18-20, 1090 Vienna, Austria
e-mail: sfshariat@gmail.com

© Springer Science+Business Media New York 2015

S.F. Shariat, E. Xylinas (eds.), *Upper Tract Urothelial Carcinoma*,
DOI 10.1007/978-1-4939-1501-9_4

multifocality, gender. The impact of obesity, smoking, and other comorbidities (ECOG, ASA) on outcomes has been recently reported but needs to be validated. The endoscopic approach of distal ureter management during radical nephroureterectomy has been shown to be at higher risk of bladder recurrence.

The incorporation of such prognosticators into clinical prediction models might help to guide decision-making with regard to timing of surveillance, type of treatment, performance of lymphadenectomy, and consideration of neoadjuvant or adjuvant systemic therapies.

Keywords Upper tract urothelial carcinoma • Radical nephroureterectomy • Prognosis • Molecular markers • Prediction

Introduction

Upper tract urothelial carcinoma (UTUC) is a rare disease and accounts for only 5 % of the urothelial carcinomas [1]. The outcomes of patients with UTUC are heterogeneous and, therefore, difficult to predict. Given the low incidence of the disease, data regarding clinicopathological predictors of outcomes are sparse. The lack of randomized trials in patients with UTUC makes decisions complex. Recently, multi-institutional collaborative studies have identified several potential outcome predictors following radical nephroureterectomy (RNU) for UTUC, improving the traditional pathologic staging system [2–9]. Accurate estimation of treatment success, complications, and long-term morbidity is essential for patients to make informed medical decisions regarding management of their disease. To this end, researchers have developed prognostic tools based on statistical models to obtain the most accurate and reliable predictions. These tools can provide predictions that are both evidence-based and individualized. Among the available decision tools, nomograms currently represent the most accurate and widely used tools for prediction of outcomes in patients with cancer [10]. Nomograms have been adopted in oncologic disciplines such as breast, colon, prostate, kidney, and bladder cancers [11].

In this review we discuss the established prognostic factors in UTUC (including clinicopathological features and molecular markers) and the currently available predictive tools. Moreover, this chapter may serve as an initial step toward a comprehensive reference guide for physicians to better understand UTUC prognosis.

Patient-Related Factors (Table 4.1)

Patient Age

Several population-based and multicenter studies have reported that advanced patient age is an independent predictor of cancer-specific mortality (CSM) after RNU [12–14]. The mean age at diagnosis is around 70 years old and thus significantly older than renal cell carcinoma. Changes in the biologic potential of the tumor, with

Table 4.1 Prognostic factors of upper tract urothelial carcinoma related to the patient

Characteristics	Comment	References
Age	Advanced chronological age is an independent predictor of DR, CSM, and OM	[12–14]
Gender	No impact of gender on outcomes	[15]
Race	Afro-American race independent predictor of CSM	[16, 17]
Comorbidities	– ECOG-PS ≥ 1 is an independent predictor of OM – ASA score independent predictor of CSM	[14, 18, 19]
Obesity	Body mass index ≥ 30 is an independent predictor of DR, CSM, and OS	[2]
Smoking exposure	Smoking status and cumulative exposure associated with DR, CSM, and OM	[20, 21]

DR disease recurrence, *CSM* cancer-specific mortality, *OM* overall mortality

UTUC being more aggressive in elderly patients, as well as to differences in care patterns (e.g., greater reluctance to perform radical surgery in these individuals) could be an explanation for this finding. Based on the evidence, age should not be an exclusion criterion for RNU as the complications of this procedure in the elderly are not excessive or much different from their young counterparts.

Patient Gender

UTUC is more common in men than in women [1]. Conversely to lower tract UC, female gender is not associated with features of aggressive disease [6] or oncologic outcomes after RNU [15]. Therefore, gender should not be considered as a predictor of survival in patients with UTUC.

Patient Race

The incidence of UTUC appears to be increasing in most racial groups, mostly because of earlier detection. While a multicenter study performed at academic centers did not show any difference between races [16], Afro-Americans have been shown to have worse outcomes compared with other racial groups [17]. As with many diseases, whether this is due to differences in biological processes or more likely due to differences in health attitudes and access to care remains to be evaluated.

Comorbidities ASA and ECOG

Eastern Cooperative Oncology Group performance status (ECOG-PS) has been shown to be independently associated with higher perioperative mortality and overall mortality (OM) after RNU, but not disease recurrence (DR) and CSM [18]. Conversely, the French collaborative group reported an association of ASA score with cancer-specific mortality after RNU [19]. In a recent study, addition of ECOG to a multivariable model including standard clinicopathological features was significantly associated with DR and CSM, while age lost its association [14]. Thus, these findings need further investigation and validation.

Obesity

The prognostic role of obesity has been demonstrated for several malignancies, such as renal cell and prostate cancer. A recent multi-institutional study examined the relationship between body mass index and oncologic outcomes in UTUC patients [2]. The authors reported that a body mass index ≥30 was associated with DR, CSM, and OM. Further studies need to investigate the biological rationale of such findings and whether this risk can be modified.

Smoking Status and Cumulative Exposure

Smoking exposure represents an established risk factor for the development of UC [20]. A recent multicenter study investigated the relationship between smoking exposure and prognosis of UTUC patients [21]. The authors showed that smoking status (current versus never) and cumulative exposure (heavy long-term smokers: >20 cigarettes per day and >20years) were associated with both DR and CSM (Fig. 4.1) [21]. Interestingly, smoking cessation of more than 10 years mitigated these detrimental effects [21]. The authors concluded that smoking cessation programs should be integral parts of the cancer care administrated to UTUC patients.

Disease-Related Factors (Table 4.2)

Hydronephrosis

Several studies explored the relationship between hydronephrosis on preoperative imaging, pathologic stage, and CSS in patients with UTUC. Presence of hydronephrosis has been associated with more advanced disease stage [22–24] and CSS [25].

Symptoms

The presence of systemic symptoms such as pain or weight loss has been associated with presence of higher-stage and higher-grade UTUC [26] and OM in patients treated with RNU for UTUC [27]. Further multi-institutional efforts are still needed to validate this predictor. With more advanced imaging studies, most of the patients with systemic symptoms will be likely identified as metastatic.

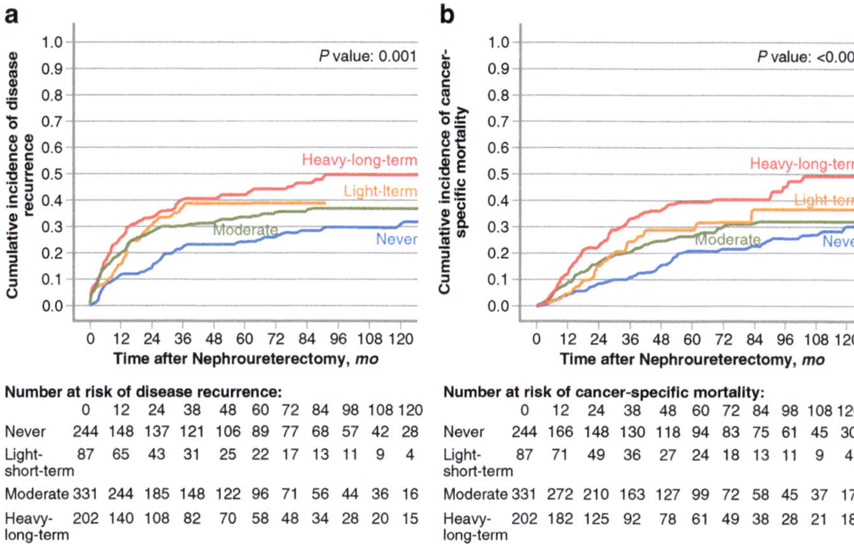

Fig. 4.1 Estimates of disease recurrence and cancer-specific mortality incidences according to the cumulative smoking intensity in 864 upper tract urothelial carcinoma patients treated with radical nephroureterectomy. Adapted from Michael Rink, Evanguelos Xylinas, Vitaly Margulis, Eugene K. Cha, Behfar Ehdaie, Jay D. Raman, et al. Impact of smoking on Oncologic Outcomes of Upper Tract Urothelial Carcinoma After Radical Nephroureterectomy. European Urology null 2012 null http://dx.doi.org/10.1016/j.eururo.2012.06.029

Table 4.2 Prognostic factors of upper tract urothelial carcinoma related to the disease

Characteristics	Comment	References
Hydronephrosis	Presence of hydronephrosis is associated with higher stage, DR, and CSM	[22–25]
Symptoms	Systemic symptoms are associated with metastatic disease	[26, 27]
Tumor location	The impact of tumor location on outcomes results in contradictory findings	[28–30]
Tumor multifocality	Presence of multifocal tumors is an independent predictor of CSM	[8, 31, 32]
Tumor size	Tumor size >3 cm is an independent predictor of DR and CSM	[33, 34]
Previous/synchronous bladder cancer	Presence of a previous or synchronous bladder cancer is an independent predictor of IVR	[37–39]

DR disease recurrence, *CSM* cancer-specific mortality, *IVR* intravesical recurrence, *OM* overall mortality

Tumor Location

The impact of tumor location (renal pelvicalyceal system compared with ureter) on the prognosis of patients with UTUC is controversial. Several single-institutional studies initially reported that ureteral location was associated with worse outcomes [28, 29]. A recent multi-institutional French study confirmed these findings [8]. On the contrary, several other population-based and multi-institutional studies found no association of tumor location with oncologic outcomes after RNU once adjusted for tumor stage [5, 30]. To conclude, the currently available retrospective studies do not permit a definitive conclusion regarding the impact of tumor location on UTUC prognosis. However, while there is a differential impact of tumor location on tumor stage, lymph node status and tumor stage are more powerful drivers of tumor biology and clinical behavior.

Tumor Multifocality

Multifocal tumors are defined as tumors with two or more distinct locations within the urinary tract. Tumor multifocality (occurring in at least 30 % of patients) in retrospective studies has been shown to be an independent predictor of CSM (Fig. 4.2) [8, 31]. Tumor presence in both the renal pelvicalyceal system and ureter is worse than either location with regard to cancer-specific outcomes [32]. Based on the current literature evidence, tumor multifocality should be routinely determined by clinicians with adequate sampling and reported by pathologists.

Tumor Size

Tumor size is an established predictor of cancer-related outcomes in several malignancies. A cutoff of tumor diameter of 3 cm and 4 cm has been associated with occurrence of metastasis [33] and intravesical recurrence after RNU [34], respectively. Both these studies need validation in studies with larger cohorts. From clinical experience, Ta tumors can reach a large size and have a low risk of becoming invasive. Whether tumor size is an accurate predictor of biological behavior of an individual tumor remains to be determined.

Clinical Tumor Grade and Stage

Endoscopic evaluation (+/–biopsy) establishes the definitive diagnosis of UTUC and helps risk stratify patients towards conservative or radical management. Biopsy grade is accurate and can help predict pathologic findings [24]. Unlike lower tract UC, the clinical staging of UTUC is difficult because biopsies that include underlying muscle are generally not possible [35]. Imaging studies can help improve clinical staging based on the presence of hydronephrosis (see above) and invasion in soft tissue [36].

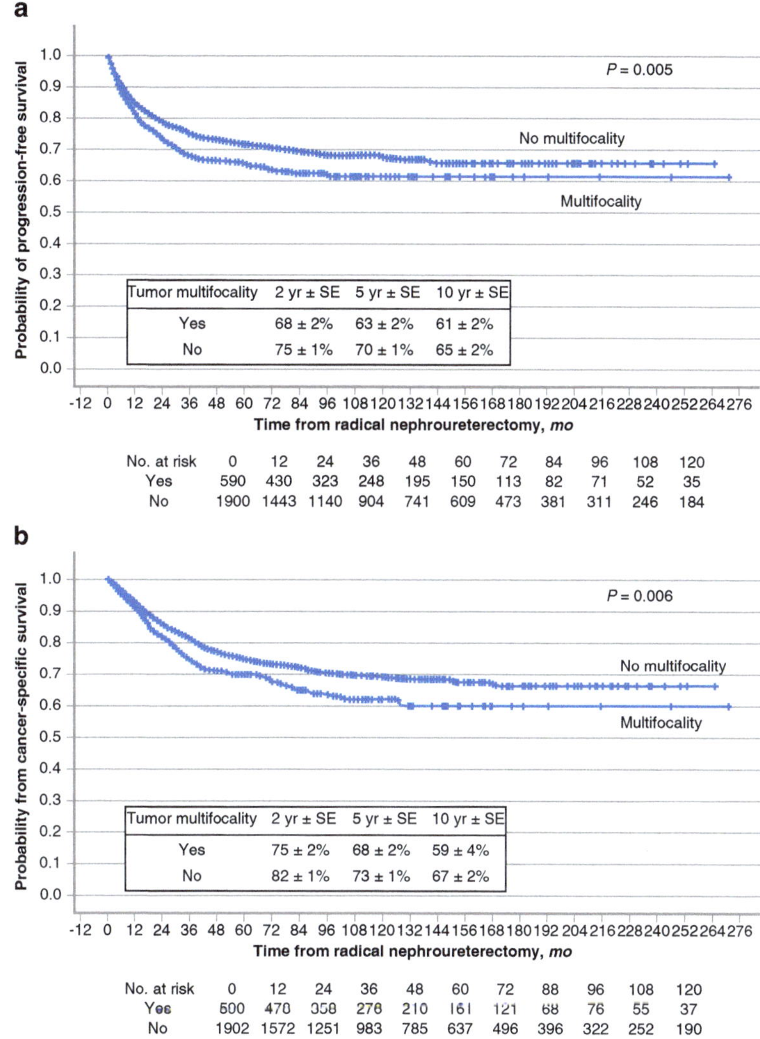

Fig. 4.2 Kaplan–Meier plots of progression-free and cancer-specific survival stratified according to tumor multifocality in 2,492 patients treated with radical nephroureterectomy for upper tract urothelial carcinoma. Adapted from Thomas F. Chromecki, Eugene K. Cha, Harun Fajkovic, Vitaly Margulis, Giacomo Novara, Douglas S. Scherr et al. The Impact of Tumor Multifocality on Outcomes in Patients Treated With Radical Nephroureterectomy. European Urology Volume 61, Issue 2 2012 245–253. http://dx.doi.org/10.1016/j.eururo.2011.09.017

Previous/Synchronous Bladder Cancer

UTUC are considered part of a pan-urothelial phenomenon that can yield multifocal tumors including lower tract UC. Previous history of bladder cancer has been associated with intravesical recurrence [37, 38], DR, and CSM after RNU [37, 39].

Surgery-Related Factors (Table 4.3)

Delayed Surgery

In lower tract UC, a delay between diagnosis and radical cystectomy (≥3 months) is considered to have a negative impact on prognosis. In UTUC, a multi-institutional study investigated the prognostic impact of the time interval between diagnosis and RNU on oncologic outcomes [40]. The study showed that a longer interval (≥3 months) was also associated with advanced pathological stage, DR, and CSM in patients with invasive disease [40]. This data together with that from the lower tract indicated that once the tumor becomes invasive, which is difficult to assess clinically in UTUC, one should proceed to definite therapy in a time-sensitive fashion.

Surgical Approach

Open RNU (ONU) with excision of a bladder cuff is considered the gold standard treatment of invasive or high-risk noninvasive UTUC regardless of the location of the tumor in the urinary tract [1]. Laparoscopic RNU (LNU) has emerged as a minimally invasive alternative to ONU, with advantages in terms of lower blood loss, shorter length of hospital stay, and shorter convalescence [41, 42]. To date, only one prospective randomized trial showed no difference in terms of DR and CSM between LNU and ONU [43]. In non-organ-confined tumors LNU was inferior to ONU. This difference could be attributed to surgeon experience and other factors such as the differential use of lymph node dissection between the two groups. A population-based study (with a propensity score matched analysis) and a meta-analysis of retrospective studies confirmed the safety of LNU with regard to oncologic outcomes when compared to ONU [41, 42]. As long that one abides to the oncologic principles, there should be no difference between the different approaches.

Table 4.3 Prognostic factors of upper tract urothelial carcinoma related to the surgery

Characteristics	Comment	References
Delay of treatment	A delay >3 months associated with higher stages in invasive UTUC	[40]
Surgical approach	Outcomes between open and laparoscopic RNU are not different	[41–43]
Distal ureter management	– Lack of complete bladder cuff removal associated with DR and CSM – Endoscopic distal ureter management associated with IVR	[9, 44]

UTUC upper tract urothelial carcinoma, *RNU* radical nephroureterectomy, *CSM*: cancer-specific survival

Distal Ureter Management

Excision of the bladder cuff is mandatory for invasive or high-risk noninvasive UTUC [1]. Moreover the procedure must comply with oncological principles, which consist of preventing tumor seeding by avoiding entry into the urinary tract during tumor resection. Resection of the distal ureter and its orifice is performed because it is a part of the urinary tract with considerable risk of tumor recurrence. After removal of the proximal part, it is almost impossible to image or approach it by endoscopy during follow-up. Recent publications on survival after RNU have concluded that removal of the distal ureter (bladder cuff) improves prognosis after RNU [44]. Moreover, endoscopic distal ureter management has been associated with a higher risk of intravesical recurrence (Fig. 4.3) [9]. While there have been a variety of techniques described for the management of the bladder cuff, complete removal is what really matters. Techniques such as ureteral stripping lead to incomplete surgery and should be avoided [1].

Lymph Node Dissection

Lymph node dissection (LND) during RNU allows for optimal staging of the disease and may have a therapeutic role [45]. However, the anatomical sites of LND have not yet been clearly defined. Specific LND templates are likely to have a greater impact on patient survival than the number of lymph nodes removed (Fig. 4.4) [45, 46]. The cumulative data from the literature on this subject suggest that a LND should be performed during RNU or distal ureterectomy for invasive UTUC [1, 45]. The templates for LND need to be defined through large multicenter template studies. Similarly to lower tract UCB, a pathological nodal staging score has been proposed in order to predict the probability of a patient staged as pN0 to be truly node negative (Fig. 4.5) [47]. However, all data are retrospective; consequently, underreporting of the true rate of node-positive disease is likely.

Pathologic Factors (Table 4.4)

Tumor Stage

Pathologic tumor stage represents the best-established predictor of survival in patients with UTUC and should always be considered in the preoperative and postoperative counseling of these patients, specifically in the determination of the intensity of postoperative surveillance and the decision-making regarding adjuvant therapies and trials (Fig. 4.6) [39, 48].

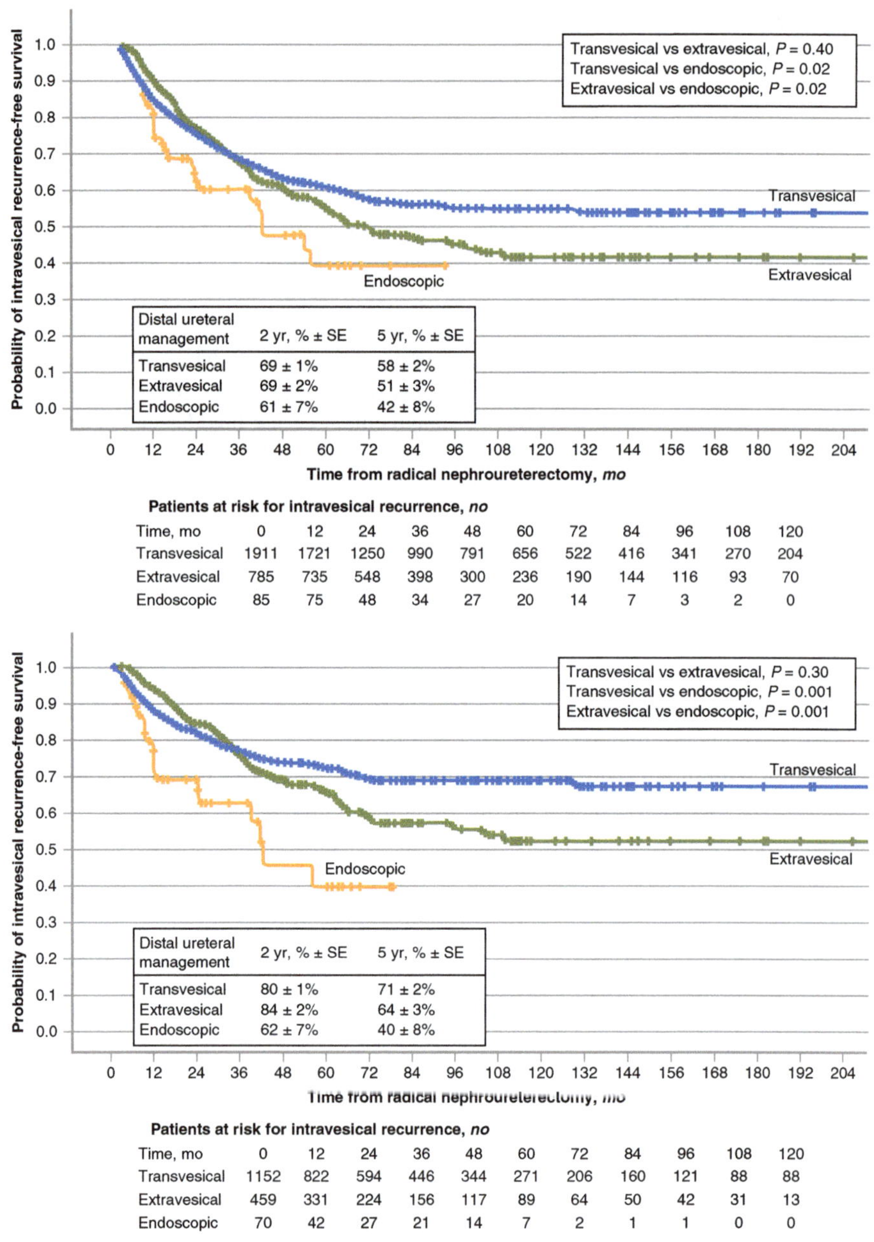

Fig. 4.3 Intravesical recurrence-free survival in 2,681 patients who underwent radical nephroureterectomy for upper tract urothelial carcinoma according to the distal ureter management. Adapted from Evanguelos Xylinas, Michael Rink, Eugene K. Cha, Thomas Clozel, Richard K. Lee, Harun Fajkovic et al. Impact of distal ureter management on oncologic outcomes following radical nephroureterectomy for upper tract urothelial carcinoma. European Urology null 2012 null. http://dx.doi.org/10.1016/j.eururo.2012.04.052

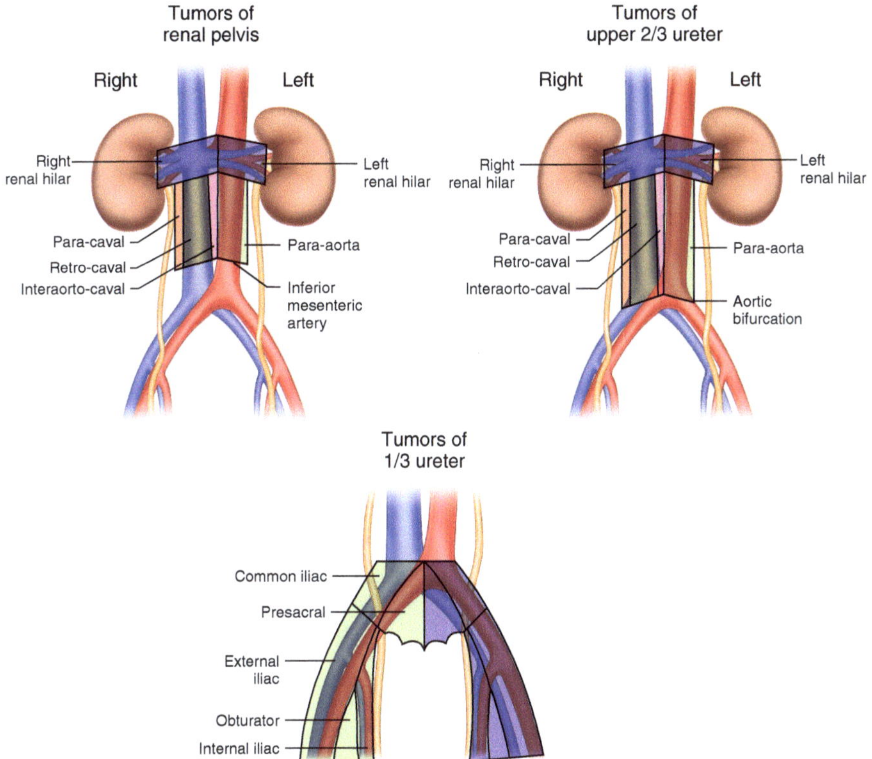

Fig. 4.4 Role of lymphadenectomy in the management of urothelial carcinoma of the bladder and the upper urinary tract. Templates of lymph node dissection for upper tract urothelial carcinoma according to tumor location. Role of lymphadenectomy in the management of urothelial carcinoma of the bladder and the upper urinary tract. Adapted from Kondo T, Tanabe K. International Journal of Urology. Volume 19, Issue 8, pages 710–721, 19 APR 2012 DOI: 10.1111/j.1442-2042.2012.03009.x http://onlinelibrary.wiley.com/doi/10.1111/j.1442-2042.2012.03009.x/full#f2

Tumor Grade

Tumor grade represents another well-established predictor of cancer-related outcomes in patients with UTUC because it is strongly related to the single cell behavior and tumor stage (Fig. 4.7). Both the 1973 and the 2004 World Health Organization (WHO) classifications are predictive of outcomes [48, 49]. Tumor grade should always be taken into account in the preoperative and postoperative counseling of these patients. Specifically in the preoperative setting, tumor grade can help guide decision regarding RNU versus endoscopic management.

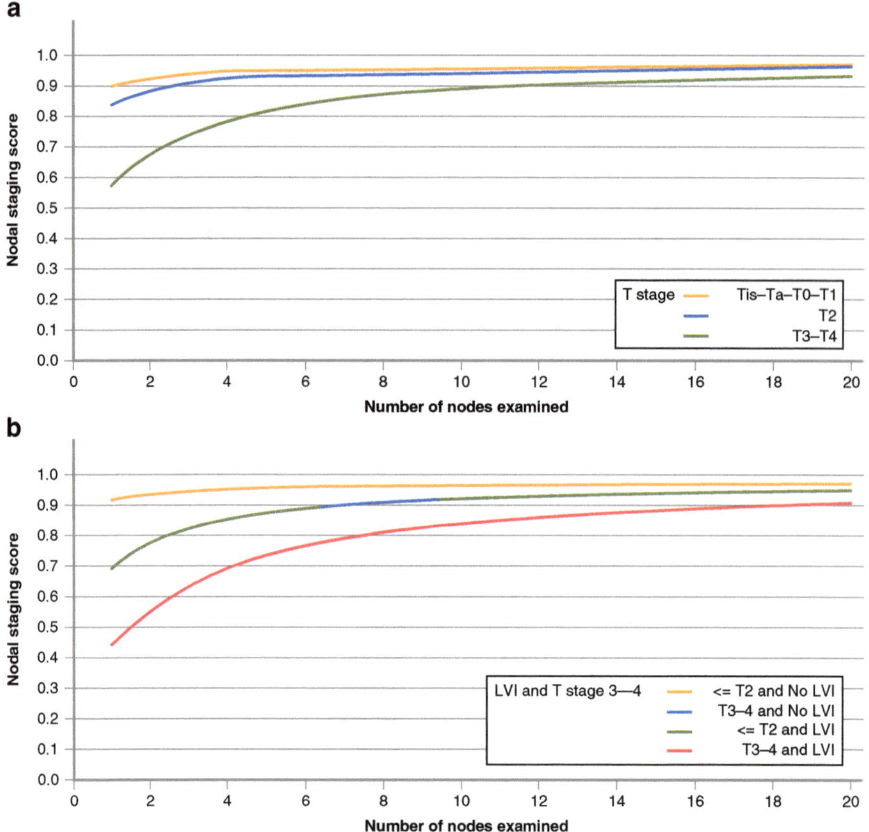

Fig. 4.5 Pathological nodal staging score in 814 patients treated with radical nephroureterectomy for upper tract urothelial carcinoma. Adapted from Evanguelos Xylinas, Michael Rink, Vitaly Margulis, Talia Faison, Evi Comploj, Giacomo Novara, et al. Prediction of true nodal status in patients with pathological lymph node negative upper tract urothelial carcinoma at radical nephroureterectomy. The Journal of Urology Volume 189, Issue 2 2013 468–473. http://dx.doi.org/10.1016/j.juro.2012.09.036

Concomitant Carcinoma In Situ

Concomitant carcinoma in situ (CIS) of the upper urinary tract represents a rare entity that is considered to be associated with DR and CSM in patients with organ-confined disease [50]. Moreover, presence of concomitant CIS is associated with intravesical recurrence after RNU [51, 52]. Therefore, the presence of concomitant CIS should always be evaluated in patients with UTUC, because they may require more aggressive surveillance regimens and strategies utilizing topical therapies.

Table 4.4 Prognostic factors of upper tract urothelial carcinoma related to pathologic features

Characteristics	Comment	References
Pathologic tumor stage	Advanced pT stage is an independent predictor of DR and CSM	[39, 48]
Pathologic Tumor Grade	– Higher tumor grade is an independent predictor of DR and CSM. – Both the 1973 and the 2004 WHO classifications of tumor grade independently predict cancer control outcomes	[48, 49]
Concomitant CIS	Concomitant CIS is associated with advanced tumor stage and grade and is an independent predictor of IVR, DR, and CSM	[50–52]
LVI	Presence of LVI associated with advanced tumor stage/grade, DR, and CSM, specifically in pN0 patients	[4, 54]
Tumor architecture	Sessile tumor associated with DR and CSM	[48, 55, 56]
Tumor necrosis	Controversial impact on oncologic outcomes	[57, 58]
LNI	Presence of LNI associated with DR and CSM	[45, 48, 53]

DR disease recurrence, *CSM* cancer-specific mortality, *CIS* concomitant carcinoma in situ, *IVR* intravesical recurrence, *LNI* lymph node involvement

Lymph Node Invasion

The presence of lymph node invasion (LNI) is considered an important prognostic factor, indicating the metastatic spread of a tumor to its lymph nodes [45, 48]. In patients with LNI, lymph node density (≥30 %) may help risk stratify patients with regard to DR and CSM [53]. Extranodal extension appears to be a powerful predictor of clinical outcomes in patients with LNI [3, 53]. LNI is an important prognostic factor in patients with UTUC. Efforts are still needed to standardize the indications and LND templates.

Lymphovascular Invasion

In retrospective studies, lymphovascular invasion (LVI) is present in approximately 20 % of UTUC and it represents an independent predictor of DR and CSS specifically adding information in patients with lymph node negative UTUC [4, 54]. LVI status should be reported in the pathologic report of all UTUC specimens [4, 54]. Consensus regarding the pathologic definition of LVI needs to be reached.

Tumor Architecture

Several studies have investigated the prognostic impact of tumor architecture (sessile compared with papillary) on the survival of patients with UTUC. Three multi-institutional studies found that a sessile/infiltrative growth pattern was associated with

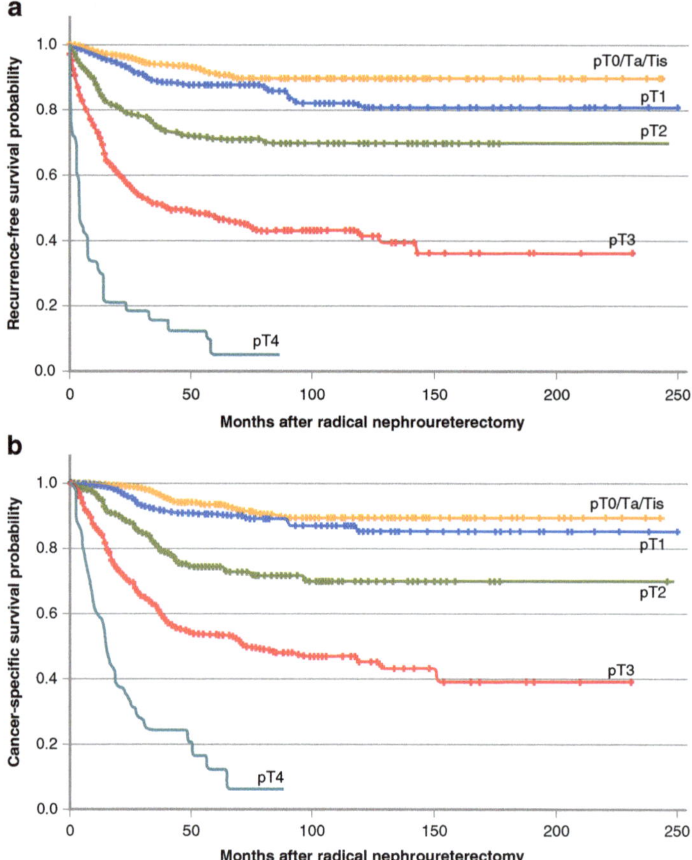

Fig. 4.6 Outcomes of radical nephroureterectomy: A series from the Upper Tract Urothelial Carcinoma Collaboration. Kaplan–Meier plots of progression-free and cancer-specific survival stratified according to tumor stage in 1,363 patients treated with radical nephroureterectomy for upper tract urothelial carcinoma. Outcomes of radical nephroureterectomy: a series from the Upper Tract Urothelial Carcinoma Collaboration. Adapted from Margulis V, Shariat SF, Matin SF, Kamat AM, Zigeuner R, Kikuchi E, et al. Cancer 2009. Volume 115, Issue 6, pages 1224–1233, 20 JAN 2009 DOI: 10.1002/cncr.24135. http://onlinelibrary.wiley.com/doi/10.1002/cncr.24135/full#fig2

features of aggressive disease, DR, and CSM [48, 55, 56]. These findings suggest that tumor architecture should always be mentioned during the endoscopic evaluation of UTUC, as well as in the gross description of the pathological reports.

Tumor Necrosis

Extensive tumor necrosis (defined as >10 % of the tumor area) is an independent predictor of oncologic outcomes in patients after RNU [57]. However, a recent multicenter international study failed to confirm these findings [58]. Thus, the prognostic

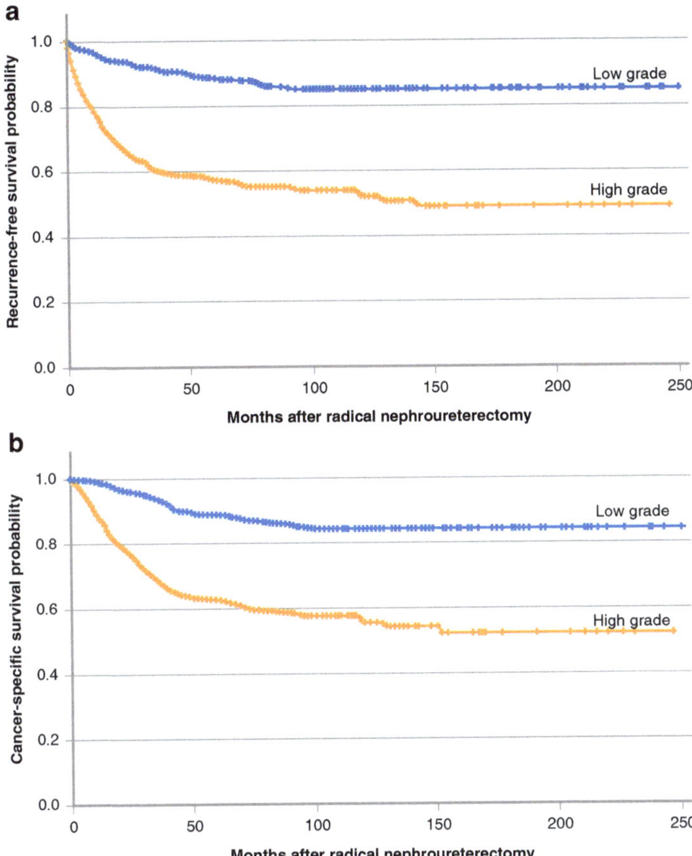

Fig. 4.7 Outcomes of radical nephroureterectomy: A series from the Upper Tract Urothelial Carcinoma Collaboration. Kaplan–Meier plots of progression-free and cancer-specific survival stratified according to tumor grade in 1,363 patients treated with radical nephroureterectomy for upper tract urothelial carcinoma. Outcomes of radical nephroureterectomy: a series from the Upper Tract Urothelial Carcinoma Collaboration. Adapted from Margulis V, Shariat SF, Matin SF, Kamat AM, Zigeuner R, Kikuchi E, et al. Cancer. 20009. Volume 115, Issue 6, pages 1224–1233, 20 JAN 2009 DOI: 10.1002/cncr.24135. http://onlinelibrary.wiley.com/doi/10.1002/cncr.24135/full#fig

role of tumor necrosis in UTUC patients needs further confirmation in larger well-designed multi-institutional studies. Whether it adds to other pathologic features thereby impacting clinical decision-making remains to be proven.

Positive Surgical Margins

The presence of positive surgical margins is reported in ≤8.5 % of RNU cases and strictly depends on the management of the bladder cuff. Presence of positive surgical margins has been associated with higher rates of DR and CSM [59]. One needs, however, to differentiate between ureteral positive margin and soft tissue positive margin. While both negatively impact outcomes of the patient, soft tissue positive margins lead to fast demise of the patient [59].

Histological Variants

In retrospective studies, almost 25 % of patients with UTUC treated with RNU harbor histological variants [60]. Variant histology was associated with features of aggressive disease [60], but not with oncologic outcomes when adjusted for the effects of standard clinicopathological features [60]. Moreover, variant histology does not seem to affect response to adjuvant systemic chemotherapy in patients treated with RNU [61]. Future studies may allow to differentiate between the different types of variant histology.

Molecular Markers (Table 4.5)

Tissue-Based Markers

Several research groups are working on UTUC oncogenesis and progression pathways. Tissue-based markers, such as cell cycle regulators (p53) [62], cell proliferation (Ki67) [63], angiogenesis (EGFR and HIF1a) [64, 65], cell adhesion (E-cadherin) [66, 67], and apoptosis (Bcl-2 and survivin) [68, 69] have been tested with promising prognostic value. The main limitations shared by these studies are their retrospective nature and their small sample size, thus requiring further validation before inclusion in clinical decision-making for the management of UTUC. More than bladder UC, we need biomarkers to improve clinical staging of UTUC.

Blood-Based Markers

Only a few blood-based markers have been investigated in UTUC patients. Increased levels of C-reactive protein and leukocytes have been associated with DR and CSM [70–73]. However, to date, the evidence is thin in order to support the role of blood-based markers as predictors of outcomes in UTUC patients.

Genetic Markers

Microsatellite instability (MSI) is defined as the presence of ubiquitous mutations in microsatellite DNA sequences and has been found to be associated with hereditary non-polyposis colorectal cancer, as well as with many sporadic human cancers.

Table 4.5 Summary of the molecular markers in the upper tract urothelial carcinoma patients

Markers	Function	Method	Comment	References
Tissue-based				
P53	Cell cycle regulation	Immunohistochemistry	Overexpression is associated with advanced T stage and higher tumor grade	[62]
Ki-67	Cell proliferation	Immunohistochemistry	Overexpression is associated with advanced T stage and higher tumor grade. It is an independent predictor of synchronous/metachronous bladder cancer	[63]
EGFR	Cell proliferation and differentiation	Immunohistochemistry	Overexpression is associated with advanced disease and metaplastic differentiation	[64]
HIF-1α	Angiogenesis	Immunohistochemistry	Overexpression is an independent marker of DR and OM.	[65]
E-cadherin	Cell adhesion	Immunohistochemistry	Lower levels are associated with advanced disease and are an independent predictor of DR and CSM	[66, 67]
Bcl-2	Apoptosis	Immunohistochemistry	Overexpression is associated with advanced T stage and higher tumor grade	[68]
Survivin	Apoptosis	Immunohistochemistry	Overexpression is associated with advanced T stage and higher tumor grade. It is an independent predictor of CSM	[69]
Blood-based				
C-reactive protein	Inflammatory response	ELISA	Elevated levels are independently associated with DR and CSM	[70–73]
Leukocytes	Inflammatory response	Cytometry	Elevated levels are independently associated with DR and CSM	[71]
Genetic				
Microsatellite instability	Defect in DNA repair process	PCR	Microsatellite instability is an independent marker of CSM	[74, 75]

DR disease recurrence, *CSM* cancer-specific mortality, *OM* overall mortality

The presence of MSI has also been demonstrated in UTUC patients [74]. Moreover, microsatellite instability (MSI) is associated with prognosis [75].

To date, no marker has fulfilled the clinical and statistical criteria necessary to support their introduction in daily clinical decision-making [76].

Prediction Tools (Table 4.6)

Nomograms have been proposed in the pre- and postoperative setting to predict different endpoints in order to improve patient counseling, follow-up scheduling, identification of the best patient for conservative management, lymph node dissection, chemotherapy administration, and risk stratification for inclusion in clinical trials. The variety of the variables incorporated into nomograms has expanded from standard clinical and pathological features to imaging techniques [36].

Preoperative Prediction of Pathologic Features at RNU

With the improvement of endoscopic tools, many UTUC patients can today be managed conservatively. Tumor staging is notoriously difficult in the preoperative setting if not impossible in many cases. Prediction tools can help identify which patients have T2 and higher stage UTUC and therefore benefit from RNU. Improved understanding of the extent of LND and thoughtful integration of systemic therapy with surgical resection may further help improve treatment outcomes of patients with advanced UTUC [45]. Neoadjuvant chemotherapy may be particularly beneficial in UTUC [77] because the loss of renal function after RNU [78] may render a patient ineligible for treatment with cisplatin-based combination chemotherapy. Unfortunately, chemotherapy and more aggressive surgery may expose patients to increased morbidity with possible overtreatment. Several studies have shown that patients with muscle-invasive UTUC benefit from LND and neoadjuvant chemotherapy, especially those with non-organ-confined (NOC) UTUC [7, 45, 77]. Thus, the accurate prediction of muscle-invasive and/or NOC UTUC can guide appropriate patient selection for these treatments as well as for inclusion in relevant clinical trials. To date, only three models have been described in the preoperative setting [36, 79, 80].

Margulis et al. developed a multivariable model for the prediction of NOC-UTUC based on easily available preoperative clinical and pathologic features ($n = 659$) [80]. Their prediction tool based on tumor location, architecture, and grade enabled the prediction of NOC disease at RNU with an accuracy of 76.6 %.

A multi-institutional study focused on the ability of hydronephrosis to predict advanced disease. Brien et al. relied on data from 172 patients who underwent RNU for UTUC at five referral centers [24]. They found that the presence of preoperative hydronephrosis was associated with advanced stage UTUC and concluded that a readily available imaging modality may improve preoperative risk stratification for

Table 4.6 Available predictive models in upper tract urothelial carcinoma

Reference	Prediction form	Setting	Endpoint	Number of patients	Variables	Accuracy	Validation
Margulis et al. (2010) [80]	Probability nomogram	Preoperative	Prediction of non-organ-confined disease after RNU	659	Tumor location, grade, and architecture	76.6 %	Internal
Favaretto et al. (2012) [36]	Risk grouping	Preoperative	Predictors of pathological stage at the time of RNU	274	High grade on ureteroscopy biopsies, tumor location, local invasion, and hydronephrosis on imaging	71 % for muscle-invasive UTUC and 70 % for non organ-confined	Not performed
Jeldres et al. (2010) [83]	Probability nomogram	Postoperative	5-year CSS	5,918	Age, T stage, LN status, grade	75.4 %	Internal
Yates et al. (2012) [84]	Probability nomogram	Postoperative	3-, 5-year CSS	667	Age, T stage, LN status, grade, tumor location	78 %	Internal
Cha et al. (2012) [85]	Probability nomogram	Postoperative	2-, 5-year RFS and CSS	2,244	Age, T stage, LN status, grade, LVI, architecture, and concomitant CIS	80.7 % for RFS and 82 % for CSS	Internal
Roupret et al. 2013 [86]	Probability nomogram	Postoperative	5-year CSS	3,387	Age, T stage, LN stage, architecture, and LVI	79 %	Internal

RNU radical nephroureterectomy, *RFS* recurrence-free survival, *CSS* cancer-specific survival, *LN* lymph node, *LVI* lymphovascular invasion, *Cis* carcinoma in situ

UTUC patients, thereby guiding use of conservative management versus extirpative surgery as well as the need for neoadjuvant chemotherapy regimens. Messer et al. confirmed these findings in a larger series of 408 patients [79].

Favaretto et al. also combined results from imaging and ureteroscopy [36] and confirmed that invasion and hydronephrosis on preoperative imaging and high-grade tumor at ureteroscopy or cytology were significantly associated with muscle-invasive UTUC on RNU specimen. The combination of these three reached an accuracy of 71 % for predicting NOC UTUC.

Further research is needed to determine whether use of these prediction models could help in patient's counseling and decision-making regarding conservative management versus RNU, administration of neoadjuvant chemotherapy, and/or performance of extended LND. The incorporation of novel biomarkers or modern imaging modalities could probably increase the accuracy of these models [81]. There is no doubt that the preoperative prediction is crucial to the appropriate management of UTUC.

Prediction of Oncological Outcomes after RNU

The rationale for postoperative assessment relies on the ability to propose adjuvant systemic therapy to patients at the highest risk experiencing DR and ultimately death from UTUC. Moreover, it allows evidence-based follow-up scheduling. Several post-operative prognostic risk factors have been identified to help in this clinical decision-making process. Currently, decisions are made based on individual attribution of risk to pathological stage [48], tumor grade [48], lymphovascular invasion [4], LNI [45, 48, 82], and extent of lymphadenectomy [82]. Several nomograms have integrated most of these features to predict DR and CSM after RNU for UTUC [83–85].

Jeldres et al. proposed the first nomogram for UTUC in the postoperative setting [83]. Within the Surveillance, Epidemiology, and End Results database, the authors identified 5,918 patients who had been treated with RNU for UTUC and randomly split them into a development (n=2,959) and external validation cohort (n=2,959). Their model based on age, tumor stage, tumor grade, and lymph node status predicted 5-year cancer-specific survival with an accuracy of 75.4 %. It was significantly more accurate ($p<0.01$) than the 2002 American Joint Committee on Cancer–International Union Against Cancer (AJCC/UICC) TNM classification (64.8 %). However, the tumor grading system they used was a historical classification [1].

Recently, three new nomograms were proposed, one from the French collaborative group [84], one from the international UTUC collaboration [85], and one combining the two datasets of patients [86]. Yates et al. combined clinical and pathological variables to give accurate predictions regarding 5-year cancer-specific survival [84]. Their cohort included 667 patients from 21 French institutions who underwent RNU for UTUC. Using five variables (age, tumor location, tumor grade, T stage, and LN status), their nomogram had a predictive accuracy of 78 %.

The international UTUC collaboration nomogram study [85] combined several more novel prognostic factors than the previous nomograms: age, T stage, tumor grade,

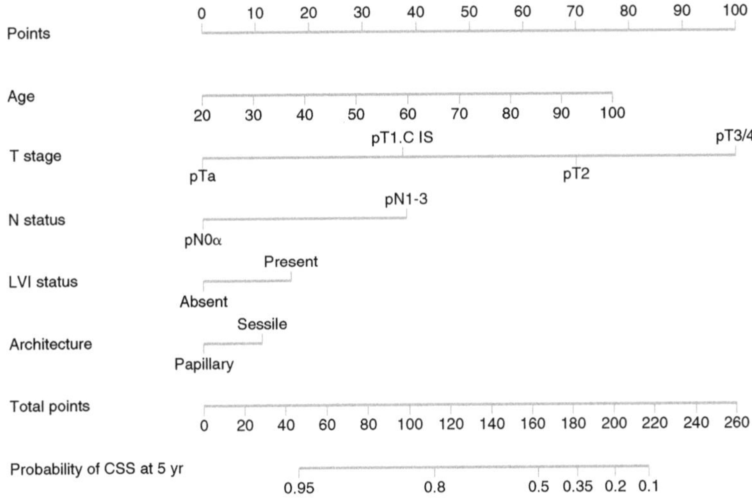

Fig. 4.8 Nomogram predicting 5-year cancer-specific survival after radical nephroureterectomy for upper tract urothelial carcinoma. Adapted from Morgan Roupret, Vincent Hupertan, Thomas Seisen, Pierre Colin, Evanguelos Xylinas, David R. Yates, et al. Prediction of cancer specific survival after radical nephroureterectomy for upper tract urothelial carcinoma: development of an optimized postoperative nomogram using decision curve analysis. The Journal of Urology Volume 189, Issue 5 2013 1662–1669. http://dx.doi.org/10.1016/j.juro.2012.10.057

LN status, lymphovascular invasion, architecture of the tumor, and concomitant Cis. Cha et al. [85] included 2,244 patients treated with RNU without neoadjuvant or adjuvant therapy at 23 international institutions. Their nomograms predicted DR and CSM with 76.8 % and 81.5 % accuracy, respectively. These models offer improvements in calibration over AJCC stage grouping.

Finally the combined nomogram study included 3,387 patients treated with RNU (Fig. 4.8) [86]. The merged study population was randomly split into development ($n = 2{,}371$) and validation ($n = 1{,}016$) cohorts. Decision curve analyses were used in order to select the most performant model, which included age, T stage, LN status, tumor architecture, and lymphovascular invasion. The discrimination of the nomogram was 79 % and it was well calibrated. While these prediction tools offer an approach towards evidence-based integration of complex data, their clinical utility remains to be proven.

Limitations

Study Design

The major limitations of all the data discussed above are the retrospective and multicenter design of the studies [1, 36, 79, 80, 83–85]. The low incidence of UTUC does only allow such an approach in the first phase. To be able to create a large cohort, national or international studies are needed with multiple institutions and surgeons. Moreover, specific model criteria, such as inclusion and exclusion criteria, do not allow the use of models for patients with different characteristics or who have been exposed to different treatment modalities.

Suboptimal Predictive Accuracy

No prediction model developed to date is perfect. This might be due to the lack of consideration of all potential risk factors and from the inability to assemble all known prognostic factors optimally. Urothelial carcinomas have a heterogeneous biologic behavior. Therefore, there is a need for novel biomarkers and imaging tools to capture the complex biological potential of UTUC and thereby enhance the predictive accuracy of current tools.

Validation

These nomograms were satisfactorily accurate (discrimination between patients with or without the outcome of interest) and well calibrated (accuracy of a prediction for an individual patient). However, before these prediction tools are put into widespread use, they need to be externally validated in populations other than the population used for their development [87]. Indeed, differences in disease and population characteristics as well as in treatment protocols and expertise may undermine the accuracy and calibration of predictive tools when they are applied to a different population. For example, prediction tools that were developed using high-volume-center databases may not be applicable to community practice. It is therefore necessary to externally validate these predictive tools.

Conclusions

Five years ago, there were no predictive tools to guide us in the management of the rare disease that is UTUC. Clinicians were basing their recommendations and decisions on their previous experience and limited literature, comprising small cohorts. The drastic increase in the quality and the quantity of UTUC research based on the power of international collaborative networks (i.e., UTUC collaboration, French database) has allowed the development of sophisticated mathematical modeling to accurately predict outcomes of each individual patient. Despite the significant added understanding and value of these information for our patients with UTUC, some limitations persist as discussed above. In the future, prospective registry studies and clinical trials are necessary to advance our understanding and improve the care delivered to UTUC patients. With the arrival of comparative effectiveness research combined with the power of personalized medicine tools such as tumor sequencing, a new era has risen, flattening the hurdles in the management of UTUC patients. More than ever before, multiple specialties need to come together to improve care for UTUC patients through comprehensive collaborative research and tumor boards [88].

References

1. Roupret M, Zigeuner R, Palou J, et al. European guidelines for the diagnosis and management of upper urinary tract urothelial cell carcinomas: 2011 update. Eur Urol. 2011;59:584–94.
2. Ehdaie B, Chromecki TF, Lee RK, et al. Obesity adversely impacts disease specific outcomes in patients with upper tract urothelial carcinoma. J Urol. 2011;186:66–72.
3. Fajkovic H, Cha EK, Jeldres C, et al. Prognostic value of extranodal extension and other lymph node parameters in patients with upper tract urothelial carcinoma. J Urol. 2012;187:845–51.
4. Kikuchi E, Margulis V, Karakiewicz PI, et al. Lymphovascular invasion predicts clinical outcomes in patients with node-negative upper tract urothelial carcinoma. J Clin Oncol. 2009;27:612–8.
5. Raman JD, Ng CK, Scherr DS, et al. Impact of tumor location on prognosis for patients with upper tract urothelial carcinoma managed by radical nephroureterectomy. Eur Urol. 2010;57:1072–9.
6. Shariat SF, Favaretto RL, Gupta A, et al. Gender differences in radical nephroureterectomy for upper tract urothelial carcinoma. World J Urol. 2011;29:481–6.
7. Lughezzani G, Burger M, Margulis V, et al. Prognostic factors in upper urinary tract urothelial carcinomas: a comprehensive review of the current literature. Eur Urol. 2012;62:100–14.
8. Ouzzane A, Colin P, Xylinas E, et al. Ureteral and multifocal tumours have worse prognosis than renal pelvic tumours in urothelial carcinoma of the upper urinary tract treated by nephroureterectomy. Eur Urol. 2011;60:1258–65.
9. Xylinas E, Rink M, Cha EK, et al. Impact of distal ureter management on oncologic outcomes following radical nephroureterectomy for upper tract urothelial carcinoma. Eur Urol. 2014;65:210–7.
10. Shariat SF, Kattan MW, Vickers AJ, et al. Critical review of prostate cancer predictive tools. Future Oncol. 2009;5:1555–84.
11. Xylinas E, Kluth L, Mangal S, et al. Predictive tools for clinical decision-making and counseling of patients with upper tract urothelial carcinoma. World J Urol. 2013;31:31–6.
12. Lughezzani G, Jeldres C, Isbarn H, et al. Nephroureterectomy and segmental ureterectomy in the treatment of invasive upper tract urothelial carcinoma: a population-based study of 2299 patients. Eur J Cancer. 2009;45:3291–7.
13. Shariat SF, Godoy G, Lotan Y, et al. Advanced patient age is associated with inferior cancer-specific survival after radical nephroureterectomy. BJU Int. 2010;105:1672–7.
14. Chromecki TF, Ehdaie B, Novara G, et al. Chronological age is not an independent predictor of clinical outcomes after radical nephroureterectomy. World J Urol. 2011;29:473–80.
15. Lughezzani G, Sun M, Perrotte P, et al. Gender-related differences in patients with stage I to III upper tract urothelial carcinoma: results from the surveillance, epidemiology, and end results database. Urology. 2010;75:321–7.
16. Matsumoto K, Novara G, Gupta A, et al. Racial differences in the outcome of patients with urothelial carcinoma of the upper urinary tract: an international study. BJU Int. 2011;108:E304–9.
17. Raman JD, Messer J, Sielatycki JA, et al. Incidence and survival of patients with carcinoma of the ureter and renal pelvis in the USA, 1973–2005. BJU Int. 2011;107:1059–64.
18. Martinez-Salamanca JI, Shariat SF, Rodriguez JC, et al. Prognostic role of ECOG performance status in patients with urothelial carcinoma of the upper urinary tract: an international study. BJU Int. 2012;109:1155–61.

19. Berod AA, Colin P, Yates DR, et al. The role of American Society of Anesthesiologists scores in predicting urothelial carcinoma of the upper urinary tract outcome after radical nephroureterectomy: results from a national multi-institutional collaborative study. BJU Int. 2012; 110:E1035–40.
20. McLaughlin JK, Silverman DT, Hsing AW, et al. Cigarette smoking and cancers of the renal pelvis and ureter. Cancer Res. 1992;52:254–7.
21. Rink M, Xylinas E, Margulis V, et al. Impact of smoking on oncologic outcomes of upper tract urothelial carcinoma after radical nephroureterectomy. Eur Urol. 2013;63:1082–90.
22. Cho KS, Hong SJ, Cho NH, et al. Grade of hydronephrosis and tumor diameter as preoperative prognostic factors in ureteral transitional cell carcinoma. Urology. 2007;70:662–6.
23. Ito Y, Kikuchi E, Tanaka N, et al. Preoperative hydronephrosis grade independently predicts worse pathological outcomes in patients undergoing nephroureterectomy for upper tract urothelial carcinoma. J Urol. 2011;185:1621–6.
24. Brien JC, Shariat SF, Herman MP, et al. Preoperative hydronephrosis, ureteroscopic biopsy grade and urinary cytology can improve prediction of advanced upper tract urothelial carcinoma. J Urol. 2010;184:69–73.
25. Ng CK, Shariat SF, Lucas SM, et al. Does the presence of hydronephrosis on preoperative axial CT imaging predict worse outcomes for patients undergoing nephroureterectomy for upper-tract urothelial carcinoma? Urol Oncol. 2011;29:27–32.
26. Raman JD, Shariat SF, Karakiewicz PI, et al. Does preoperative symptom classification impact prognosis in patients with clinically localized upper-tract urothelial carcinoma managed by radical nephroureterectomy? Urol Oncol. 2011;29:716–23.
27. Inman BA, Tran VT, Fradet Y, et al. Carcinoma of the upper urinary tract: predictors of survival and competing causes of mortality. Cancer. 2009;115:2853–62.
28. Park J, Ha SH, Min GE, et al. The protective role of renal parenchyma as a barrier to local tumor spread of upper tract transitional cell carcinoma and its impact on patient survival. J Urol. 2009;182:894–9.
29. Zigeuner RE, Hutterer G, Chromecki T, et al. Bladder tumour development after urothelial carcinoma of the upper urinary tract is related to primary tumour location. BJU Int. 2006;98:1181–6.
30. Favaretto RL, Shariat SF, Chade DC, et al. The effect of tumor location on prognosis in patients treated with radical nephroureterectomy at Memorial Sloan-Kettering Cancer Center. Eur Urol. 2010;58:574–80.
31. Chromecki TF, Cha EK, Fajkovic H, et al. The impact of tumor multifocality on outcomes in patients treated with radical nephroureterectomy. Eur Urol. 2012;61:245–53.
32. Yafi FA, Novara G, Shariat SF, et al. Impact of tumour location versus multifocality in patients with upper tract urothelial carcinoma treated with nephroureterectomy and bladder cuff excision: a homogeneous series without perioperative chemotherapy. BJU Int. 2012;110:E7–13.
33. Simone G, Papalia R, Loreto A, et al. Independent prognostic value of tumour diameter and tumour necrosis in upper urinary tract urothelial carcinoma. BJU Int. 2009;103:1052–7.
34. Pieras E, Frontera G, Ruiz X, et al. Concomitant carcinoma in situ and tumour size are prognostic factors for bladder recurrence after nephroureterectomy for upper tract transitional cell carcinoma. BJU Int. 2010;106:1319–23.
35. Guarnizo E, Pavlovich CP, Seiba M, et al. Ureteroscopic biopsy of upper tract urothelial carcinoma: improved diagnostic accuracy and histopathological considerations using a multi-biopsy approach. J Urol. 2000;163:52–5.
36. Favaretto RL, Shariat SF, Savage C, et al. Combining imaging and ureteroscopy variables in a preoperative multivariable model for prediction of muscle-invasive and non-organ confined disease in patients with upper tract urothelial carcinoma. BJU Int. 2012;109:77–82.
37. Mullerad M, Russo P, Golijanin D, et al. Bladder cancer as a prognostic factor for upper tract transitional cell carcinoma. J Urol. 2004;172:2177–81.
38. Xylinas E, Colin P, Audenet F, et al. Intravesical recurrence after radical nephroureterectomy for upper tract urothelial carcinomas: predictors and impact on subsequent oncological outcomes from a national multicenter study. World J Urol. 2013;31:61–8.

39. Novara G, De Marco V, Dalpiaz O, et al. Independent predictors of contralateral metachronous upper urinary tract transitional cell carcinoma after nephroureterectomy: multi-institutional dataset from three European centers. Int J Urol. 2009;16:187–91.
40. Waldert M, Karakiewicz PI, Raman JD, et al. A delay in radical nephroureterectomy can lead to upstaging. BJU Int. 2010;105:812–7.
41. Ni S, Tao W, Chen Q, et al. Laparoscopic versus open nephroureterectomy for the treatment of upper urinary tract urothelial carcinoma: a systematic review and cumulative analysis of comparative studies. Eur Urol. 2012;61:1142–53.
42. Hanna N, Sun M, Trinh QD, et al. Propensity-score-matched comparison of perioperative outcomes between open and laparoscopic nephroureterectomy: a national series. Eur Urol. 2012;61:715–21.
43. Simone G, Papalia R, Guaglianone S, et al. Laparoscopic versus open nephroureterectomy: perioperative and oncologic outcomes from a randomised prospective study. Eur Urol. 2009;56:520–6.
44. Lughezzani G, Sun M, Perrotte P, et al. Should bladder cuff excision remain the standard of care at nephroureterectomy in patients with urothelial carcinoma of the renal pelvis? A population-based study. Eur Urol. 2010;57:956–62.
45. Roscigno M, Brausi M, Heidenreich A, et al. Lymphadenectomy at the time of nephroureterectomy for upper tract urothelial cancer. Eur Urol. 2011;60:776–83.
46. Kondo T, Tanabe K. Role of lymphadenectomy in the management of urothelial carcinoma of the bladder and the upper urinary tract. Int J Urol. 2012;19:710–21.
47. Xylinas E, Rink M, Margulis V, et al. Prediction of true nodal status in patients with pathological lymph node negative upper tract urothelial carcinoma at radical nephroureterectomy. J Urol. 2013;189:468–73.
48. Margulis V, Shariat SF, Matin SF, et al. Outcomes of radical nephroureterectomy: a series from the Upper Tract Urothelial Carcinoma Collaboration. Cancer. 2009;115:1224–33.
49. Lopez-Beltran A, Bassi P, Pavone-Macaluso M, et al. Handling and pathology reporting of specimens with carcinoma of the urinary bladder, ureter, and renal pelvis. Eur Urol. 2004;45:257–66.
50. Wheat JC, Weizer AZ, Wolf Jr JS, et al. Concomitant carcinoma in situ is a feature of aggressive disease in patients with organ confined urothelial carcinoma following radical nephroureterectomy. Urol Oncol. 2012;30:252–8.
51. Otto W, Shariat SF, Fritsche HM, et al. Concomitant carcinoma in situ as an independent prognostic parameter for recurrence and survival in upper tract urothelial carcinoma: a multicenter analysis of 772 patients. World J Urol. 2011;29:487–94.
52. Xylinas E, Rink M, Margulis V, et al. Multifocal carcinoma in situ of the upper tract is associated with high risk of bladder cancer recurrence. Eur Urol. 2012;61:1069–70.
53. Bolenz C, Shariat SF, Fernandez MI, et al. Risk stratification of patients with nodal involvement in upper tract urothelial carcinoma: value of lymph-node density. BJU Int. 2009;103:302–6.
54. Novara G, Matsumoto K, Kassouf W, et al. Prognostic role of lymphovascular invasion in patients with urothelial carcinoma of the upper urinary tract: an international validation study. Eur Urol. 2010;57:1064–71.
55. Remzi M, Haitel A, Margulis V, et al. Tumour architecture is an independent predictor of outcomes after nephroureterectomy: a multi-institutional analysis of 1363 patients. BJU Int. 2009;103:307–11.
56. Fritsche HM, Novara G, Burger M, et al. Macroscopic sessile tumor architecture is a pathologic feature of biologically aggressive upper tract urothelial carcinoma. Urol Oncol. 2012;30:666–72.
57. Zigeuner R, Shariat SF, Margulis V, et al. Tumour necrosis is an indicator of aggressive biology in patients with urothelial carcinoma of the upper urinary tract. Eur Urol. 2010;57:575–81.
58. Seitz C, Gupta A, Shariat SF, et al. Association of tumor necrosis with pathological features and clinical outcome in 754 patients undergoing radical nephroureterectomy for upper tract urothelial carcinoma: an international validation study. J Urol. 2010;184:1895–900.

59. Colin P, Ouzzane A, Yates DR, et al. Influence of positive surgical margin status after radical nephroureterectomy on upper urinary tract urothelial carcinoma survival. Ann Surg Oncol. 2012;19:3613–20.
60. Rink M, Robinson BD, Green DA, et al. Impact of histological variants on clinical outcomes of patients with upper urinary tract urothelial carcinoma. J Urol. 2012;188:398–404.
61. Xylinas E, Rink M, Margulis V, et al. Histologic variants of upper tract urothelial carcinoma do not affect response to adjuvant chemotherapy after radical nephroureterectomy. Eur Urol. 2012;62:e25–6.
62. Ku JH, Byun SS, Jeong H, et al. The role of p53 on survival of upper urinary tract urothelial carcinoma: a Systematic review and meta-analysis. Clin Genitourin Cancer. 2013;11:221–8.
63. Jeon HG, Jeong IG, Bae J, et al. Expression of Ki-67 and COX-2 in patients with upper urinary tract urothelial carcinoma. Urology. 2010;76:513. e7–12.
64. Leibl S, Zigeuner R, Hutterer G, et al. EGFR expression in urothelial carcinoma of the upper urinary tract is associated with disease progression and metaplastic morphology. APMIS. 2008;116:27–32.
65. Nakanishi K, Hiroi S, Tominaga S, et al. Expression of hypoxia-inducible factor-1alpha protein predicts survival in patients with transitional cell carcinoma of the upper urinary tract. Clin Cancer Res. 2005;11:2583–90.
66. Inoue K, Slaton JW, Karashima T, et al. The prognostic value of angiogenesis factor expression for predicting recurrence and metastasis of bladder cancer after neoadjuvant chemotherapy and radical cystectomy. Clin Cancer Res. 2000;6:4866–73.
67. Fromont G, Roupret M, Amira N, et al. Tissue microarray analysis of the prognostic value of E-cadherin, Ki67, p53, p27, survivin and MSH2 expression in upper urinary tract transitional cell carcinoma. Eur Urol. 2005;48:764–70.
68. Nakanishi K, Tominaga S, Hiroi S, et al. Expression of survivin does not predict survival in patients with transitional cell carcinoma of the upper urinary tract. Virchows Arch. 2002; 441:559–63.
69. Jeong IG, Kim SH, Jeon HG, et al. Prognostic value of apoptosis-related markers in urothelial cancer of the upper urinary tract. Hum Pathol. 2009;40:668–77.
70. Saito K, Kawakami S, Ohtsuka Y, et al. The impact of preoperative serum C-reactive protein on the prognosis of patients with upper urinary tract urothelial carcinoma treated surgically. BJU Int. 2007;100:269–73.
71. Lehmann J, Suttmann H, Kovac I, et al. Transitional cell carcinoma of the ureter: prognostic factors influencing progression and survival. Eur Urol. 2007;51:1281–8.
72. Tanaka N, Kikuchi E, Shirotake S, et al. The predictive value of c-reactive protein for prognosis in patients with upper tract urothelial carcinoma treated with radical nephroureterectomy: a multi-institutional study. Eur Urol. 2014;65:227–34.
73. Stein B, Schrader AJ, Wegener G, et al. Preoperative serum C- reactive protein: a prognostic marker in patients with upper urinary tract urothelial carcinoma. BMC Cancer. 2013;13:101.
74. Roupret M, Catto J, Coulet F, et al. Microsatellite instability as indicator of MSH2 gene mutation in patients with upper urinary tract transitional cell carcinoma. J Med Genet. 2004;41:e91.
75. Roupret M, Fromont G, Azzouzi AR, et al. Microsatellite instability as predictor of survival in patients with invasive upper urinary tract transitional cell carcinoma. Urology. 2005;65:1233–7.
76. Bensalah K, Montorsi F, Shariat SF. Challenges of cancer biomarker profiling. Eur Urol. 2007;52:1601–9.
77. Matin SF, Margulis V, Kamat A, et al. Incidence of downstaging and complete remission after neoadjuvant chemotherapy for high-risk upper tract transitional cell carcinoma. Cancer. 2010;116:3127–34.
78. Lane BR, Smith AK, Larson BT, et al. Chronic kidney disease after nephroureterectomy for upper tract urothelial carcinoma and implications for the administration of perioperative chemotherapy. Cancer. 2010;116:2967–73.
79. Messer JC, Terrell JD, Herman MP, et al. Multi-institutional validation of the ability of preoperative hydronephrosis to predict advanced pathologic tumor stage in upper-tract urothelial carcinoma. Urol Oncol. 2013;31:904–8.

80. Margulis V, Youssef RF, Karakiewicz PI, et al. Preoperative multivariable prognostic model for prediction of nonorgan confined urothelial carcinoma of the upper urinary tract. J Urol. 2010;184:453–8.
81. Shariat SF, Chade DC, Karakiewicz PI, et al. Combination of multiple molecular markers can improve prognostication in patients with locally advanced and lymph node positive bladder cancer. J Urol. 2010;183:68–75.
82. Roscigno M, Shariat SF, Margulis V, et al. The extent of lymphadenectomy seems to be associated with better survival in patients with nonmetastatic upper-tract urothelial carcinoma: how many lymph nodes should be removed? Eur Urol. 2009;56:512–8.
83. Jeldres C, Sun M, Lughezzani G, et al. Highly predictive survival nomogram after upper urinary tract urothelial carcinoma. Cancer. 2010;116:3774–84.
84. Yates DR, Hupertan V, Colin P, et al. Cancer-specific survival after radical nephroureterectomy for upper urinary tract urothelial carcinoma: proposal and multi-institutional validation of a post-operative nomogram. Br J Cancer. 2012;106:1083–8.
85. Cha EK, Shariat SF, Kormaksson M, et al. Predicting clinical outcomes after radical nephroureterectomy for upper tract urothelial carcinoma. Eur Urol. 2012;61:818–25.
86. Roupret M, Hupertan V, Seisen T, et al. Prediction of cancer-specific survival after radical nephroureterectomy for upper tract urothelial carcinoma: development of an optimized post-operative nomogram using decision curve analysis. J Urol. 2013;189:1662–9.
87. Nuhn P, May M, Fritsche HM, et al. External validation of disease-free survival at 2 or 3 years as a surrogate and new primary endpoint for patients undergoing radical cystectomy for urothelial carcinoma of the bladder. Eur J Surg Oncol. 2012;38:637–42.
88. Xylinas E, Roupret M, Kluth L, et al. Collaborative research networks as a platform for virtual multidisciplinary, international approach to managing difficult clinical cases: an example from the Upper Tract Urothelial Carcinoma Collaboration. Eur Urol. 2012;62:943–5.

Chapter 5
Conservative Management of Low-Risk UTUC

Fatima Z. Husain, Mesut Remzi, Vitaly Margulis, Sima P. Porten, and Surena F. Matin

Abstract Conservative management of upper tract urothelial cancer (UTUC) treats tumor, prevents disease progression, lowers potential morbidity, and avoids unnecessary loss of renal function by avoiding nephroureterectomy. Limitations associated with conservative therapies include the potential for undetected disease progression. Patients with UTUC are more difficult to stage clinically than in bladder cancer. Endoscopic management can be performed ureteroscopically or percutaneously. Ideal indications include a unifocal tumor, small tumor size, and low-grade disease. A positive selective cytology suggests the presence of higher grade disease and potentially more advanced pathological T stage. Endoscopic technique is critical both for accurate diagnostic purposes and for safe performance of the procedure. The results of endoscopic therapy are highly dependent on tumor factors, with low-grade tumors having much better results than high-grade tumors. The use of adjuvant topical therapy after complete endoscopic tumor control remains unclear. The strongest role for topical therapy for UTUC is for CIS, when it is used as primary therapy. The use of segmental or distal ureterectomy and partial nephrectomy for UTUC has narrow indications with the latter needing to be applied extremely selectively. Nephroureterectomy remains the gold standard treatment, but comes at the cost of significant loss of renal function. Single-dose treatment of the bladder after nephroureterectomy is considered a new standard of care, and could be considered an option by extension of this logic, to single-dose treatment after endoscopic therapy of the upper tracts.

F.Z. Husain, MD • S.P. Porten, MD • S.F. Matin, MD (✉)
Department of Urology, UT MD Anderson Cancer Center,
1515 Holcombe Blvd, Unit 1373, Houston, TX 77030, USA
e-mail: fatimazhusain@gmail.com; sporten@mdanderson.org; surmatin@mdanderson.org

M. Remzi, MD
Department of Urology, Ladesklinikum Korneuburg, Korneuburg, Austria
e-mail: mremzi@gmx.at

V. Margulis, MD
Department of Urology, UT Southwestern Medical Center,
5323 Harry Hines Blvd, Dallas, TX 75390, USA
e-mail: Vitally.margulis@utsouthwestern.edu

© Springer Science+Business Media New York 2015
S.F. Shariat, E. Xylinas (eds.), *Upper Tract Urothelial Carcinoma*,
DOI 10.1007/978-1-4939-1501-9_5

Keywords Ureteral cancer • Renal pelvis cancer • Urothelial cancer • Survival • Surgical treatments

Introduction

The goal of conservative management of upper tract urothelial cancer (UTUC) is to treat tumor, prevent disease progression, lower potential morbidity, and avoid unnecessary loss of renal function by avoiding nephroureterectomy. This approach is primarily driven by imperative and elective indications for renal preservation or to decrease morbidity in the patient. But there are limitations associated with conservative therapies, the potential for undetected disease progression in UTUC, and the mounting evidence that many of these cases represent an aggressive phenotype distinct from bladder disease. Patients with UTUC are more difficult to stage clinically than in bladder cancer, as invasion is not easily assessed on biopsy nor easily seen on imaging unless it is in the extreme, such as with parenchymal renal or perinephric fat invasion, or lymphadenopathy, all associated with a grim survival [1, 2]. Patients managed with endoscopic approaches are thus often highly selected, requiring specialized and long-term follow-up care.

Urothelial carcinomas of the upper tract, which includes the renal calyces, pelvis, and ureter, account for only about five percent of all urothelial malignancies, even though the incidence of upper tract disease is increasing [3, 4]. Although renal pelvic tumors account for a majority of upper tract urothelial carcinomas (UTUC), the incidence of ureteral malignancy is increasing. Review of Surveillance, Epidemiology, and End Results (SEER) data from 1973 to 1996 showed an increase in incidence of ureteral tumors from 0.69 to 0.73 per 100,000 person-years, but no significant increase in the incidence of renal pelvis tumors. Additionally, it showed a 5-year disease-specific survival of 75 % for urothelial carcinoma of the upper tract [4].

Urothelial carcinoma of the upper tract is rare, which leaves management and treatment of this diagnosis an evolving topic. While the gold standard of therapy remains radical nephroureterectomy with excision of bladder cuff, the promotion for more conservative, nephron-sparing management options, including endoscopic resection, topical therapy, ureterectomy, and partial nephrectomy, has become more apparent. These methods are especially advantageous in cases of bilateral disease, solitary kidney, and poor renal function overall, and even for individuals who have a normal contralateral kidney with low-grade disease [4, 5]. The key to these alternatives to treatment is the advancement of technology, including imaging and surgical instruments, allowing for better visualization and identification of these areas.

Prior to determining the method of management for UTUC, it is critical to review the prognostic predictors of outcomes. Lughezzani et al. [6] described two categories of clinical prognostic factors, including patient, such as age, race, ECOG performance status (Eastern Cooperative Oncology Group), obesity, and smoking

Table 5.1 Prognostic patient and tumor factors

	Risk	References
Patient factors		
Age*	Increasing age associated with worse disease survival	[7, 8]
Race	Disease-specific annual mortality greater in black than in white individuals	[9]
Gender	Females are more likely to have more advanced pathologic stage and higher tumor grade, but gender is not an independent predictor of outcomes	[10, 11]
Obesity	Body mass index ≥30 is an independent predictor of higher recurrence and worse survival	[6]
ECOG performance status	ECOG-PS ≥1 is an independent predictor of worse overall survival	[6]
Smoking status	Active smokers with higher risk of: (1) bladder recurrence (2) advanced stage disease, disease recurrence, and cancer-specific mortality	[12–14]
Tumor factors		
Biopsy grade*	High grade associated with worse survival and higher recurrence	[15, 16]
Multifocality (number)	Associated with worse survival	[15]
Tumor size*	Tumors >3–4 cm associated with higher stage, reduced survival, and greater bladder recurrence risk	[17–19]
Presence of hydronephrosis*	Independently predicts worse stage and survival	[20–22]
Bladder cancer history	Independently predicts higher recurrence and lower survival	[6]
Tumor architecture*	Sessile architecture associated with more invasive disease	[23]
Symptoms	Systemic symptoms more indicative of advanced disease than local symptoms	[6]

Items identified with asterisks are those shown to have significant independent impact on recurrence and survival

status, and disease characteristics such as tumor location, tumor size, clinical grade, hydronephrosis, symptoms, and previous and/or synchronous bladder cancer. Patient characteristics inconsistent with advanced disease, absent obvious adverse radiologic findings, are age, tumor architecture, cytology, tumor grade on biopsy, and the presence of hydronephrosis. Table 5.1 lists the factors considered with the most relevant, independent prognosticators highlighted. Ultimately, the method of management is based not only on these factors but as well as on surgeon experience and available equipment. Evidence-based treatment and algorithms are difficult for this disease given that most data originate from retrospective single-institution or multi-institutional efforts in very selected patients, and very little to none in prospective fashion.

Endoscopic Management

Ureteroscopy was first introduced in the 1950s, with the first flexible ureteroscopy performed in 1964 by Marshall; however, due to limitations in optics the use of ureteroscopy did not become more popular and common until the 1980s. With advances in technology, including diameter and size of ureteroscopes, flexibility, and other recent refinements including percutaneous access and the introduction of access sheaths allowing multiple biopsies [16]. This approach is now increasingly used to treat many urologic conditions, including UTUC [9]. It was not until 1985 that the first treatment of renal pelvic cancer was performed endoscopically [24]. Ureteroscopy not only can be used to identify the location and extent of tumor, but can also be used as a curative option in select patients, providing the added advantage of a nephron-sparing technique.

Indications

Indications for endoscopic management, as delineated by the European Association of Urology's Guidelines on Upper Tract Carcinomas in 2013 and summarized in Table 5.2, include unifocal tumor, tumor size (less than 1 cm), low-grade tumors, and no evidence of invasive or advanced disease on imaging [25]. Ideally, cytology should also be negative to rule out the possibility of high-grade disease, as this has been associated with a higher chance of lymphovascular invasion and advanced pathological T stage; however the value of cytology in UTUC is not well investigated [26]. Patients selected for this endoscopic intervention thus must be carefully selected, and demonstrate an understanding that compliance to a close follow-up and surveillance protocol will be essential.

Ureteroscopy can be performed through the retrograde or antegrade fashion, depending on ease of access to the tumor location. With retrograde ureteroscopy, ureteral lesions are easily accessed, versus the use of antegrade (percutaneous) ureteropyeloscopy for renal pelvis lesions that are difficult to access from below, and lower pole calyx lesions, which are also difficult to access through a retrograde approach [24, 27].

Percutaneous therapy has been shown to be safe and effective treatment of low-grade small tumors and it usually requires a second look procedure to assess for any residual disease. It is associated with somewhat higher morbidity than a ureteroscopic

Table 5.2 Ideal indications for endoscopic management of UTUC

1.	Unifocal tumor
2.	<1 cm size
3.	Low grade
4.	Negative selective cytology
5.	No evidence of invasion on imaging

approach given its greater invasiveness, and as it is technically more involved, overall this modality is used less frequently than a ureteroscopic approach [25, 28]. However, it has the advantage of being able to debulk larger tumors, as well as easier access to the lower pole collecting system.

Endoscopic Treatment and Limitations

Depending on the size of the tumor, these can be biopsied using biopsy forceps or a stone basket, or may be fulgurated using a laser [29]. Because the ureter and renal pelvis is thin walled, caution must be taken not to resect too deeply, as perforation easily occurs. Lasers can then be used for the purposes of achieving hemostasis, to fulgurate the tumor bed, and as resection devices as well. The tissue penetration of the holmium YAG (Ho:YAG) laser is less than 0.5 mm, which provides a decreased risk of thermal damage, and is better suited to treat more superficial tumors. The neodymium:yttrium-aluminum-garnet (Nd:YAG) laser has deeper penetration (5–10 mm), which is helpful in treating larger lesions, especially in the renal pelvis [29, 30].

Endoscopic technique is critical for staging purposes prior to definitive therapy such as with surgical intervention or multimodality therapy with neoadjuvant chemotherapy. Although there have been advancements in endoscopic instruments, there are prognostic factors that are nearly impossible to assess endoscopically, including primary tumor stage and presence of lymphovascular invasion [3].

Some of the limitations to this technique include ureteral perforation and strictures. Ureteral perforation has been reported in approximately 10 % and is managed by discontinuing the procedure, ureteral stenting, or percutaneous nephrostomy tube drainage. Similarly, ureteral strictures are noted to be the most common complication of endoscopic management, at approximately 14 %, which are managed by balloon dilatation, laser incision, or surgical reconstruction [30]. As well, there have been concerns raised regarding the risk of understaging and undergrading [31]. Up to 45 % of cases have been found to be upstaged at nephroureterectomy, although how patients are selected for surgery and how accurately patients are staged clinically radically alter this expectation [32].

Results of Endoscopic Management

Results of endoscopic management are generally evaluated in the context of not only disease survival and recurrence (which should clarify bladder, local, and distant locations), but as well rates of renal preservation and disease progression. Published results of ureteroscopic management have to be considered carefully given the retrospective nature of reports and the highly selected patients they represent. Nevertheless certain consistent results are seen. Patients undergoing endoscopic management generally have a higher local recurrence rate, varying between 15 and 90 %, with an average in these reports of about 61 %. Local recurrence is highly related to tumor grade, with low-grade tumors recurring 14–52 %, and high-grade tumors 40–76 % of the time [33]. Thus, close invasive surveillance is mandatory, given the high recurrence rate of UTUC. Similar data exist with percutaneous therapy, with low-grade tumors recurring 23–35 %, and high-grade tumors 40–42 % of the time, but in this review even more limited number of patients were considered [33].

Bladder recurrences after endoscopic therapy occur between 15 and 70 % in published studies, and these are likely influenced by prior or concurrent bladder disease. Recent data showing a reduction of bladder recurrences after nephroureterectomy with single-dose instillation of chemotherapy would suggest that instituting this practice immediately after endoscopic management may have the same effect [34].

In regard to renal preservation and progression, patient selection affects the results. Nevertheless renal preservation rates for both ureteroscopic and percutaneous therapy are generally favorable, ranging from 50 to 100 % [35]. It should be noted, however, that this is usually associated with multiple procedures. Progression is strongly dependent on tumor grade, with very few well-sampled low-grade tumors progressing, whereas high-grade tumors have a higher likelihood of progression [17].

There have also been concerns about causing metastatic disease by pyelovenous or pyelolymphatic seeding with instrumentation, but this has not been substantiated by several studies which have investigated this issue [36, 37]. Similarly, concerns exist about seeding a percutaneous tract if treatment is performed through this technique, but this is rarely reported and unlikely with proper patient selection with those with low-grade tumors. There is, however, a substantiated and real risk of bladder recurrence, as noted above and likely influenced by a prior history of bladder cancer [38, 39]. Thus patients require lifelong bladder surveillance.

Topical Therapy

While the role of adjuvant intracavitary (topical) therapy is well established for bladder urothelial carcinoma, its role for UTUC remains unclear, and is hindered not only by the rarity of the disease and absence of any prospective trials, but as well due to the difficulty of access to the renal pelvis and ureter for instillation of treatment and absence of a reservoir in these areas to allow for proper dwell time. Topical therapy would theoretically prevent tumor implantation and reduce recurrence rates. As well, for cases of CIS of the upper tract, it could act as primary therapy. Table 5.3

Table 5.3 Options for topical therapy of UTUC

Choice of agent	Mode of delivery
BCG	Antegrade via nephrostomy tube
Mitomycin-c	Retrograde via ureteral catheter
Reduced dose BCG + Interferon-alpha	
Gemcitabine	

lists the potential choices of agents and modes of delivery. Placement of a stent and relying on reflux is not a reliable method and is not recommended.

The greatest experience with topical therapy is with the use of BCG via nephrostomy tube, with the largest experience from the Swiss group. In their series of 55 patients, the best results were obtained for patients with CIS, who had a 5 % risk of progression, whereas as adjuvant therapy after endoscopic ablation of presumed Ta/T1 papillary tumors, progression occurred in 41 % [40]. In regard to chemotherapy agents, the greatest experience is with mitomycin-c, but given the small number of patients and variable selection criteria, definitive conclusions are difficult to reach, with the exception that it appears to be very well tolerated with minimal toxicity or adverse events [41].

Distal or Segmental Ureterectomy

Distal ureterectomy represents a viable kidney-sparing approach when there are isolated tumors in the lower ureter, and no evidence of multifocality more proximally (which is seen in 20–30 % of cases), particularly when renal preservation is desired. The entire lower ureter and bladder cuff are resected, and reimplementation is performed with the aid of a psoas hitch or Boari flap. It should be noted that the reimplanted ureter is located more anteriorly, and further away from the bladder neck, making future endoscopic surveillance potentially more difficult.

A more rarely indicated procedure is segmental ureterectomy. While popular in the days before advances in endoscopic instrumentation, the ability to manage most low-risk tumors without a surgical incision has rendered the utility of this procedure much less relevant, and particularly in light of the risk of multifocality as well as significant risk of recurrence in the distal ureter. Indications for segmental ureterectomy include isolated small tumors in the proximal or mid-ureter (where sufficient mobilization of the ureter for a tension-free anastomosis may be performed). The two most concerning adverse outcomes of this approach include tumor spillage, positive margins with incomplete tumor resection, inability to perform anastomosis in a tension-free manner, and stricture formation.

Overall, the oncological, retrospectively reported outcomes in selected patients with low-risk disease can be favorable, with recurrence rates similar to radical nephroureterectomy [42–45].

Partial Nephrectomy

The literature is sparse about the application of partial nephrectomy for UTUC. Goel et al. (2006) described the use of partial nephrectomy in 12 patients with a solitary kidney, chronic renal insufficiency, or bilateral synchronous tumors [46]. Endoscopic technique was not used because of tumor size, location, or stage/grade which did not allow for endoscopic management. Recurrence developed in 5

(42 %) of 12 patients and progression occurred in 6 (50 %). The factors affecting recurrence were stage, grade, multifocality, positive surgical margins, and the pathologic tumor stage. High-grade and positive surgical margins were found to be important risk factors. The risk of recurrence or progression was related to the tumor stage and grade [46].

From a technical perspective, partial nephrectomy for UTUC is a challenging endeavor. As opposed to partial nephrectomy for renal cell carcinoma, additional care must be taken in regard to the urothelial margin, which is difficult to determine before or during the actual partial nephrectomy itself, as it may not correspond to any of the surface landmarks. In these rare cases, the authors copiously utilize intraoperative ultrasonography to plan the resection margins. Similar to segmental ureterectomy, the indications for this procedure are extremely narrow and include the presence of a unifocal tumor and a significant desire to preserve renal function. Appropriate patients are those with imperative indications, not amenable to endoscopic approaches, and those with polar tumors, where upper or lower pole calyces are excised en bloc with overlying renal parenchyma.

Nephroureterectomy

Nephroureterectomy with excision of bladder cuff remains the gold standard treatment for UTUC. Adibi et al. recently reviewed the oncological outcomes after radical nephroureterectomy for UTUC in 1,462 patients between 1982 and 2007 [3]. Interestingly, over the decades they noted a progression of technique and management of UTUC. In the 1980s, open surgery was the standard, followed in the 1990s by the increased use of laparoscopic technique. After the first decade of the new century, there is a growing interest in the use of preoperative chemotherapy. Despite this, there were no statistically significant differences in disease-free survival and cancer-specific survival over the three decades [3].

With the advances in technology, now the possibilities of laparoscopic and robotic-assisted laparoscopic approaches exist. These approaches also allow for a lymph node dissection. These minimally invasive techniques provide the benefit of decreased postoperative pain and length of hospitalization. The approach to this procedure depends on preoperative assessment of the patient and surgeon experience and comfort. There are basic oncological principles that apply and which must be adhered to regardless of the approach. These include the inviolable edicts to prevent tumor spillage, prevent positive margins (strongly linked to recurrence as well as survival), and completely resect the distal ureter and bladder cuff.

From a technical perspective radical nephroureterectomy is similar to radical nephrectomy for kidney cancer, which includes early ligation of the renal vessels and mobilization of the kidney outside Gerota's fascia, but also includes early clipping of the ureter to prevent unnecessary tumor spillage into the bladder, and complete resection of the ureter to include a bladder cuff. Important technical nuances unique to this disease are that in cases of ureteral tumors, copious periureteral tissue should be taken to avoid a positive margin, which for tumors in the intramural ureter may include a need to perform a partial cystectomy if there is a question of possible invasion present.

Routine removal of the adrenal gland is unnecessary. The role of lymphadenectomy remains unclear, but given the accumulating evidence for its therapeutic benefit in bladder cancer many experts are reconsidering this application for patients with high-risk UTUC, which is not the focus of this chapter. While retrospective in nature, the current data suggest that those with truly low-risk, noninvasive disease appear to have little to benefit from lymphadenectomy [47].

Take-home Points

1. Clinical risk stratification for UTUC remains poor, but the combination of biopsy grade, tumor architecture, cytology, hydronephrosis, and tumor size can be used to help refine patient selection for conservative management.
2. Endoscopy plays a pivotal role in diagnosis and risk stratification and planning of subsequent intervention, if needed.
3. Endoscopy can play an important role for conservative management of small volume (unifocal) low-grade disease, when renal preservation is desired.
4. The role of topical therapy to the upper tracts remains unproven, but retrospective data suggest utility in those with CIS, and holds promise for reducing recurrences as adjuvant therapy after total endoscopic control of papillary tumors.
5. Distal ureterectomy may be applied for select patients with isolated tumors in the distal ureter.
6. The role of segmental ureterectomy in the current era of advanced endoscopic instrumentation has diminished but may be a viable option in select cases.
7. Indications for partial nephrectomy for UTUC are extremely narrow and patient selection and technical approach should be critically considered.
8. Radical nephroureterectomy is still considered the standard of care, precluding the need for intensive surveillance of a conserved organ and the possibility of unmonitored tumor progression, but at the price of significant renal functional loss.
9. Single-dose treatment of the bladder after nephroureterectomy could be considered a new standard of care based on two randomized prospective studies showing a benefit and little harm [34, 48].
10. Single-dose treatment of the bladder after endoscopic treatment can be considered based on the above data, but this has not been specifically evaluated in the setting of endoscopic therapy.

Acknowledgments Kaylynn Brooks provided editorial assistance.

References

1. Brown GA, Busby JE, Wood CG, et al. Nephroureterectomy for treating upper urinary tract transitional cell carcinoma: Time to change the treatment paradigm? BJU Int. 2006;98:1176.
2. Margulis V, Shariat SF, Matin SF, et al. Outcomes of radical nephroureterectomy: a series from the Upper Tract Urothelial Carcinoma Collaboration. Cancer. 2009;115:1224.
3. Adibi M, Youssef R, Shariat SF, et al. Oncological outcomes after radical nephroureterectomy for upper tract urothelial carcinoma: comparison over the three decades. Int J Urol. 2012;19:1060.
4. Raman JD, Messer J, Sielatycki JA, et al. Incidence and survival of patients with carcinoma of the ureter and renal pelvis in the USA, 1973–2005. BJU Int. 2011;107:1059.
5. Gerber GS, Steinberg GD. Endourologic treatment of renal pelvic and ureteral transitional cell carcinoma. Tech Urol. 1999;5:77.
6. Lughezzani G, Burger M, Margulis V, et al. Prognostic factors in upper urinary tract urothelial carcinomas: a comprehensive review of the current literature. Eur Urol. 2012;62:100.
7. Shariat SF, Godoy G, Lotan Y, et al. Advanced patient age is associated with inferior cancer-specific survival after radical nephroureterectomy. BJU Int. 2010;105:1672.
8. Hall MC, Womack S, Sagalowsky AI, et al. Prognostic factors, recurrence, and survival in transitional cell carcinoma of the upper urinary tract: a 30-year experience in 252 patients. Urology. 1998;52:594.
9. Munoz JJ, Ellison LM. Upper tract urothelial neoplasms: incidence and survival during the last 2 decades. J Urol. 2000;164:1523.
10. Lughezzani G, Sun M, Perrotte P, et al. Gender-related differences in patients with stage I to III upper tract urothelial carcinoma: results from the Surveillance, Epidemiology, and End Results database. Urology. 2010;75:321.
11. Fernandez MI, Shariat SF, Margulis V, et al. Evidence-based sex-related outcomes after radical nephroureterectomy for upper tract urothelial carcinoma: results of large multicenter study. Urology. 2009;73:142.
12. Rink M, Xylinas E, Margulis V, et al. Impact of smoking on oncologic outcomes of upper tract urothelial carcinoma after radical nephroureterectomy. Eur Urol. 2013;63:1082.
13. Raman JD, Ng CK, Boorjian SA, et al. Bladder cancer after managing upper urinary tract transitional cell carcinoma: predictive factors and pathology. BJU Int. 2005;96:1031.
14. Hagiwara M, Kikuchi E, Tanaka N, et al. Impact of smoking status on bladder tumor recurrence after radical nephroureterectomy for upper tract urothelial carcinoma. J Urol. 2013;189:2062.
15. Brown GA, Matin SF, Busby JE, et al. Ability of clinical grade to predict final pathologic stage in upper urinary tract transitional cell carcinoma: implications for therapy. Urology. 2007;70:252.
16. Guarnizo E, Pavlovich CP, Seiba M, et al. Ureteroscopic biopsy of upper tract urothelial carcinoma: improved diagnostic accuracy and histopathological considerations using a multi-biopsy approach. J Urol. 2000;163:52.
17. Grasso M, Fishman AI, Cohen J, et al. Ureteroscopic and extirpative treatment of upper urinary tract urothelial carcinoma: a 15-year comprehensive review of 160 consecutive patients. BJU Int. 2012;110:1618.
18. Pieras E, Frontera G, Ruiz X, et al. Concomitant carcinoma in situ and tumour size are prognostic factors for bladder recurrence after nephroureterectomy for upper tract transitional cell carcinoma. BJU Int. 2010;106:1319.
19. Simone G, Papalia R, Loreto A, et al. Independent prognostic value of tumour diameter and tumour necrosis in upper urinary tract urothelial carcinoma. BJU Int. 2009;103:1052.
20. Cho KS, Hong SJ, Cho NH, et al. Grade of hydronephrosis and tumor diameter as preoperative prognostic factors in ureteral transitional cell carcinoma. Urology. 2007;70:662.
21. Ito Y, Kikuchi E, Tanaka N, et al. Preoperative hydronephrosis grade independently predicts worse pathological outcomes in patients undergoing nephroureterectomy for upper tract urothelial carcinoma. J Urol. 2011;185:1621.

22. Ng CK, Shariat SF, Lucas SM, et al. Does the presence of hydronephrosis on preoperative axial CT imaging predict worse outcomes for patients undergoing nephroureterectomy for upper-tract urothelial carcinoma? Urol Oncol. 2011;29:27.
23. Remzi M, Haitel A, Margulis V, et al. Tumour architecture is an independent predictor of outcomes after nephroureterectomy: a multi-institutional analysis of 1363 patients. BJU Int. 2009;103:307.
24. Ristau BT, Tomaszewski JJ, Ost MC. Upper tract urothelial carcinoma: current treatment and outcomes. Urology. 2012;79:749.
25. Roupret M, Babjuk M, Comperat E, et al. European guidelines on upper tract urothelial carcinomas: 2013 update. Eur Urol. 2013;63:1059–71.
26. Comploj E, Babjuk M, Capitanio U, et al. Role of conventional cytology in the treatment of upper tract urothelial carcinoma (OSS-UTUC): results from the multi-institutional organ-sparing-UTUC collaboration. Eur Urol Suppl. 2013;12:e601.
27. Raman JD, Sosa RE, Vaughan Jr ED, et al. Pathologic features of bladder tumors after nephroureterectomy or segmental ureterectomy for upper urinary tract transitional cell carcinoma. Urology. 2007;69:251.
28. Palou J, Piovesan LF, Huguet J, et al. Percutaneous nephroscopic management of upper urinary tract transitional cell carcinoma: recurrence and long-term followup. J Urol. 2004;172:66.
29. Bagley DH, Grasso 3rd M. Ureteroscopic laser treatment of upper urinary tract neoplasms. World J Urol. 2010;28:143.
30. Raman JD, Scherr DS. Management of patients with upper urinary tract transitional cell carcinoma. Nat Clin Pract Urol. 2007;4:432.
31. Roupret M, Babjuk M, Comperat E, et al. European guidelines on upper tract urothelial carcinomas: 2013 update. Eur Urol. 2013;63:1059.
32. Smith AK, Stephenson AJ, Lane BR, et al. Inadequacy of biopsy for diagnosis of upper tract urothelial carcinoma: implications for conservative management. Urology. 2011;78:82.
33. Cutress ML, Stewart GD, Zakikhani P, et al. Ureteroscopic and percutaneous management of upper tract urothelial carcinoma (UTUC): systematic review. BJU Int. 2012;110:614.
34. O'Brien T, Ray E, Singh R, et al. Prevention of bladder tumours after nephroureterectomy for primary upper urinary tract urothelial carcinoma: a prospective, multicentre, randomised clinical trial of a single postoperative intravesical dose of mitomycin C (the ODMIT-C Trial). Eur Urol. 2011;60:703.
35. Gadzinski AJ, Roberts WW, Faerber GJ, et al. Long-term outcomes of nephroureterectomy versus endoscopic management for upper tract urothelial carcinoma. J Urol. 2010;183:2148.
36. Boorjian S, Ng C, Munver R, et al. Impact of delay to nephroureterectomy for patients undergoing ureteroscopic biopsy and laser tumor ablation of upper tract transitional cell carcinoma. Urology. 2005;66:283.
37. Hendin BN, Streem SB, Levin HS, et al. Impact of diagnostic ureteroscopy on long-term survival in patients with upper tract transitional cell carcinoma. J Urol. 1999;161:783.
38. Grasso M, Fraiman M, Levine M. Ureteropyeloscopic diagnosis and treatment of upper urinary tract urothelial malignancies. Urology. 1999;54:240.
39. Roupret M, Hupertan V, Traxer O, et al. Comparison of open nephroureterectomy and ureteroscopic and percutaneous management of upper urinary tract transitional cell carcinoma. Urology. 2006;67:1181.
40. Giannarini G, Kessler TM, Birkhauser FD, et al. Antegrade perfusion with bacillus Calmette-Guerin in patients with non-muscle-invasive urothelial carcinoma of the upper urinary tract: who may benefit? Eur Urol. 2011;60:955.
41. Audenet F, Traxer O, Bensalah K, et al. Upper urinary tract instillations in the treatment of urothelial carcinomas: a review of technical constraints and outcomes. World J Urol. 2013;31:45.
42. Lughezzani G, Jeldres C, Isbarn H, et al. Nephroureterectomy and segmental ureterectomy in the treatment of invasive upper tract urothelial carcinoma: a population-based study of 2299 patients. Eur J Cancer. 2009;45:3291.
43. Colin P, Ouzzane A, Pignot G, et al. Comparison of oncological outcomes after segmental ureterectomy or radical nephroureterectomy in urothelial carcinomas of the upper urinary tract: results from a large French multicentre study. BJU Int. 2012;110:1134.

44. Jeldres C, Lughezzani G, Sun M, et al. Segmental ureterectomy can safely be performed in patients with transitional cell carcinoma of the ureter. J Urol. 2010;183:1324.
45. Murphy DM, Zincke H, Furlow WL. Primary grade 1 transitional cell carcinoma of the renal pelvis and ureter. J Urol. 1980;123:629.
46. Goel MC, Matin SF, Derweesh I, et al. Partial nephrectomy for renal urothelial tumors: clinical update. Urology. 2006;67:490.
47. Kondo T, Tanabe K. The role of lymph node dissection in the management of urothelial carcinoma of the upper urinary tract. Int J Clin Oncol. 2011;16:170.
48. Ito A, Shintaku I, Satoh M, et al. Prospective randomized phase II trial of a single early intravesical instillation of pirarubicin (THP) in the prevention of bladder recurrence after nephroureterectomy for upper urinary tract urothelial carcinoma: the THP Monotherapy Study Group Trial. J Clin Oncol. 2013;31:1422.

Chapter 6
Surgical Management of High-Risk Upper Tract Urothelial Carcinoma

Georgios Gakis, Ashish M. Kamat, Vitaly Margulis, Seth P. Lerner, and Arnulf Stenzl

Abstract The definition of high-risk UTUC comprises the risk of progression, and not merely the risk of intracavitary recurrence. In this respect, open radical nephroureterectomy is the standard treatment for high-risk UTUC, which consists of the removal of the entire kidney and ureter along with excision of the bladder cuff. Laparoscopic approaches have been shown to provide similar outcomes in terms of lymph node yield and completeness of resection, but these techniques have to be considered investigational.

Kidney-sparing surgery for the management of high-risk UTUC is an acceptable alternative to RNU in selected patients with elective or imperative indications. Close and lifelong surveillance of the remaining urothelium is mandatory in all patients undergoing kidney-sparing surgery for high-risk UTUC. Adjuvant intracavitary instillation of BCG is an effective option in patients with pure or concomitant CIS of the upper tract while its benefit remains questionable in Ta-T1 disease. Perioperative single-dose intravesical chemotherapy following RNU has shown to reduce the risk of intravesical recurrence following RNU.

Increasing evidence suggests a prognostic role of regional lymph node dissection during RNU as the presence of positive nodes is associated with an increased risk of recurrence. However, its extent has not been investigated in depth so far.

G. Gakis, MD, FEBU • A. Stenzl (✉)
Department of Urology, University Hospital Tübingen, Hoppe-Seyler Strasse 3, 72076 Tübingen, Germany
e-mail: Gcorgios.Gakis@med.uni tuebingen.de; arnulf.stenzl@med.uni-tuebingen.de

A.M. Kamat, MD
Department of Urology, M. D. Anderson Cancer Center, Houston, TX, USA
e-mail: akamat@mdanderson.org

V. Margulis, MD
Department of Urology, University of Texas Southwestern Medical Centre, Dallas, TX, USA
e-mail: vitaly.margulis@utsouthwestern.edu

S.P. Lerner, MD
Scott Department of Urology, Baylor College of Medicine, Houston, TX, USA
e-mail: slerner@bcm.edu

© Springer Science+Business Media New York 2015
S.F. Shariat, E. Xylinas (eds.), *Upper Tract Urothelial Carcinoma*,
DOI 10.1007/978-1-4939-1501-9_6

Keywords High-risk • Upper tract urothelial carcinoma • Radical nephroureterectomy • Lymph node dissection • Kidney-sparing • Ureterectomy • Laparoscopy • Perioperative instillation • Intracavitary instillation • Bladder cuff excision

Introduction

The surgical treatment of high-risk upper tract urothelial carcinoma (UTUC) is one of the most challenging management issues in uro-oncology. The definition of high-risk UTUC comprises the risk of progression, and not merely the risk of intracavitary recurrence. In this respect, radical nephroureterectomy is considered the gold standard treatment for high-risk UTUC [1]. However, a recent surge in the number of publications on prognostic factors has improved our understanding of this rare oncologic disease [2]. The range of surgical approaches to the upper tract involves open, endoscopic, and laparoscopic procedures. Histological determinants for high-risk UTUC are tumor grade (high vs. low grade) and depth of tumor infiltration (≥T1 vs. Ta) [1]. In this respect, staging before planning the surgical approach in high-risk UTUC is critical in order to accurately assess the local tumor extent, renal function, involvement of regional lymph nodes, and distant sites. The focus of book chapter is to provide a comprehensive overview on the current status of the surgical management options in high-risk UTUC.

Extent of Radical Nephroureterectomy

The indication of performing radical nephroureterectomy (RNU) in high-risk UTUC is based on various preoperative clinical and pathologic risk factors and patient-centered, non-oncologic parameters. With increasing evidence of the significance of renal function on overall survival in other cancer entities (i.e., in renal cell carcinoma) [3] kidney-sparing surgery has come to the fore of clinicians to maximally preserve renal function in patients with high-risk UTUC [4]. While prognostic factors for survival after RNU have been extensively studied, only a few reports have addressed the role of predictive factors for the oncologic efficacy of nephron-sparing procedures [5]. By contrast to non-muscle-invasive bladder cancer in which endoscopic ablative procedures and the administration of intravesical instillation regimens can easily be performed to preserve the bladder [6] the sometimes elaborate accessibility to the upper tract significantly hampers a priori any attempt to study in depth the role of endoscopic methods in high-risk UTUC. Furthermore, effective intraluminal instillation regimens with BCG, which have been successfully used in high-risk bladder cancer, require a minimum of contact time to allow the agent to interact with the urothelium which is limited by the natural peristalsis of the renal pelvis and ureter [7].

For these reasons, RNU is still considered the gold standard treatment in high-risk UTUC [1]. The extent of RNU consists of the removal of the entire kidney and ureter, excision of the bladder cuff, and regional lymphadenectomy [1]. The "radicality" of surgery aims to avoid the risk of local failure which is associated with dismal prognosis [1]. All these procedures can be performed with either open or laparoscopic approach while excision of the bladder cuff can be also performed endoscopically [1].

Lymph Node Dissection in High-Risk UTUC

Lymphatic Distribution in the Retroperitoneum

In patients with muscle-invasive urothelial carcinoma of the bladder, performance of an extended lymph node dissection (LND) at radical cystectomy increases node yield and identifies more node metastases in patients with positive nodes. While a survival benefit is suggested, this important clinical question is being addressed in ongoing Phase III randomized trials [8]. There is controversy around the performance and extent of pelvic and retroperitoneal LND in high-risk UTUC [1]. There are three factors which limit our understanding of the therapeutic role of LND in high-risk UTUC. One important factor is the scant knowledge of the lymphatic distribution in the retroperitoneum [9]. As lymphatic drainage patterns of the renal pelvis and ureter vary considerably, defining specific LND templates according to the primary tumor location may enable anatomic LND in patients at high risk for lymph node-positive disease. A study of 181 patients treated with RNU recorded location of metastatic nodes according to the primary tumor location. In tumors of the right renal pelvis, the primary metastatic sites were preferentially the right renal hilar, paracaval, and retrocaval nodes. Tumors of the upper two-thirds of the right ureter primarily metastasized to the retrocaval and inter-aortocaval nodes. In tumors of the left renal pelvis, the primary sites were the left renal hilar and para-aortic nodes. Tumors of the upper two-thirds of the left ureter primarily metastasized to the para-aortic nodes. Importantly, tumors of the lower ureter primarily metastasized to nodes inferior to the aortic bifurcation [10]. These data may form the basis for future prospective research to better understand the lymphatic spread to the retroperitoneum.

Oncological Significance of Lymph Node Dissection at RNU

Due to the paucity of data on the prognostic benefit of LND in high-risk UTUC the performance of LND at RNU is most often surgeon dependent [11]. This translates into a considerable selection bias in terms of the reported rates of lymph node involvement at RNU. Open RNU series have demonstrated an equally inconsistent use of regional LND compared to laparoscopic techniques. Some series reported that only 50 % of patients underwent an LND at RNU with wide variations in the extent of the LND used [12]. One negative consequence of the inconsistent use of LND may be an underestimation of LN tumor involvement in high-risk UTUC. In a large combined series of 44 institutions 62 % of patients did not undergo any lymph node dissection [12]. Due to this, the selection of patients for LND at RNU includes those with bulky or infiltrative lymph node pattern, obvious LN tumor involvement on preoperative imaging, or lymphadenopathy identified at the time of surgery.

The surgeon's decision on the operative technique used to remove the primary tumor may also influence the indication of performing LND at RNU. Several studies have investigated whether open or laparoscopic techniques influence lymph node yield. While laparoscopic nephroureterectomy (LNU) has been shown to achieve similar LN yields compared to open RNU some comparative series suggest patients undergoing LNU are less likely to receive a LN dissection [13–18].

However, the diagnosis of positive nodes at RNU dramatically affects disease-specific outcomes. Node-negative disease is independently associated with an improved disease-specific survival compared to node-positive with an increase in the relative risk of death of approximately 2–3 [19–21]. Consequently, it has to be borne in mind that a proportion of patients who do not receive a regional lymph node dissection (pNx) will harbor LN involvement and as such are at risk for recurrence. In this respect, the prognostic benefit of LND at RNU in terms of removing micrometastatic awaits further elucidation.

Despite the absence of completed randomized studies on the necessity and extent of LND at RNU it can be hypothesized from the literature on high-risk bladder cancer [8] that LND in high-risk UTUC may improve the accuracy of lymph node staging and locoregional control of the disease. Yet, as lymphatic spread of UTUC in the retroperitoneum and pelvis from urothelial cancer has not been clearly established, it seems more sensible to define the anatomic limits of LND based on tumor location and a minimum number of lymph nodes identified by the pathologist in order to ensure accurate lymph node staging that will guide decision-making regarding the need for adjuvant treatment. In this respect, one of largest multicenter series to date reported on staging accuracy based on the number of retrieved lymph nodes. Among 551 patients treated with RNU and regional LND in a 15-year period, positive lymph nodes were present in 25 % of the patients. The removal of eight nodes resulted in a 75 % probability to detect at least one positive node while a more extensive LND with 13 removed nodes yielded a probability of 90 % [22]. These data stress the importance of a meticulous regional LND in UTUC to ensure accurate nodal staging. The pivotal question, however, remains whether a more meticulous LND will also translate into an improved survival. Another study based on the same cohort of patients found that the number of removed lymph nodes independently predicted cancer-specific mortality. A cutoff of eight nodes was the most informative value to predict cancer-specific mortality [23].

Nonetheless, as in the last years the definition of an adequate LND in muscle-invasive bladder cancer has shifted from a minimum number of lymph nodes need to be removed to the definition of LND templates [8] it seems reasonable to address this issue in high-risk UTUC as well. In addition, increasing evidence suggests a hypothesis that the anatomical extent of regional LND may play a critical role for survival in lymph node-positive UTUC. A single-center, retrospective series evaluated lymph node metastatic patterns as well the underlying anatomical templates in 81 patients treated with RNU for non-metastatic UTUC of the renal pelvis and/or ureter [24]. Regional lymph nodes were considered adequately resected when the incidence of positive nodes was higher than 30 %. Thus, an LND was retrospectively defined as being complete when all primary lymphatic metastatic sites were removed. Conversely, it was considered incomplete when the removal of all primary metastatic sites was incomplete. Survival depended significantly on the extent of LND with stage ≥ pT3 patients to derive the highest prognostic benefit from the procedure. Likewise, patient survival improved when the number of removed lymph nodes increased.

Indeed, growing evidence suggests that tumor stage may guide clinicians to perform a more extended LND at RNU. According to smaller series, performance of LND is associated with a lower risk of local recurrence but does not appear to influence disease-specific survival [25–27]. However, in those with lymph node-positive disease [27] lymph node density (defined as the ratio of the number of tumor-bearing vs. removed nodes) was critical for outcome as patients with an LND threshold value of >20 % showed decreased recurrence-free survival [27]. Importantly, in patients with clinically node-negative pT1-T4 UTUC a "complete" LND, defined as outlined above [10], improved cancer-specific survival after adjusting for adjuvant chemotherapy while the number of removed nodes did not [28]. Another multicenter series retrospectively compared outcomes in 1,130 patients with stage pT1-T4 UTUC. While in stage pT1 disease a significant difference between patients staged pN0 and pNx was not noted, LND in the group of patients with pT2-T4N0 UTUC resulted in improved cancer-specific survival compared to those in whom LND was omitted (pNx) [29]. These results were also confirmed in a retrospective, multicenter series of 785 patients treated with RNU in which patients with pN0 disease displayed significantly improved cancer-specific survival in the presence of pathologically advanced tumor stages (pT2-T4) [30]. In summary, besides improved nodal staging, the current body of evidence suggests that LND at the time of RNU impacts survival in high-risk UTUC.

In conclusion, the burden of retrospective studies suggests that LND improves local staging influences survival in patients with high-risk UTUC. Therefore, lymph node dissection in patients with high-risk (clinically infiltrative, high-grade, or pathologically muscle-invasive) UTUC should be recommended at the time of surgical resection while its extent needs further investigation.

Management of the Distal Ureter at Radical Nephroureterectomy

Radical nephroureterectomy for UTUC includes also the excision of the ipsilateral bladder cuff [1, 31] as its omission at RNU represents a significant risk factor for local recurrence in up to two-thirds of the patients [32–34]. During bladder cuff resection, it is imperative to prevent tumor seeding by avoiding tumor cell spilling outside the resected renoureteral unit [1, 35]. Multiple techniques have been established for bladder cuff excision, which are based on different surgical approaches. These include extravesical, transvesical, and endoscopic techniques. The standard technique of bladder cuff resection is the open, en bloc excision together with the ipsilateral kidney and ureter. The open approach can be performed either transvesically or extravesically [31].

Extravesical Approach

The advantage of extravesical excision of the distal ureter is the avoidance of an anterior cystotomy which reduces the risk of tumor cell spilling at RNU and prolonged hospitalization due to postoperative catheterization. By this approach, a complete removal of the bladder cuff removal is more difficult than with a transvesical or endoscopic technique as the extravesical approach necessitates a "blind" clamping of the ureteral hiatus with a right-angle clamp or a stapler while placing simultaneously traction on the ureter. Moreover, this approach may compromise contralateral ureteral integrity [31, 36]. To facilitate the performance of extravesical approach in laparoscopic radical nephroureterectomy gentle traction needs to be simultaneously applied to the ureter to "tent up" the wall of the bladder for placement of a laparoscopic GIA tissue stapler [31, 36, 37]. This can be preceded by cystoscopic unroofing of the intramural ureter [37]. Nevertheless, this technique is surgically challenging and has been therefore associated with a higher rate of positive surgical margins and a trend towards inferior disease-free survival [36, 38].

Transvesical Approach

During transvesical resection of the bladder cuff, an anterior cystotomy is performed, the contralateral ureteral office is visualized, and the affected ipsilateral ureter is circumferentially dissected around its orifice to remove a cuff of bladder with the specimen. A thorough preoperative cystoscopic evaluation is therefore necessary to exclude the presence of concomitant urothelial bladder cancer. A pure laparoscopic transvesical approach is technically demanding approach as it needs the use of traction sutures on the bladder cuff to guide the area of excision [39]. Combining the laparoscopic approach with transvesical cystoscopic Collin's knife incision for detachment of the distal ureter may facilitate the laparoscopic management of the bladder cuff resection [40]. As experience with the robotic surgical approaches in uro-oncologic surgery increases, the increased range of motion with the robot may alleviate transvesical laparoscopic nephroureterectomy.

Endoscopic Approach

As has been shown decades ago, the bladder cuff can be also managed endoscopically at RNU [41]. Major concerns of this technique include tumor spillage from extravasated urine (although techniques for endoscopic ligation of the distal ureter stump have been described [42]) as well as the risk for incomplete resection of the intramural ureter due to avulsion of the specimen [42, 43]. As such, this technique should be avoided for distal ureteral tumors [43, 44].

By using either electrocautery or a Collins's knife, first transurethral resection of the ureteral orifice is carried out and the intramural ureter is excised until perivesical fat is visualized [42, 45, 46]. After this, the patient is repositioned for the remainder of the nephroureterectomy, which can be performed with either an open or laparoscopic approach [42]. Once the kidney is dissected free and the renal hilum is divided, the distal ureter dissection is completed meeting up with the endoscopic resection in order to ensure complete removal of the distal ureter and bladder cuff. The bladder is closed primarily. Applying gentle traction to separate the specimen from the bladder (so-called "pluck" technique) is associated with a risk of incomplete removal of the intramural ureter and bladder cuff [45].

Oncological Efficacy of Different Bladder Cuff Resection Techniques

Investigators from the population-based Surveillance, Epidemiology, and End Results (SEER) database evaluated outcomes in 4,210 patients treated with nephroureterectomy and different bladder cuff resection techniques between 1988 and 2006. The omission of bladder cuff resection at RNU was associated with a significantly increased risk of cancer-specific mortality among patients with locally advanced tumor stages (pT3-T4N0/x or pTany pN1-3 [47]. These results stress the importance of bladder cuff excision for optimizing cancer control in patients with high-risk UTUC.

While comparative randomized trials are lacking in terms of the oncologic efficacy of these three different techniques, recent data from retrospective series have given some insight into the efficacy of different bladder cuff resection techniques. Of 301 patients undergoing RNU, 43 % underwent an extravesical approach, 27 % a transvesical excision of the distal ureter, and 30 % an endoscopic transurethral incision [48]. After a median follow-up of 33 months, the respective bladder recurrence rates did not differ between the applied techniques (24 % vs 24 % vs 18 %, respectively; $p=0.48$). Similar results were reported from a large, multicenter study, wherein bladder cuff excision was likewise not found to be significantly associated with cancer-specific mortality [18].

However, in terms of intravesical bladder cancer recurrence, a multicenter retrospective study of 2,681 patients who underwent nephroureterectomy over a 20-year

Table 6.1 Select series reporting on intravesical recurrence for different bladder cuff excision techniques

Study	N pat.	Median F/U [mo.]	N (EV)	N (IV)	N (TUI)	5-year bladder RFS [%] (EV)	5-year bladder RFS [%] (IV)	5-year bladder RFS [%] (TUI)
Li et al. [48]	301	33	129	81	91	24	24	18
Xylinas et al. [49]	2,681	58	785	1,811	85	58	51	42

EV extravesical, *IV* intravesical, *TUI* transurethral incision, *RFS* recurrence-free survival, *F/U* follow-up, *mo* months)

period reported significant differences between the three methods. In this study patients underwent either transvesical ($n = 1{,}811$), extravesical ($n = 785$), or endoscopic ($n = 85$) approaches to the distal ureter [49]. Patients who were subjected to an endoscopic approach had a significantly lower 5-year intravesical recurrence-free survival (42 %) than patients who underwent either a transvesical (58 %) or extravesical (51 %) approach to the distal ureter, although no significant difference in intravesical recurrence was found between the transvesical and extravesical approach. On multivariable analysis, the endoscopic approach to the distal ureter remained associated with a significantly increased risk of subsequent intravesical tumor recurrence [49]. Nevertheless, as shown in other studies [47, 48], no differences were reported for cancer-specific and overall survival for the three surgical approaches to the distal ureter [49].

Altogether, while the optimal approach to management of the distal ureter remains to be determined within randomized studies, the burden of retrospective series, as outlined above, supports the assumption that all approaches to the distal ureter (either transvesical, extravesical, or endoscopic) are valid options as long as complete excision of the bladder cuff is achieved and intraoperative tumor spillage is avoided. In addition, early clipping of the distal ureter proximally located upper tract tumors may reduce the risk of intravesical recurrence [35]. Table 6.1 provides an overview on the largest series evaluating intravesical recurrence-free survival according to the different bladder cuff excision techniques.

Kidney-Sparing Surgery in High-Risk UTUC

Patient Selection for KSS in High-Risk UTUC

In select patients with imperative or elective indication, kidney-sparing surgery (KSS) is an option for the treatment of patients with high-risk UTUC as an alternative to upfront RNU [50]. Similar to conservative treatment of early invasive bladder cancer (staged pT1), a major concern of conducting kidney-sparing treatment in high-risk UTUC is the risk of progression in case of treatment failure, which may have a negative impact on survival. Imperative indications for nephron-sparing surgery include patients with solitary kidneys, bilateral disease, or severe renal insufficiency who would be rendered functionally or anatomically anephric after RNU. Following demonstration of the technical feasibility with acceptable oncologic outcomes in patients with imperative indication, investigators have expanded the indication for KSS to elective cases aiming to ensure maximum kidney function after treatment [51–53].

One critical aspect of KSS in high-risk UTUC is proper patient selection to avoid the risk of treatment failure. Another issue is the accuracy of pathologic staging and grading given the currently available endoscopic techniques. In this respect, a detailed diagnostic ureterorenoscopy using flexible instruments is imperative prior to consideration of any nephron-sparing approach in high-risk UTUC to evaluate the extent of the tumor lesion and obtain representative biopsies as well as a cytology of the tumor-affected renoureteral unit [54, 55, 56–58]. However, the accurate clinical and pathological staging of upper tract tumors can be difficult as with the current available endoscopic equipment it is often not possible to obtain a full-thickness biopsy to evaluate for muscle invasion. In this respect, a high degree of concordance has been observed between tumor grade assessed on endoscopically obtained upper tract biopsies compared to tumor grade (84–91 %) [59–61] and stage at the time of RNU [62]. Therefore, tumor grade at biopsy is considered a strong surrogate marker for stage and, thus, for the final clinical decision-making for a kidney-sparing approach. Omission to perform a biopsy at diagnostic ureterorenoscopy inherits the risk of understaging as macroscopic tumor appearance does not reliably predict tumor grade. In this respect, Thompson et al. demonstrated that 21 % of tumors thought to be low grade on visual inspection were subsequently found to be high grade on pathologic review of RNU specimen [53].

Notably, in patients with elective or imperative indication opting for a kidney-sparing approach lifelong surveillance of the upper tracts and bladder is obligatory as the risk of recurrence ranges considerably (3–63 %) [63, 64] and may even occur after more than 15 years of follow-up [65].

Kidney-Sparing Surgical Techniques for the Treatment of High-Risk UTUC

Variations in primary tumor size, location, and grade decide on the surgical method for nephron-sparing treatment in high-risk UTUC. Basically, KSS in UTUC includes either endoscopic resection or segmental/total ureterectomy. Endoscopic resection and laser-based ablative techniques can be performed via either retrograde or antegrade manipulation. Ureterectomy is feasible for high-grade, infiltrative ureteral lesions and carcinoma in situ (CIS) of the ureter.

Technique of Partial and Total Ureterectomy

In patients with high-risk UTUC in the proximal, mid, and/or distal part of the ureter a segmental or total ureterectomy is a feasible option for carefully selected patients with imperative or elective indications in order to maintain renal function. The approach is highly dependent on the location of the tumor and available reconstructive options.

Tumors located in the distal ureter that are not amenable to endoscopic management can be treated with a segmental resection of the distal ureter and an appropriate bladder cuff. Access to the distal ureter can be gained by either an open or laparoscopic approach or in combination. For distal ureterectomy and bladder cuff excision, a lower midline or Gibson incision allows for excellent exposure of the distal ureter and bladder. Small series have reported successful cases of laparoscopic and robotic-assisted distal ureterectomy with psoas hitch reimplantation [66–69]. A major concern with these techniques includes prolonged operative time (averaging 4 h) and complications including anastomotic strictures and port-site recurrences [68, 70]. Therefore, to ensure maximum oncological safety special attention has to be paid to the risk of tumor spillage as local recurrence due to residual tumor is often associated with a dismal prognosis [71].

After distal ureterectomy, reconstruction of the upper tract can be performed by different methods. Direct reimplantation at the dome of the can be performed if the remaining ureter is long enough. If a significant portion of the distal ureter needs to be removed to provide tumor-free margins and additional length is required, the bladder can be mobilized using the psoas-hitch or boari-flap technique to substitute for the resected ureteral length. Ureters can be reimplanted into the bladder via a refluxing versus non-refluxing anastomosis. While a non-refluxing anastomosis may theoretically limit infection and seeding of tumor cells in the upper tract, stricture rates may be higher and endoscopic surveillance may be more difficult [72]. Given the lack of data to guide urologists either way, the choice of a reflexive technique should be left to the discretion of the treating surgeon. In case of tumor location in the mid ureter the appendix can also be used to bridge the ureteric gap [73]. In cases of subtotal ureterectomy, ileal substitution is necessary. In the presence of preexisting renal dysfunction, the segment of ileum can be tapered and a psoas hitch performed to minimize sequelae from urinary reabsorption through the bowel mucosa. Renal autotransplantation to the iliac vessels following total ureterectomy has also been described, although this should only be considered as a last resort given the potential for loss of the kidney [74].

Survival After Distal and Segmental Ureterectomy

The long-term results of distal ureterectomy in high-grade distal UTUC have shown to be comparable to RNU series [75]. A study by Simonato et al. on 73 patients with distal UTUC used different reconstruction techniques including psoas hitch (52 %), end-to-end anastomosis (29 %), direct ureteroneocystostomies (15 %), and Boari flap reconstruction (4 %). Of the 73 patients, 42 (58 %) had infiltrative stages (pT1-T4) while the remaining 31 patients displayed only pTa stage disease at final examination. After a median follow-up of 87 months, the overall 5-year bladder RFS was 82 % and cancer-specific survival 94 %. None of the patients with pTa stage died from disease while those with pT2 and pT3 stages showed acceptable survival rates at 5 years of 78 % and 75 %, respectively. Presence of high-grade disease was found to contribute to worse survival in infiltrative stages (≥pT1) but not in pTa disease [64].

A large multi-institutional study retrospectively reviewed outcomes of 52 patients who were treated with segmental ureterectomy compared to 416 patients who were subjected to upfront RNU. After a median follow-up of 26 months, no significant differences were noted for 5-year CSS and RFS with 88 % and 37 % at 5 years after segmental ureterectomy compared to 86 % and 48 % after RNU, respectively [63]. These results were confirmed in an analysis of the Surveillance, Epidemiology, and End Results database. Of a total of 2,044 patients with T1-T4 ureteral carcinoma, 569 (28 %) underwent segmental ureterectomy while 1,222 (60 %) patients who underwent RNU with bladder cuff removal and 253 patients (12 %) without bladder cuff removal. Five-year disease-specific mortality was similar among the three groups (87 %, 82 %, and 81 %, respectively). Multivariable analysis showed no significant effect of the type of surgery on cancer outcomes. Similarly authors found that, apart from pT and pN stage neither tumor location nor type of surgery were independent prognostic factors [76]. These results suggest that essentially all patients (including even those with advanced T stage) can safely undergo segmental resection in ureteral carcinoma; however, selection bias and possible inconsistencies have to be taken into account [77]. Table 6.2 provides an overview of selected series reporting outcomes after segmental or distal ureterectomy.

Endoscopic KSS in High-Risk UTUC

For endoscopic management of high-risk UTUC access to the tumor can be established via either an antegrade or retrograde approach. Using semirigid or flexible instruments tumors can be easily visualized and ablation of the tumor can be

Table 6.2 Select series reporting outcomes after segmental or distal ureterectomy

Study	N pat. (Ux)	N (RNU with bladder cuff excision)	Median Follow-up (in months)	Technique of Ux	N pat. (≥pT1)	5-year bladder RFS (%)	5-year CSS (Ux) (%)	5 year CSS (RNU) (%)
Simonato et al. [71]	73	–	87	Distal	42	82	94	–
Colin et al.[a] [63]	52	416	26	Segmental	–	–	86	88
Lughezzani et al.[a] [76]	569	1,222	–	Segmental	–	–	87	82

Ux ureterectomy, *RFS* recurrence-free survival, *CSS* cancer-specific survival, *RNU* radical nephroureterectomy

[a]Compared to RNU series

performed using electrocautery, holmium:YAG, or neodymium:YAG lasers. The main benefits of the retrograde approach include maintaining a closed urinary system and less morbidity than the antegrade approach. In cases of larger tumors, lesions in the lower renal calyces not accessible by retrograde ureteroscopy, and in patients with urinary diversions creating difficult retrograde access, an antegrade approach may be more sensible as larger instruments can be used and direct access to the affected calyx can be easily gained.

Outcomes After Endoscopic KSS in High-Risk UTUC

Select series reporting outcomes after endoscopic KSS for high-risk UTUC are outlined in Table 6.3. As disease-specific mortality in UTUC has been shown to be independently associated only with grade and body mass index which have been

Table 6.3 Select series of patients undergoing endoscopic management for high-risk UTUC

Study	N (RU)	HG, biopsy confirmed, N (%),	Follow-up (in months)	Overall UTUC recurence, N (%)	RNU, N (%)	DSM
Ureteroscopic						
Daneshmand et al. [62]	30	14 (47)]	Median: 31	27 (90 %)	4 (13 %)	1 (3 %)
Roupret et al.[a,b] [80]	27	8 (33)	Median: 52	4 (15 %)	7 (26 %)	19 %
Thompson et al.[c] [53]	83	8 (10)	Median: 55	46 (55 %)	27 (33 %)	9 (11 %)
Lucas et al.[a,b] [81]	39 (41)	12 (29)	Median: 33	17 (46 %)	11 (28 %)	LG 14 %, HG 33 %
Grasso et al.[a,b] [82]	80	14 (18)	Mean: 38	LG 51 (77 %) HG 14 (100 %)	LG 11 (17 %), HG 4 (29 %)	LG 8 (12.1 %), HG 12
Cutress et al.[a,b] [78]	73	6 (8)	Median: 54	50 (69 %)	14 (19 %)	7(10 %)
Percutaneous						
Lee et al.[a] [84]	50	13 (26)	Mean: 47	6 (12 %)	–	4 (8 %)
Rastinehad et al. [85]	82 (89)	39(44)	Mean: 61	30 (33 %)	12 (13.5 %)	–
Combination Ureteroscopy and Percutaneous						
Suh et al. [5]	27	8 (33 %)	Median: 21	23 (85 %)	7 (26 %)	–
Gadzinski et al.[a] [79]	33 (34)	8 (24)	Mean: 58	27 (84)	12 (35 %)	6 % LG, 25 % HG

RU renal units, *RNU* radical nephroureterectomy, *HG* high grade, *DSM* disease-specific mortality, *LG* low grade)

[a]Comparative to RNU

[b]Stratified by grade

[c]Pure elective indications

identified as predictors of DSM [78–80] it seems promising to take a closer look to the reported survival rates based on the type of treatment in high-risk UTUC. Yet, studies on outcomes after ureterorenoscopic treatment of high-risk UTUC are scarce and subjected to selection biases and small patient numbers. One study reported that among 48 patients with low-grade UTUC disease-specific survival rates between those treated with ureterorenoscopy and RNU for low-grade tumors did not differ significantly at 5 years (86 % vs. 87 %). Among the 68 patients with high-grade tumors only 12 underwent endoscopic treatment while the remaining 56 were subjected to upfront RNU. No significant differences were noted between both groups (68 % vs. 75 %, respectively; $p=0.52$), but conclusions relating to high-grade tumors are limited due to the low number of included patients treated with ureteroscopic ablation [81].

High rates of upper tract recurrence after ureterorenoscopic treatment for high-risk UTUC have been reported with grade-related 5-year recurrence-free survival of 63 %, 34 %, and 17 % in G1, G2, and G3, respectively ($p=0.011$) [78, 82]. These results show that recurrence rates in patients undergoing NSS for high-grade UTUC are ultimately high which underscore the importance of close and lifelong follow-up. The need for salvage RNU in patients stratified by grade is a higher rate of RNU for high rather than low-grade tumors (25 % vs. 17 %). Similarly, Cutress et al. demonstrated 5-year renal unit survival of 96 %, 71 %, and 20 % in G1, G2, and G3, respectively ($p<0.001$) [82]. Complications related to ureteroscopic treatment include distal ureteral strictures with rates up to 17 %, sepsis in up to 11 %, and ureteral perforation in up to 9 % of cases. Care must be taken during ablation with electrocautery or lasers to prevent perforation of the ureter, as the thickness is less than the bladder. Therefore, it is important to maintain good visualization during ablation as poor intraoperative vision may lead to difficulties in achieving complete tumor ablation endoscopically, with the potential of leaving residual tumor behind, thereby possibly resulting in high rates of recurrence [83].

Outcomes After Percutaneous Nephroscopy

Percutaneous management of high-risk UTUC may be an option for larger tumors in the renal calyces as larger instruments can be inserted into a particular renal calyx. Additionally, in patients with urinary diversions or when access in a retrograde fashion is difficult to be achieved, percutaneous treatment may be an option.

As with other series on KSS in high-risk UTUC, results on percutaneous treatment are poorly stratified by grade which limits meaningful conclusions. Recurrence rates in the upper urinary tract range significantly from 12 to 66 % with one study demonstrating higher rates in high- vs low-grade disease (31 % vs 5 %) [84]. The most recent and largest study consisted of 89 renal units treated by percutaneous nephroscopy (PCN) of which 39 tumors were high grade. A second look nephroscopy was routinely performed within 1 week with re-resection if necessary, and a third look nephroscopy done at 3 months to reevaluate for recurrence. Authors reported a recurrence rate of 33 % with higher rates in high- (38 %) vs. low-grade (30 %) tumors [85].

Main complications following percutaneous management of UTUC include blood transfusions due to hemorrhage (13 %) and risk of stricture formation (5 %). Additionally, tumor seeding along the percutaneous nephrostomy tract has been described [85–87].

Intracavitary Instillation Therapy in High-Risk UTUC

In patients with high-risk UTUC some studies have demonstrated the clinical feasibility of intracavitary adjuvant instillation therapy. In one study of 89 patients with low- and high-grade UTUC who were treated with PCN, 50 patients received a 6-week course of BCG and 39 patients with no adjuvant therapy. No difference was noted in recurrence when stratified by stage and grade [88]. Although study numbers were small, the results of this study suggest no significant role for adjuvant BCG in patients with Ta/T1 UTUC and no evidence of CIS, regarding prevention of recurrence or progression. This may be due to inherent differences in the biology between UTUC and urothelial bladder cancer, or incomplete resection of UTUC, thereby leaving residual tumor behind. Positive response rates (defined as negative cytology on follow-up) to a 6-week course of BCG were noted to range from 64 to 100 % with subsequent rates of recurrence noted in 9–50 % of patients. In a case series reporting outcomes in 11 patients with pure CIS of the upper tract treated with BCG compared to five patients treated with immediate RNU, no difference in 5-year RFS (78 % vs 67 %) and 5-year DSS (91 vs. 80 %) was noted [89]. Therefore, these good response rates suggest that BCG should be evaluated in clinical trials in patients with pure or concomitant CIS of the upper tract. Table 6.4 provides an overview of selected series reporting outcomes after intracavitary treatment for UTUC.

Perioperative Intravesical Chemotherapy for Prevention of Bladder Cancer Recurrence Following RNU

Metachronous bladder cancer has been reported in up to 50 % of patients undergoing RNU for UTUC. In retrospective series, risk factors for intravesical recurrence have been found to be upper tract tumor multifocality and a prior history of bladder cancer. Interestingly, correlation studies have shown a high degree of concordance (~90 %) for tumor grade between upper tract and metachronous bladder tumors [91]. Although intravesical recurrences are often superficial and most often occur within the first 2 years after RNU, patients remain at lifelong risk of recurrence.

To avert the negative consequences of intraoperative tumor spillage during RNU, a prospective, non-blinded trial (OMDIT-c) randomized 244 patients to receive either single-dose mitomycin-C (40 mg; $N=144$) or saline ($N=140$). In the per-protocol

Table 6.4 Select series reporting outcomes after intracavitary treatment for UTUC

Study	N (RU)	HG	Follow-up (in months)	Type of treatment	Route of instillation/endoscopic treatment	UT recurrence	RNU	DSM
Ta/T1								
Rastinehad et al.[a] [85]	(50)	39	Mean: 61	BCG	Anterograde/PCN	18 (36 %)	9 (50 %)	–
Cutress et al.[a] [78]	18	–	Median: 54	Mitomycin	Anterograde or retrograde/URS or PCN	46 %	–	–
Giannarini et al. [90]	(22)	–	Median: 42	BCG	Anterograde/-	13 (59 %)	5 (23 %)	5 (23 %)
CIS						PR	Recurrence	DSM
Kojima et al.[a] [89]	11		Median: 58	BCG	Retrograde	9 (82 %)	3 (27 %)	1
Giannarini et al. [90]	(42)		42	BCG	Anterograde	–	17 (40 %)	–

RU renal units, *HG* high grade, *UT* upper tract, *RNU* radical nephroureterectomy, *DSM* disease-specific mortality, *PR* positive response

[a]Comparative to control

analysis, patients in the treatment arm were at significantly lower risk of intravesical recurrence in the first postoperative year as determined by regular cystoscopic examinations. The investigators found that the number of patients needed to be treated to prevent one intravesical recurrence was 9 and no serious events are reported as a result of mitomycin instillation. The data from this trial support the performance of prophylactic single-dose, intravesical chemotherapy to reduce the risk of intravesical recurrence following RNU [92].

Summary

- Open radical nephroureterectomy is the gold standard treatment for high-risk UTUC which consists of the removal of the entire kidney and ureter along with excision of the bladder cuff.
- Regional lymph node dissection is an integral part of RNU as the presence of positive nodes predicts increased risk of recurrence. The extent of LND at RNU has not been investigated so far.
- Laparoscopic approaches have been shown to provide similar outcomes in terms of lymph node yield and completeness of resection, but these techniques have to be considered investigational in light of lack of long-term data.
- Kidney-sparing surgery for the management of high-risk UTUC is an acceptable alternative to RNU in select patients with elective or imperative indications. Close and lifelong surveillance is mandatory in all patients undergoing kidney-sparing surgery for high-risk UTUC.
- A delay to RNU has not been shown to result in worse survival in patients undergoing nephron-sparing surgery if close surveillance is performed.
- Careful ureterorenoscopic examination with cross-sectional imaging should be conducted prior to consideration of any kidney-sparing approach.
- Tumor location, size, multiplicity, and tumor grade are key determinants for effective cancer control in patients undergoing nephron-sparing surgical approaches.
- High-grade UTUC in the distal, mid, or proximal part of the ureter can be successfully managed with segmental or total ureterectomy with bladder or ileal reconstruction techniques to bridge the ureteral gap.
- Patients with imperative reasons for kidney preservation (solitary kidney, bilateral UUTUC, or renal insufficiency), who have high-grade tumors within the renal pelvis or calyces, and would be rendered to hemodialysis following RNU, can be managed endoscopically.
- Adjuvant intracavitary instillation of BCG is an effective option in patients with pure or concomitant CIS of the upper tract while its benefit remains questionable in Ta-T1 disease.

Disclosure All authors have nothing to disclose.

References

1. Rouprêt M, Babjuk M, Compérat E, Zigeuner R, Sylvester R, Burger M, Cowan N, Böhle A, Van Rhijn BW, Kaasinen E, Palou J, Shariat SF. European guidelines on upper tract urothelial carcinomas: 2013 update. Eur Urol. 2013;63:1059–71.
2. Green DA, Rink M, Xylinas E, Matin SF, Stenzl A, Roupret M, Karakiewicz PI, Scherr DS, Shariat SF. Urothelial carcinoma of the bladder and the upper tract: disparate twins. J Urol. 2013;189:1214–21.
3. Badalato GM, Kates M, Wisnivesky JP, Choudhury AR, McKiernan JM. Survival after partial and radical nephrectomy for the treatment of stage T1bN0M0 renal cell carcinoma (RCC) in the USA: a propensity scoring approach. BJU Int. 2012;109:1457–62.
4. Smith P, Mandel J, Raman JD. Conservative nephron-sparing treatment of upper-tract tumors. Curr Urol Rep. 2013;14:102–8.
5. Suh RS, Faerber G, Wolf Jr JS. Predictive factors for applicability and success with endoscopic treatment of upper tract urothelial carcinoma. J Urol. 2003;170:2209–16.
6. Babjuk M, Burger M, Zigeuner R, Shariat SF, van Rhijn BW, Compérat E, Sylvester RJ, Kaasinen E, Böhle A, Palou Redorta J, Rouprêt M. EAU guidelines on non-muscle-invasive urothelial carcinoma of the bladder: update 2013. Eur Urol. 2013;64:639–53. doi:10.1016/j.eururo.2013.06.003.
7. Maurice MJ, Madi R, Chuang DY, Abouassaly R. Retrograde chemoinfusion of the upper tract: standardizing the delivery of topical adjuvant therapy. J Endourol. 2013;27:540–4.
8. Gakis G, Efstathiou J, Lerner SP, Cookson MS, Keegan KA, Guru KA, Shipley WU, Heidenreich A, Schoenberg MP, Sagaloswky AI, Soloway MS, Stenzl A, International Consultation on Urologic Disease-European Association of Urology Consultation on Bladder Cancer 2012. ICUD-EAU International Consultation on Bladder Cancer 2012: Radical cystectomy and bladder preservation for muscle-invasive urothelial carcinoma of the bladder. Eur Urol. 2013;63:45–57.
9. Miocinovic R, Gong MC, Ghoneim IA, Fergany AF, Hansel DE, Stephenson AJ. Presacral and retroperitoneal lymph node involvement in urothelial bladder cancer: results of a prospective mapping study. J Urol. 2011;186:1269–73.
10. Kondo T, Nakazawa H, Ito F, Hashimoto Y, Toma H, Tanabe K. Primary site and incidence of lymph node metastases in urothelial carcinoma of upper urinary tract. Urology. 2007;69:265–9.
11. Secin FP, Koppie TM, Salamanca JI, Bokhari S, Raj GV, Olgac S, Serio A, Vickers A, Bochner BH. Evaluation of regional lymph node dissection in patients with upper urinary tract urothelial cancer. Int J Urol. 2007;14:26–32.
12. Fairey AS, Kassouf W, Estey E, Tanguay S, Rendon R, Bell D, Izawa J, Chin J, Kapoor A, Matsumoto E, Black P, So A, Lattouf JB, Saad F, Drachenberg D, Cagiannos I, Lacombe L, Fradet Y, Jacobsen NE. Comparison of oncological outcomes for open and laparoscopic radical nephroureterectomy: results from the Canadian Upper Tract Collaboration. BJU Int. 2012;112:791–7. doi:10.1111/j.1464-410X.2012.11474.x.
13. Favaretto RL, Shariat SF, Chade DC, Godoy G, Kaag M, Cronin AM, Bochner BH, Coleman J, Dalbagni G. Comparison between laparoscopic and open radical nephroureterectomy in a contemporary group of patients: are recurrence and disease-specific survival associated with surgical technique? Eur Urol. 2010;58:645–51.
14. Hsueh TY, Huang YH, Chiu AW, Shen KH, Lee YH. A comparison of the clinical outcome between open and hand-assisted laparoscopic nephroureterectomy for upper urinary tract transitional cell carcinoma. BJU Int. 2004;94:798–801.
15. Manabe D, Saika T, Ebara S, Uehara S, Nagai A, Fujita R, Irie S, Yamada D, Tsushima T, Nasu Y, et al. Comparative study of oncologic outcome of laparoscopic nephroureterectomy and standard nephroureterectomy for upper urinary tract transitional cell carcinoma. Urology. 2007;69:457–61.
16. Roupret M, Hupertan V, Sanderson KM, Harmon JD, Cathelineau X, Barret E, Vallancien G, Rozet F. Oncologic control after open or laparoscopic nephroureterectomy for upper urinary tract transitional cell carcinoma: a single center experience. Urology. 2007;69:656–61.

17. Waldert M, Remzi M, Klingler HC, Mueller L, Marberger M. The oncological results of laparoscopic nephroureterectomy for upper urinary tract transitional cell cancer are equal to those of open nephroureterectomy. BJU Int. 2009;103:66–70.
18. Capitanio U, Shariat SF, Isbarn H, Weizer A, Remzi M, Roscigno M, Kikuchi E, Raman JD, Bolenz C, Bensalah K, et al. Comparison of oncologic outcomes for open and laparoscopic nephroureterectomy: a multi-institutional analysis of 1249 cases. Eur Urol. 2009;56:1–9.
19. Cha EK, Shariat SF, Kormaksson M, Novara G, Chromecki TF, Scherr DS, Lotan Y, Raman JD, Kassouf W, Zigeuner R, et al. Predicting clinical outcomes after radical nephroureterectomy for upper tract urothelial carcinoma. Eur Urol. 2012;61:818–25.
20. Isbarn H, Jeldres C, Shariat SF, Liberman D, Sun M, Lughezzani G, Widmer H, Arjane P, Pharand D, Fisch M, et al. Location of the primary tumor is not an independent predictor of cancer specific mortality in patients with upper urinary tract urothelial carcinoma. J Urol. 2009;182:2177–81.
21. Favaretto RL, Shariat SF, Chade DC, Godoy G, Adamy A, Kaag M, Bochner BH, Coleman J, Dalbagni G. The effect of tumor location on prognosis in patients treated with radical nephroureterectomy at Memorial Sloan-Kettering Cancer Center. Eur Urol. 2010;58:574–80.
22. Roscigno M, Shariat SF, Freschi M, Margulis V, Karakiewizc P, Suardi N, Remzi M, Zigeuner R, Bolenz C, Kikuchi E, Weizer A, Bensalah K, Sagalowsky A, Koppie TM, Raman J, Fernández M, Ströbel P, Kabbani W, Langner C, Wheat J, Guo CC, Kassouf W, Haitel A, Wood CG, Montorsi F. Assessment of the minimum number of lymph nodes needed to detect lymph node invasion at radical nephroureterectomy in patients with upper tract urothelial cancer. Urology. 2009;74:1070–4.
23. Roscigno M, Shariat SF, Margulis V, Karakiewicz P, Remzi M, Kikuchi E, Zigeuner R, Weizer A, Sagalowsky A, Bensalah K, Raman JD, Bolenz C, Kassou W, Koppie TM, Wood CG, Wheat J, Langner C, Ng CK, Capitanio U, Bertini R, Fernández MI, Mikami S, Isida M, Ströbel P, Montorsi F. The extent of lymphadenectomy seems to be associated with better survival in patients with nonmetastatic upper-tract urothelial carcinoma: how many lymph nodes should be removed? Eur Urol. 2009;56:512–8.
24. Kondo T, Nakazawa H, Ito F, Hashimoto Y, Toma H, Tanabe K. Impact of the extent of regional lymphadenectomy on the survival of patients with urothelial carcinoma of the upper urinary tract. J Urol. 2007;178:1212–7.
25. Lughezzani G, Jeldres C, Isbarn H, Shariat SF, Sun M, Pharand D, Widmer H, Arjane P, Graefen M, Montorsi F, Perrotte P, Karakiewicz PI. A critical appraisal of the value of lymph node dissection at nephroureterectomy for upper tract urothelial carcinoma. Urology. 2010;75:118–24.
26. Ouzzane A, Colin P, Ghoneim TP, Zerbib M, De La Taille A, Audenet F, Saint F, Hoarau N, Adam E, Azemar MD, Bensadoun H, Cormier L, Cussenot O, Houlgatte A, Karsenty G, Maurin C, Nouhaud FX, Phe V, Polguer T, Roumiguié M, Ruffion A, Rouprêt M. The impact of lymph node status and features on oncological outcomes in urothelial carcinoma of the upper urinary tract (UTUC) treated by nephroureterectomy. World J Urol. 2013;31:189–97.
27. Mason RJ, Kassouf W, Bell DG, Lacombe L, Kapoor A, Jacobsen N, Fairey A, Izawa J, Black P, Tanguay S, Chin J, So A, Lattouf JB, Saad F, Matsumoto E, Drachenberg D, Cagiannos I, Fradet Y, Rendon RA. The contemporary role of lymph node dissection during nephroureterectomy in the management of upper urinary tract urothelial carcinoma: the Canadian experience. Urology. 2012;79:840–5.
28. Kondo T, Hashimoto Y, Kobayashi H, Iizuka J, Nakazawa H, Ito F, Tanabe K. Template-based lymphadenectomy in urothelial carcinoma of the upper urinary tract: impact on patient survival. Int J Urol. 2010;17:848–54.
29. Roscigno M, Shariat SF, Margulis V, Karakiewicz P, Remzi M, Kikuchi E, Langner C, Lotan Y, Weizer A, Bensalah K, Raman JD, Bolenz C, Guo CC, Wood CG, Zigeuner R, Wheat J, Kabbani W, Koppie TM, Ng CK, Suardi N, Bertini R, Fernández MI, Mikami S, Isida M, Michel MS, Montorsi F. Impact of lymph node dissection on cancer specific survival in patients with upper tract urothelial carcinoma treated with radical nephroureterectomy. J Urol. 2009;181:2482–9.

30. Burger M, Shariat SF, Fritsche HM, Martinez-Salamanca JI, Matsumoto K, Chromecki TF, Ficarra V, Kassouf W, Seitz C, Pycha A, Tritschler S, Walton TJ, Novara G. No overt influence of lymphadenectomy on cancer-specific survival in organ-confined versus locally advanced upper urinary tract urothelial carcinoma undergoing radical nephroureterectomy: a retrospective international, multi-institutional study. World J Urol. 2011;29:465–72.
31. Phé V, Coussenot O, Bitker MO, Rouprêt M. Does the surgical technique for management of the distal ureter influence the outcome after nephroureterectomy? BJU Int. 2011;108:130–8.
32. Kakizoe T, Fujita J, Murase T, Matsumoto K, Kishi K. Transitional cell carcinoma of the bladder in patients with renal pelvic and ureteral cancer. J Urol. 1980;124:17–9.
33. Strong DW, Pearse HD, Tank Jr ES, Hodges CV. The ureteral stump after nephroureterectomy. J Urol. 1976;115:654–5.
34. Strong DW, Pearse HD. Recurrent urothelial tumors following surgery for transitional cell carcinoma of the upper urinary tract. Cancer. 1976;38:2173–83.
35. Zigeuner R, Pummer K. Urothelial carcinoma of the upper urinary tract: surgical approach and prognostic factors. Eur Urol. 2008;53:720–31.
36. Matin SF, Gill IS. Recurrence and survival following laparoscopic radical nephroureterectomy with various forms of bladder cuff control. J Urol. 2005;173:395–400.
37. Shalhav AL, Dunn MD, Portis AJ, Elbahnasy AM, McDougall EM, Clayman RV. Laparoscopic nephroureterectomy for upper tract transitional cell cancer: the Washington University experience. J Urol. 2000;163:1100–4.
38. Romero FR, Schaeffer EM, Muntener M, Trock B, Kavoussi LR, Jarrett TW. Oncologic outcomes of extravesical stapling of distal ureter in laparoscopic nephroureterectomy. J Endourol. 2007;21:1025–7.
39. Hattori R, Yoshino Y, Komatsu T, Matsukawa Y, Ono Y, Gotoh M. Pure laparoscopic complete excision of distal ureter with a bladder cuff for upper tract urothelial carcinoma. World J Urol. 2009;27:253–8.
40. Gill IS, Soble JJ, Miller SD, Sung GT. A novel technique for management of the en bloc bladder cuff and distal ureter during laparoscopic nephroureterectomy. J Urol. 1999;161:430–4.
41. McDonald HP, Upchurch W, Sturdevant CE. Nephro-ureterectomy: a new technique. J Urol. 1952;67:804–9.
42. Agarwal DK, Khaira HS, Clarke D, Tong R. Modified transurethral technique for the management of distal ureter during laparoscopic assisted nephroureterectomy. Urology. 2008;71:740–3.
43. Azémar MD, Comperat E, Richard F, Cussenot O, Rouprêt M. Bladder recurrence after surgery for upper urinary tract urothelial cell carcinoma: frequency, risk factors, and surveillance. Urol Oncol. 2011;29:130–6.
44. Steinberg JR, Matin SF. Laparoscopic radical nephroureterectomy: dilemma of the distal ureter. Curr Opin Urol. 2004;14:61–5.
45. Laguna MP, de la Rossette JJ. The endoscopic approach to the distal ureter in nephroureterectomy for upper urinary tract tumor. J Urol. 2001;166:2017–22.
46. Palou J, Caparros J, Orsola A, Xavier B, Vicente J. Transurethral resection of the intramural ureter as the first step of nephroureterectomy. J Urol. 1995;154:43–4.
47. Lughezzani G, Sun M, Perrotte P, Shariat SF, Jeldres C, Budaus L, Alasker A, Duclos A, Widmer H, Latour M, Guazzoni G, Montorsi F, Karakiewicz PI. Should bladder cuff excision remain the standard of care at nephroureterectomy in patients with urothelial carcinoma of the renal pelvis? A population-based study. Eur Urol. 2010;57:956–62.
48. Li WM, Shen JT, Li CC, Ke HL, Wei YC, Wu WJ, Chou YH, Huang CH. Oncologic outcomes following three different approaches to the distal ureter and bladder cuff in nephroureterectomy for primary upper urinary tract urothelial carcinoma. Eur Urol. 2010;57:963–9.
49. Xylinas E, Rink M, Cha EK, Clozel T, Lee RK, Fajkovic H, Comploj E, Novara G, Margulis V, Raman JD, Lotan Y, Kassouf W, Fritsche HM, Weizer A, Martinez-Salamanca JI, Matsumoto K, Zigeuner R, Pycha A, Scherr DS, Seitz C, Walton T, Trinh QD, Karakiewicz PI, Matin S, Montorsi F, Zerbib M, Shariat SF, for the Upper Tract Urothelial Carcinoma Collaboration. Impact of distal ureter management on oncologic outcomes following radical nephroureterectomy

for upper tract urothelial carcinoma. Eur Urol. 2012;65:210–7. doi:10.1016/j.eururo.2012.04.052.
50. Roupret M, Zigeuner R, Palou J, Boehle A, Kaasinen E, Sylvester R, Babjuk M, Oosterlinck W. European guidelines for the diagnosis and management of upper urinary tract urothelial cell carcinomas: 2011 update. Eur Urol. 2011;59:584–94.
51. Chen GL, Bagley DH. Ureteroscopic management of upper tract transitional cell carcinoma in patients with normal contralateral kidneys. J Urol. 2000;164:1173–6.
52. Elliott DS, Segura JW, Lightner D, Patterson DE, Blute ML. Is nephroureterectomy necessary in all cases of upper tract transitional cell carcinoma? Long-term results of conservative endourologic management of upper tract transitional cell carcinoma in individuals with a normal contralateral kidney. Urology. 2001;58:174–8.
53. Thompson RH, Krambeck AE, Lohse CM, Elliott DS, Patterson DE, Blute ML. Endoscopic management of upper tract transitional cell carcinoma in patients with normal contralateral kidneys. Urology. 2008;71:713–7.
54. Bian Y, Ehya H, Bagley DH. Cytologic diagnosis of upper urinary tract neoplasms by ureteroscopic sampling. Acta Cytol. 1995;39:733–40.
55. Keeley Jr FX, Bibbo M, Bagley DH. Ureteroscopic treatment and surveillance of upper urinary tract transitional cell carcinoma. J Urol. 1997;157:1560–5.
56. Valeri A, et al. The oncologic impact of a delay between diagnosis and radical nephroureterectomy due to diagnostic ureteroscopy in upper urinary tract urothelial carcinomas: results from a large collaborative database. World J Urol. 2013;31:69–76.
57. Hendin BN, Streem SB, Levin HS, Klein EA, Novick AC. Impact of diagnostic ureteroscopy on long-term survival in patients with upper tract transitional cell carcinoma. J Urol. 1999;161:783–5.
58. Boorjian S, Ng C, Munver R, Palese MA, Vaughan Jr ED, Sosa RE, Del Pizzo JJ, Scherr DS. Impact of delay to nephroureterectomy for patients undergoing ureteroscopic biopsy and laser tumor ablation of upper tract transitional cell carcinoma. Urology. 2005;66:283–7.
59. Keeley FX, Kulp DA, Bibbo M, McCue PA, Bagley DH. Diagnostic accuracy of ureteroscopic biopsy in upper tract transitional cell carcinoma. J Urol. 1997;157:33–7.
60. Murphy DM, Zincke H, Furlow WL. Primary grade 1 transitional cell carcinoma of the renal pelvis and ureter. J Urol. 1980;123:629–31.
61. Brown GA, Matin SF, Busby JE, Dinney CP, Grossman HB, Pettaway CA, Munsell MF, Kamat AM. Ability of clinical grade to predict final pathologic stage in upper urinary tract transitional cell carcinoma: implications for therapy. Urology. 2007;70:252–6.
62. Daneshmand S, Quek ML, Huffman JL. Endoscopic management of upper urinary tract transitional cell carcinoma: long-term experience. Cancer. 2003;98:55–60.
63. Colin P, Ouzzane A, Pignot G, Ravier E, Crouzet S, Ariane MM, Audouin M, Neuzillet Y, Albouy B, Hurel S, et al. Comparison of oncological outcomes after segmental ureterectomy or radical nephroureterectomy in urothelial carcinomas of the upper urinary tract: results from a large French multicentre study. BJU Int. 2012;110:1134–41.
64. Simonato A, Varca V, Gregori A, Benelli A, Ennas M, Lissiani A, Gacci M, De Stefani S, Rosso M, Benvenuto S, et al. Elective segmental ureterectomy for transitional cell carcinoma of the ureter: long-term follow-up in a series of 73 patients. BJU Int. 2012;110:744–9.
65. Herr HW, Cookson MS, Soloway SM. Upper tract tumors in patients with primary bladder cancer followed for 15 years. J Urol. 1996;156:1286–7.
66. Uberoi J, Harnisch B, Sethi AS, Babayan RK, Wang DS. Robot-assisted laparoscopic distal ureterectomy and ureteral reimplantation with psoas hitch. J Endourol. 2007;21:368–73. discussion 372-3.
67. Basiri A, Karami H, Mehrabi S, Javaherforooshzadeh A. Laparoscopic distal ureterectomy and Boari flap ureteroneocystostomy for a low-grade distal ureteral tumor. Urol J. 2008;5:120–2.
68. Glinianski M, Guru KA, Zimmerman G, Mohler J, Kim HL. Robot-assisted ureterectomy and ureteral reconstruction for urothelial carcinoma. J Endourol. 2009;23:97–100.
69. McClain PD, Mufarrij PW, Hemal AK. Robot-assisted reconstructive surgery for ureteral malignancy: analysis of efficacy and oncologic outcomes. J Endourol. 2012;26:1614–7.

70. Naderi N, Nieuwenhuijzen JA, Bex A, Kooistra A, Horenblas S. Port site metastasis after laparoscopic nephro-ureterectomy for transitional cell carcinoma. Eur Urol. 2004;46:440–1.
71. Rink M, Sjoberg D, Comploj E, Margulis V, Xylinas E, Lee RK, Hansen J, Cha EK, Raman JD, Remzi M, Bensalah K, Novara G, Matin SF, Chun FK, Kikuchi E, Kassouf W, Martinez-Salamanca JI, Lotan Y, Seitz C, Pycha A, Zigeuner R, Karakiewicz PI, Scherr DS, Vickers AJ, Shariat SF. Risk of cancer-specific mortality following recurrence after radical nephroureterectomy. Ann Surg Oncol. 2012;19:4337–44.
72. Casale P, Grady RW, Lee RS, Joyner BD, Mitchell ME. Symptomatic refluxing distal ureteral stumps after nephroureterectomy and heminephroureterectomy. What should we do? J Urol. 2005;173:204–6.
73. Ashley MS, Daneshmand S. Re: Appendiceal substitution following right proximal ureter injury. Int Braz J Urol. 2009;35:90–1.
74. Pettersson S, Brynger H, Henriksson C, Johansson SL, Nilson AE, Ranch T. Treatment of urothelial tumors of the upper urinary tract by nephroureterectomy, renal autotransplantation, and pyelocystostomy. Cancer. 1984;54:379–86.
75. Lieber MM, Lupu AN. High grade invasive ureteral transitional cell carcinoma with a congenital solitary kidney: long-term survival after ureterectomy and radiation therapy. J Urol. 1978;120:368–9.
76. Lughezzani G, Jeldres C, Isbarn H, Sun M, Shariat SF, Alasker A, Pharand D, Widmer H, Arjane P, Graefen M, et al. Nephroureterectomy and segmental ureterectomy in the treatment of invasive upper tract urothelial carcinoma: a population-based study of 2299 patients. Eur J Cancer. 2009;45:3291–7.
77. Jeldres C, Lughezzani G, Sun M, Isbarn H, Shariat SF, Budaus L, Lattouf JB, Widmer H, Graefen M, Montorsi F, et al. Segmental ureterectomy can safely be performed in patients with transitional cell carcinoma of the ureter. J Urol. 2010;183:1324–9.
78. Cutress ML, Stewart GD, Wells-Cole S, Phipps S, Thomas BG, Tolley DA. Long-term endoscopic management of upper tract urothelial carcinoma: 20-year single-centre experience. BJU Int. 2012;110:1608–17.
79. Gadzinski AJ, Roberts WW, Faerber GJ, Wolf Jr JS. Long-term outcomes of nephroureterectomy versus endoscopic management for upper tract urothelial carcinoma. J Urol. 2010;183:2148–53.
80. Roupret M, Hupertan V, Traxer O, Loison G, Chartier-Kastler E, Conort P, Bitker MO, Gattegno B, Richard F, Cussenot O. Comparison of open nephroureterectomy and ureteroscopic and percutaneous management of upper urinary tract transitional cell carcinoma. Urology. 2006;67:1181–7.
81. Lucas SM, Svatek RS, Olgin G, Arriaga Y, Kabbani W, Sagalowsky AI, Lotan Y. Conservative management in selected patients with upper tract urothelial carcinoma compares favourably with early radical surgery. BJU Int. 2008;102:172–6.
82. Grasso M, Fishman AI, Cohen J, Alexander B. Ureteroscopic and extirpative treatment of upper urinary tract urothelial carcinoma: a 15-year comprehensive review of 160 consecutive patients. BJU Int. 2012;110:1618–26.
83. Babjuk M. What are the limitations of endoscopic management of urothelial carcinoma of the upper urinary tract? Eur Urol. 2011;60:961–3.
84. Lee BR, Jabbour ME, Marshall FF, Smith AD, Jarrett TW. 13-year survival comparison of percutaneous and open nephroureterectomy approaches for management of transitional cell carcinoma of renal collecting system: equivalent outcomes. J Endourol. 1999;13:289–94.
85. Rastinehad AR, Ost MC, Vanderbrink BA, Greenberg KL, El-Hakim A, Marcovich R, Badlani GH, Smith AD. A 20-year experience with percutaneous resection of upper tract transitional carcinoma: is there an oncologic benefit with adjuvant bacillus Calmette Guerin therapy? Urology. 2009;73:27–31.
86. Huang A, Low RK, deVere White R. Nephrostomy tract tumor seeding following percutaneous manipulation of a ureteral carcinoma. J Urol. 1995;153:1041–2.
87. Treuthardt C, Danuser H, Studer UE. Tumor seeding following percutaneous antegrade treatment of transitional cell carcinoma in the renal pelvis. Eur Urol. 2004;46:442–3.

88. Rastinehad AR, Smith AD. Bacillus Calmette-Guerin for upper tract urothelial cancer: is there a role? J Endourol. 2009;23:563–8.
89. Kojima Y, Tozawa K, Kawai N, Sasaki S, Hayashi Y, Kohri K. Long-term outcome of upper urinary tract carcinoma in situ: effectiveness of nephroureterectomy versus bacillus Calmette-Guerin therapy. Int J Urol. 2006;13:340–4.
90. Giannarini G, Kessler TM, Birkhäuser FD, Thalmann GN, Studer UE. Antegrade perfusion with bacillus Calmette-Guerin in patients with non-muscle invasive urothelial carcinoma of the upper urinary tract: who may benefit? Eur Urol. 2011;60:955–60.
91. Azemar MD, Comperat E, Richard F, Cussenot O, Roupret M. Bladder cancer recurrence after surgery for upper tract urothelial cell carcinoma: frequency, risk factors, and surveillance. Urol Oncol. 2011;29:130–6.
92. O'Brien T, Ray E, Singh R, Coker R, Beard T, et al. Prevention of bladder tumours after nephroureterectomy for primary upper tract urothelial carcinoma: a prospective, multicenter, randomized trial of single postoperative intravesical dose of mitomycin C (the OMDIT-C Trial). Eur Urol. 2011;60:703–10.

Chapter 7
The Role of Lymphadenectomy in the Management of Urothelial Carcinoma of the Upper Urinary Tract

Tsunenori Kondo, Bernard H. Bochner, Siamak Daneshmand, and Alexandre R. Zlotta

Abstract Lymphadenectomy is considered as an integral part of radical surgery for urologic malignancies. Many studies have been conducted to confirm its benefit in improving staging accuracy or survival, including in patients with renal cell carcinoma, prostate cancer, and urothelial carcinoma of the bladder. In renal cell carcinoma, the European Organization for Research and Treatment of Cancer (EORTC) randomized phase 3 Trial 30881 failed to show any therapeutic benefit of lymphadenectomy. However, this trial has been criticized for enrolling patient at a low risk of lymph node metastases. Other studies have supported the hypothesis that lymphadenectomy may be beneficial in patients with high-risk renal cell carcinoma.

Keywords Lymph Node • Lymphadenectomy • Urothelial Carcinoma • Upper Urinary Tract • Management

---

T. Kondo, MD
Department of Urology, Tokyo Women's Medical University 8-1, Kawada-cho, Shinjuku-ku, Tokyo 162-8666, Japan
e-mail: tkondo@kc.twmu.ac.jp

B.H. Bochner, MD, FACS
Urology Service, Memorial Sloan-Kettering Cancer Center, 353 E. 68th Street, New York, NY 10065, USA
e-mail: bochnerb@MSKCC.ORG

S. Daneshmand, MD
Urologic Oncology, Institute of Urology, University of Southern California, Los Angeles, CA, USA
e-mail: daneshma@med.usc.edu

A.R. Zlotta, MD, PhD, FRCSC (✉)
Division of Urology, Department of Surgery and Division of Urology, Department of Surgical Oncology, Mount Sinai Hospital, Princess Margaret Cancer Centre/University Health Network and University of Toronto, Toronto, ON, Canada
e-mail: azlotta@mtsinai.on.ca

© Springer Science+Business Media New York 2015
S.F. Shariat, E. Xylinas (eds.), *Upper Tract Urothelial Carcinoma*, DOI 10.1007/978-1-4939-1501-9_7

Introduction

Lymphadenectomy is considered as an integral part of radical surgery for urologic malignancies [1]. Many studies have been conducted to confirm its benefit in improving staging accuracy or survival, including in patients with renal cell carcinoma [2], prostate cancer [3], and urothelial carcinoma of the bladder [4]. In renal cell carcinoma, the European Organization for Research and Treatment of Cancer (EORTC) randomized phase 3 Trial 30881 failed to show any therapeutic benefit of lymphadenectomy [5] . However, this trial has been criticized for enrolling patient at a low risk of lymph node metastases. Other studies have supported the hypothesis that lymphadenectomy may be beneficial in patients with high-risk renal cell carcinoma [2, 6].

A limited benefit in staging has been anticipated with extended lymphadenectomy in patients with locally advanced disease [6].

The relatively low incidence of lymphatic metastases in renal cell carcinoma or in prostate cancer may explain the reason for the lack of consensus on the therapeutic role for the use of lymphadenectomy in these diseases [2, 7, 8]. Another explanation is that a multi-modality approach for combining surgery and effective systemic therapy like chemotherapy is likely to explain improvements in survival rather than lymphadenectomy by itself.

In contrast, urothelial carcinoma arising from the upper urinary tract (UCUT) of the urinary bladder develops lymphatic metastases at a relatively higher incidence (20–40 %) compared to the other urologic malignancies possibly given its anatomical specificities (thin wall and lymphovascular supply) [9, 10]. Moreover, a stage and grade migration over time towards more aggressive disease has been reported in UCUT when comparing cases from 1983 to 2004 [11]. Recent reports on bladder cancer support a staging and therapeutic role for extended lymphadenectomy including the common iliac and presacral nodes [12, 13]. The level of evidence in guidelines supporting the use of an extended lymphadenectomy remains low (level 3) though, due to the lack of randomized studies or standardization of the optimal extent of lymphadenectomy [14, 15].

Because of the biological similarity between UC of the upper and lower urinary tract, a possible role and benefit of lymphadenectomy in UCUT makes some sense.

In this chapter, we will describe the current status regarding the role of regional lymphadenectomy in UCUT. Although many questions remain unanswered about the role of lymphadenectomy during nephroureterectomy, we will focus on the boundaries of regional lymph node dissection (LND), its staging and therapeutic benefit, and the role of lymph node measurements (i.e. LN counts, number of positive LNs and LN density).

The History of Lymphadenectomy in UCUT

Lymphatic metastases are commonly found in UCUT with an incidence of 30–40 % [11, 16]. Thus, lymphadenectomy was suggested as an essential part of radical nephroureterectomy from the 1970s [17]. However, the extent and template for lymphadenectomy was not clearly described. Some mapping studies were conducted in the 1980s showing that lymphatic metastatic spread from UCUT was primarily to the para-aortic and para-caval nodes and that from the distal ureter spread to the pelvic nodes [11, 18, 19]. However until the 1990s, the optimal extent of dissection was not established and it was not clear whether lymphadenectomy had any role in improving the staging accuracy or patient survival.

In the 1990s, two studies were published examining the role of lymphadenectomy. Komatsu et al. reported that cancer-specific survival (CSS) was higher in patients without lymphatic metastases (pN0) than those with lymph node involvement (pN+), demonstrating that prognostic information was gained by properly staging the regional LNs by lymphadenectomy [20]. However, any therapeutic benefit for lymphadenectomy was unclear from this study. Miyake et al. suggested that lymphadenectomy may improve CSS in selected patients without lymph vessel invasion [21]. These studies raised a discussion about the therapeutic role of lymphadenectomy in patients with UCUT, but a major limitation was their small sample size.

The Boundary of Regional Lymph Nodes

As mentioned above, early mapping studies conducted in the 1980s showed that lymphatic spread from the renal pelvis and the upper/mid ureter primarily reached to the renal hilar, abdominal para-aortic, and para-caval nodes while the drainage of the distal ureter was primarily to the intrapelvic nodes [11, 18, 19]. This description is still referenced in the latest TNM classification [22].

In 2007, Kondo et al. reported detailed mapping studies of lymph nodes from 42 patients with lymph node metastases by using surgical specimens or radiological findings [23]. They examined the nodal sites of primary metastases according to the location of the tumors (renal pelvis, upper and middle ureter, and lower ureter). They showed that the primary metastatic sites encompassed a wider area for tumors of the right renal pelvis and the upper two-thirds of the right ureter as compared with what was previously assumed [23]. The updated results of this mapping study were published later on, increasing the number of patients up to 75 (Table 7.1) [24]. The primary sites of lymphatic metastases were the right renal hilar, para-caval, retro-caval, and interaorto-caval nodes for tumors of the right renal pelvis. Those of the upper and middle ureter also spread primarily to the right renal hilar, retro-caval, and interaorto-caval nodes. The left renal hilar and para-aortic nodes were the primary metastatic sites from the tumors of the left renal pelvis, as well as for the upper and middle ureter. The lower boundary was at the level of the inferior mesenteric artery for tumors of the renal pelvis and that of the aortic bifurcation for tumors of the upper and middle ureter. Ipsilateral pelvic nodes including the common iliac, external iliac, obturator, internal iliac, and presacral nodes were the primary sites of nodal involvement in tumors of the lower ureter. Strong and definitive conclusions have to been tempered though because of the reduced number of tumors evaluated at each site.

Table 7.1 Summary of the primary sites of nodal involvement according to the location of the tumor

Location of the primary tumor (no. of patients with nodal metastasis)		Suprahilar	Hilar	Para-caval	Retro-caval	Interaorto-caval	Para-aortic	Common iliac	External iliac	Obturator	Internal iliac	Presacral
Right	RP (22)	–	14 (84 %)	8 (36 %)	9 (41 %)	3 (14 %)	–	–	–	–	–	
	UU (3)	–	1 (33 %)	–	1 (33 %)	2 (66 %)	–	–	–	–	–	
	MU (5)	–	–	–	1 (20 %)	4 (80 %)	–	–	–	–	–	
	LU (7)	–	–	–	–	–	–	4 (57 %)	1 (14 %)	5 (71 %)	2 (29 %)	1 (14 %)
Left	RP (25)	–	20 (80 %)	–	–	1 (4 %)	11 (44 %)	–	–	–	–	
	UU (0)	–	–	–	–	–	–	–	–	–	–	
	MU (5)	–	–	–	–	–	5 (100 %)	–	–	–	–	
	LU (8)	–	–	–	–	–	–	4 (50 %)	2 (25 %)	3 (38 %)	1 (13 %)	

R-RP right renal pelvis, *R-UU* right upper ureter, *R-MU* right middle ureter, *R-LU* right lower ureter, *L-RP* left renal pelvis, *L-UU* left upper ureter, *L-MU* left middle ureter, *L-LU* left lower ureter

From Kondo T, Tanabe K. Role of lymphadenectomy in the management of urothelial carcinoma of the bladder and the upper urinary tract. Int J Urol. 2012:19:710–21

Assouad et al. reported on the lymphatic drainage from the kidney using adult cadavers [25]. The lymphatic flow from the right kidney travels through both the anterior and posterior aspect of the inferior vena cava whereas on the left it connects to the left renal hilar and/or the para-aortic nodes. The results from their basic studies are very similar to those of the mapping study in the clinical setting reported by Kondo.

Based on the findings from these two studies, Kondo et al. currently propose dissecting the regional lymph nodes within a defined anatomical extent in which the incidence of metastasis is in the 10 % or more range (Fig. 7.1) [24]. They recently reported the results of a prospective study confirming the survival benefit of lymphadenectomy in tumors of the renal pelvis using this anatomical template [26]. The rationale of the template for renal pelvic cancer appears to be supported by this study. However, this template needs to be validated by other studies examining lymph node mapping in UCUT.

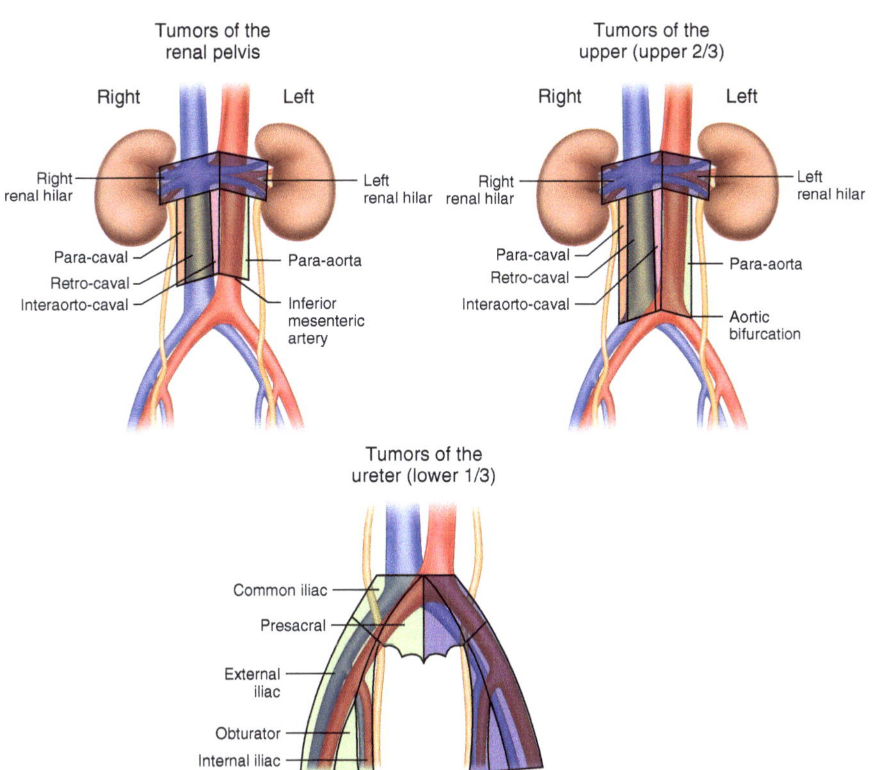

Fig. 7.1 Template of the anatomical lymph node dissection extent

Staging Benefits of Lymphadenectomy in UCUT

Improved staging is one of the expected advantages of lymphadenectomy. It may provide more accurate stratification of patients according to lymph node metastases status. In bladder cancer, the staging benefit of extending the template of lymphadenectomy has been thoroughly studied. The incidence of node-positive disease increases as the number of lymph nodes retrieved becomes higher by extending the cranial boundary of lymphadenectomy from below the bifurcation of the common iliac artery to that of the aortic bifurcation [14, 27–29]. Thus, extended lymphadenectomy is likely to improve the staging accuracy in bladder cancer although the optimal template remains debated and the extent of the benefit probably limited. Indeed a more thorough PLND and subsequently more LNs evaluated improve staging; however mapping data suggests that LN spread to the common arteries or above in the absence of LN involvement in the lower packets is a rare event, likely no more than 6–7 %.

In UCUT, Komatsu et al. examined the efficacy of a wide template of lymphadenectomy in the improvement of staging accuracy in 36 patients [20]. They used a wide template for lymphadenectomy similar to that proposed by Kondo and colleagues [24]. A clear stratification of patients with nodal involvement (pN+) was observed, with lower CSS than those without nodal metastases (pN0) [18]. Roscigno et al. reported that patients with pN0 confirmed by lymphadenectomy had a higher 5-year CSS than those without lymphadenectomy (pNx) (73 % versus 48 %, $p<0.001$) [30]. They also used a similar template in their study. Five-year CSS did not significantly differ between patients with pNx and those with pN+(48 % versus 39 %, $p=0.476$).

Results from several multi-institutional studies have been published, as shown in Table 7.2. Roscigno et al. collected data from 13 institutions and conducted a similar analysis, showing that the 5-year CSS increases incrementally from pN+to pNx to pN0 (35 % vs 69 % vs 71 %, $p<0.001$ and $p=0.032$) in an analysis of 1,130 patients with pT1 or higher [31]. This difference became more obvious when they analyzed 813 patients with pT2 stage or higher (5-year CSS: 33 vs 58 vs 70 %, $p<0.001$ and $p=0.017$). Abe et al. also showed that survival free from any recurrence, including locoregional or distant recurrences, was significantly higher in patients with pN0 than those with pNx in patients with pT2 or higher [32]. In contrast, there was no significant difference in any recurrence-free survival between pN0 and pNx in patients with pT1. In patients with advanced disease, these two multi-institutional studies showed significantly higher survival of patients with pN0 than those with pNx (Fig. 7.2).

Other studies could not find an improvement in survival in patients with pN0, but reported worse survival rates in those with pN+than those with pNx. Burger et al. also examined the influence of lymph node status on patient survival in 785 patients from nine institutions [33]. They showed that lymphadenectomy can identify patients with pN+who have significantly lower CSS in both organ-confined disease and those with locally advanced disease. Stratification of the patients with pN0 in

Table 7.2 Reports on staging benefit of lymphadenectomy in UCUT

Authors	Year	Institute	Subject	No. of patients	Template of LND	Results	Staging benefits	References
Roscigno	2008	Single	≥pT2	132	Described	5y-CSS: pN0 73 % > pNx 48 % ($p<0.001$) = pN+39 % ($p=0.476$)	Yes	[30]
Roscigno	2009	Multi	≥pT1	1130	Not well described	5y-CSS: pN0 77 % > pNx 69 % ($p=0.032$) > pN+35 % ($p<0.001$)	Yes	[31]
			≥pT2	813		5y-CSS: pN0 70 % > pNx 58 % ($p=0.017$) > pN+33 % ($p<0.001$)		
Abe	2010	Multi	pT1	66	Not well described	RFS: pN0=pNx ($p=0.702$)	Yes in ≥pT2	[32]
			≥pT2	227		RFS: pN0>pNx ($p<0.001$) =pN+ ($p=0.134$)		
Burger	2011	Multi	Organ-confined	519	Not well described	CSS: pN0=pNx=pN+	Yes In locally advanced disease	[33]
			Locally advanced	266		CSS: pN0=pNx ($p=0.633$) >pN+ ($p<0.001$)		
Lughezzani	2010	Multi	pT1, pT2	1324	Not described	CSS: T1 pN0=pNx ($p=0.4$)=pN+ ($p=0.1$) T2 pN0=pNx ($p=0.8$)=pN+ ($p=0.1$)	Yes In ≥pT3	[34]
			pT3, pT4	1382		CSS: T3 pN0=pNx ($p=0.9$)>pN+ ($p<0.001$) T4 pN0=pNx ($p=0.3$)>pNx ($p<0.001$)		
Mason	2012	Multi	All patients	1029	Not described	OS: pN0 66.1 % = pNx 66.0 % ($p=0.617$) > pN+22.3 % ($p<0.01$)	Yes	[35]
Ouzzane	2013	Multi	All patients	714	Not described	5y-CSS: pN0 81 % = pNx 85 % ($p=0.6$) >pN+47 % ($p<0.001$)	Yes but in T1 ?	[36]
			≥pT2	337		CSS: pN0=pNx ($p=0.44$) =pN+ ($p<0.15$)		

LND lymphadenectomy, *CSS* cancer-specific survival, *RFS* recurrence-free survival, *LNs* lymph nodes, *CompLND* complete lymphadenectomy, *DFS* disease-free survival, *OS* overall survival

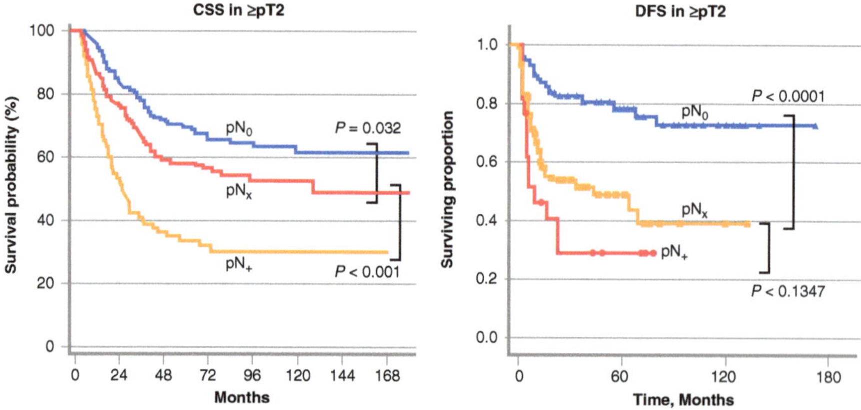

Fig. 7.2 Staging benefit of lymphadenectomy by stratification of patients with pN0 vs pNx. Adapted from Roscigno. J Urol. 2009: 181:2482 and Abe. Eur J Surg Oncol. 2010: 36:1085

terms of survival from those with pNx was possible only in locally advanced disease. Lughezzani et al. conducted a population-based study by using a surveillance, epidemiology, and end results (SEER) database [34]. Lymphadenectomy could not discriminate between patients with pN0 and those with pNx at any stage of the disease. Both in uni- (HR: 1.19; $p=.09$) and multivariate analysis pN(x) vs pN(0) status was not associated with worse survival (HR: 0.99; $p=.9$). Mason et al. collected data from 1,029 patients treated in ten institutions in Canada [35]. The number of positive nodes and the number of nodes removed were not associated with survival although it provided more accurate staging. Ouzzane et al. reported the multi-institutional results of 714 patients in France [36]. A better stratification through lymphadenectomy in patients with pN+was observed, but not in those with pN0 when they analyzed all patients. In contrast to other studies, CSS was not significantly different among these three groups in patients with pT2 or higher. It is unclear whether their results mean that a staging benefit is observed in patients with pT1 or lower. Representative results from Lughezzani et al. and Bergur et al. are shown in Fig. 7.3.

When summarizing these results in Table 7.2, two important points should be emphasized. The first is that all reports support a staging benefit. The results can be divided into two categories: those reporting a better patient stratification of pN0 from pNx, and those stratifying only pN+but not pN0 from pNx. In the studies reporting the latter results, the extent of lymphadenectomy was not described. The extent of lymphadenectomy may have influenced their results, but this remains to be determined. The second point is that this staging benefit appears to be more prominent in patients with muscle-invasive disease. Guidelines currently support a role for lymphadenectomy in the optimal staging of high-grade UCUT [37, 38]. However, it remains unknown what the minimally required extent of lymphadenectomy is for adequate staging purposes since the template of lymphadenectomy was not standardized in most of these studies. Of note, Xylinas et al. developed a pathological

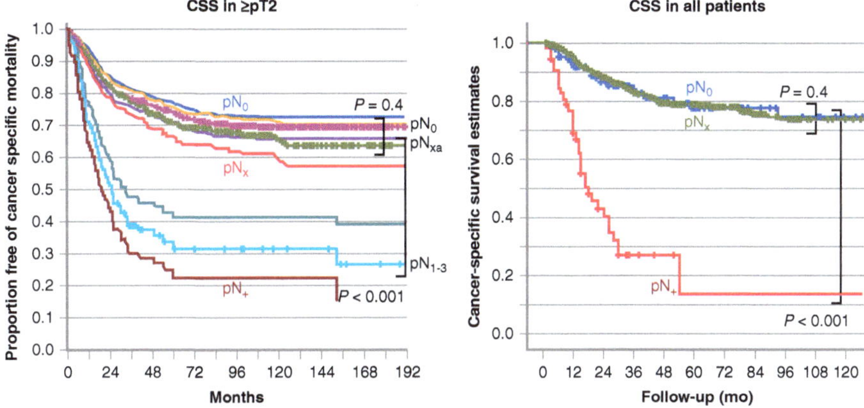

Fig. 7.3 Staging benefit of lymphadenectomy by stratification of patients with pN+vs pNx. Adapted from Lughezzani. Urology. 2010: 75:118 and Burger. World J Urol. 2011: 29:465

nodal staging model that allows quantification of the likelihood that a patient with pathologically node-negative disease has, indeed, no lymph node metastasis. This is the prediction of the true nodal status in patients with pathological lymph node-negative upper tract urothelial carcinoma at radical nephroureterectomy. The probability of missing lymph node metastasis decreased as the number of nodes examined increased. Even when five nodes were examined, 12 % of patients would have been misclassified. The proportion of those with a positive node increased with advancing pathological T stage and lymphovascular invasion [39].

Therapeutic Benefits of Lymphadenectomy in UCUT

In contrast to the staging benefit supported by most of the studies, the role of lymphadenectomy in UCUT in improving patient survival still remains controversial. One reason behind the difficulties in proving the therapeutic benefits of lymphadenectomy is that in patients with micro-metastatic disease captured by lymph node dissection, a major part of the benefit is likely driven by adjuvant chemotherapy, not necessarily the surgical removal of the nodes themselves, which serves as a staging procedure. Extrapolating evidence obtained from experience with multimodal therapy of patients with urothelial bladder cancer, additional improvements in oncological outcomes for patients with UTUC are likely to be achieved through integration of effective systemic chemotherapy in addition to the local control and staging provided by surgery [40]. In addition, especially for patients suffering from advanced tumor stages, survival rates have not dramatically improved over the last decades with distant metastases being one of the main reasons for treatment failure. Chemotherapy in an adjuvant or neoadjuvant setting seems therefore to be a promising approach worth exploring which may further blur the true survival benefit of lymphadenectomy in UTUC [41].

Several studies from single institutions have suggested an improvement in patient survival by performing lymphadenectomy.

Kondo et al. compared patient survival according to lymphadenectomy status [42]. They first determined that regional node metastases were observed in 30 % or more of patients based on their mapping study [23]. They divided their retrospective cohort into three subgroups, including patients for whom the regional nodes were all dissected (complete lymphadenectomy (CompLND)); those in whom lymphadenectomy did not include all regional sites (incomplete lymphadenectomy (IncompLND)); and those without lymphadenectomy (No-LND). CSS was not significantly different among the three groups when all patients were included. But the survival rate increased incrementally from No-LND to IncompLND to CompLND in 88 patients with pT3 or higher (Fig. 7.4). The difference in CSS between CompLND and No-LND was statistically significant. Moreover, CompLND was found to be a significant independent factor to reduce the risk of cancer-specific mortality. They conducted their revised analysis by increasing the number of the patients to 191 with pT2 or higher and 140 with pT3 or higher [24]. CompLND significantly improved CSS compared to IncompLND or No-LND in patients with pT2 or higher ($p=0.03$) and in those with pT3 or higher ($p=0.01$) (Fig. 7.4). Brausi et al. examined the influence of lymphadenectomy on a relatively wide scale in 82 patients with pT2 or higher [43]. The extent of lymphadenectomy they used was as follows: the para-aorta or para-caval between the renal hilus and the inferior mesenteric artery for renal pelvis or upper ureteric cancers; the para-aorta or para-caval, between the renal hilus and bifurcation of the common iliac artery for mid-ureteric cancers; and the pelvic nodes on the ipsilateral side for lower ureteric cancers. The disease-specific survival (DFS) of 40 patients with lymphadenectomy was higher than in those with No-LND (81.6 % versus 44.8 %, $p=0.007$) (Fig. 7.5). They also showed LND as a significant independent factor to reduce the risk of

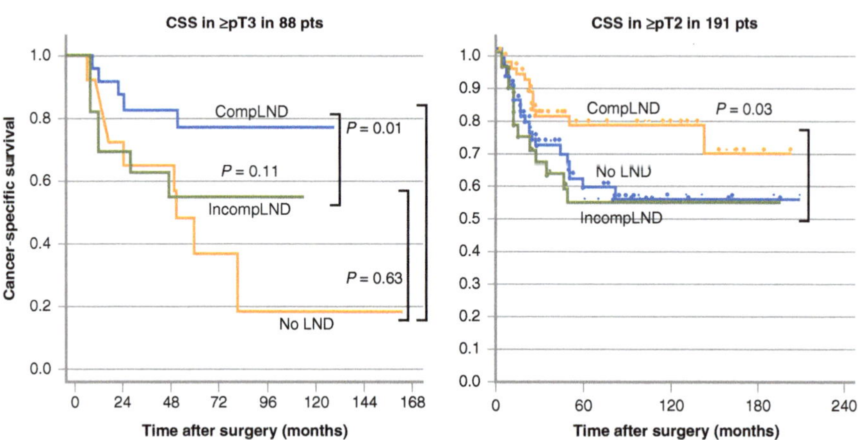

Fig. 7.4 Cancer-specific survival according to the status of lymphadenectomy. Adapted from Kondo. J Urol. 2007: 178:1212 and Kondo. Int J Urol. 2012: 19:710

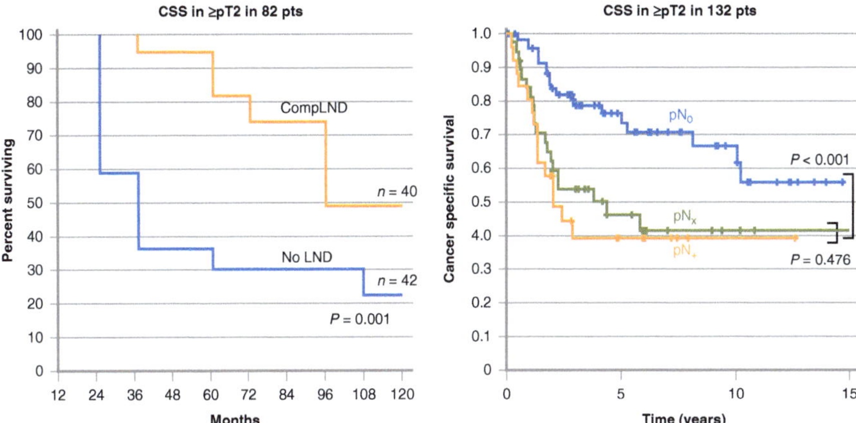

Fig. 7.5 Survival benefit of lymphadenectomy in advanced disease. Adapted from Brausi. Eur Urol. 2007: 52:1414 and Roscigno. Eur Urol. 2008: 53:794

cancer-specific mortality. It should be mentioned though that these studies were non-randomized, therefore preventing strong and definitive conclusions. Roscigno et al. conducted a similar study in the retrospective cohort of 132 patients with pT2 or higher [30, 44]. The extent of lymphadenectomy was also similar to that used in the study by Brausi [43]. Lymphadenectomy significantly improved CSS of the patients compared to those with No-LND (5 year CSS: 57 % versus 40 %, $p=0.01$). They also showed a higher 5-year CSS in patients with pN0 than in those with pNx (72 % versus 39 %, $p<0.001$), emphasizing the prognostic disadvantage of omitting lymphadenectomy (Figure 7.5). Multivariate analysis showed that lymphadenectomy and pN0 status were significant independent predictors for CSS.

Several multi-institutional studies have been published on this very topic with diverging results. Multi-institutional studies have an advantage in that the results are confirmed with a large number of patients. On the other hand, the drawback is the lack of standardization of the extent of lymphadenectomy. Therefore results should be interpreted with caution. The results of a study involving 1,130 patients from 13 international institutes reported by Roscigno showed no therapeutic benefit from LND. Five-year CSS did not significantly differ between the patients with LND and those without (66 % vs 69 %, $p=0.23$) [31]. They further examined the influence of the extent of lymphadenectomy on patient survival in patients with ≥ pT1pN0 using the same data set [44]. In 552 patients who underwent lymphadenectomy, CSS was significantly higher in patients for whom 8 or more LNs were removed than for those with an LN yield of less than 8 (84 % versus 73 %, $p=0.038$), and the number of LNs removed independently influenced the CSS of patients (Fig. 7.6). This could also represent stage migration due to improved LN staging and not necessarily be related to a real therapeutic benefit.

In addition, the risk of cancer-specific mortality continued to decrease as the number of the lymph nodes removed increased (Fig. 7.6).

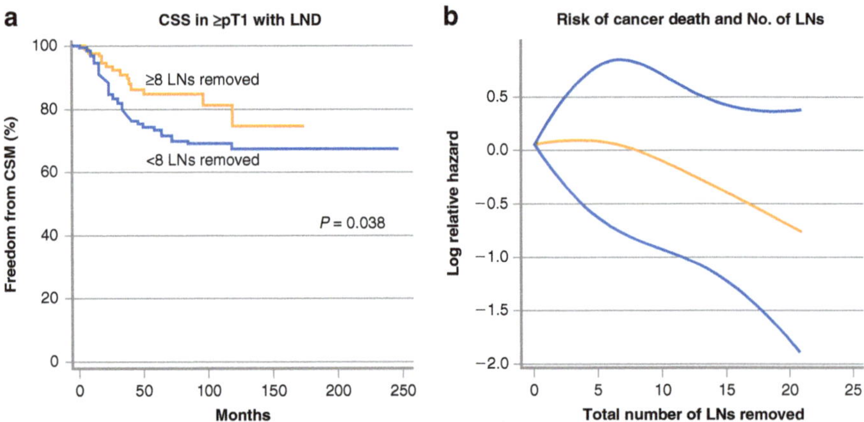

Fig. 7.6 Influence of LND extent influencing on patient survival. Adapted from Roscigno. Eur Urol. 2009: 56:512

Abe et al. also examined the influence of lymph node status in 293 patients from multiple institutions [32]. These authors reported a staging benefit of lymphadenectomy in patients with pT2 or higher by showing an improved CSS in patients with pN0 than those with pNx (Fig. 7.2). They also performed multivariate analyses and showed that pNx was an adverse factor not only for locoregional recurrence (HR 3.96, $p=0.0026$), but also for distant relapse recurrence (HR 2.86, $p=0.0024$). The study by Burger also demonstrated that patients with pN0 disease presented with a lower risk of recurrence (HR 0.3, $p<0.001$) and death (HR: 0.3; $p<0.001$) compared to pNx disease on multivariate analysis in locally advanced disease [33]. It should be mentioned though that these results should be interpreted with caution as there is no proof a better staging translate into improved survival.

In contrast to the abovementioned studies, other multi-institutional studies failed to support a therapeutic role for lymphadenectomy. Lughezzani reported the results of a population-based study of 2,824 patients in the SEER database [34]. They failed to show any therapeutic benefit of lymphadenectomy. No difference in CSS between pN0 and pNx even in patients with muscle-invasive disease ($p=0.4$) was reported (Fig. 7.3). Multivariate analysis also showed that omitting lymphadenectomy (pNx) had no influence on cancer-specific mortality. Similar results were reported by Ouzzane from 786 patients in a French multi-institutional study [36] and by Mason from 1,029 patients in Canada [35]. The latter two studies showed no difference between patients with pN0 and those with pNx, and pNx did not reduce the risk of cancer-specific mortality after adjusting for other clinical parameters by multivariate analysis. Again, the extent of lymphadenectomy was not described in the latter studies due to the nature of the multi-institutional studies.

The jury is therefore still out and it should be outlined that improved staging does not mean therapeutic advantage at the present time. All these above studies were retrospective, but one prospective study was recently reported. Kondo and colleagues

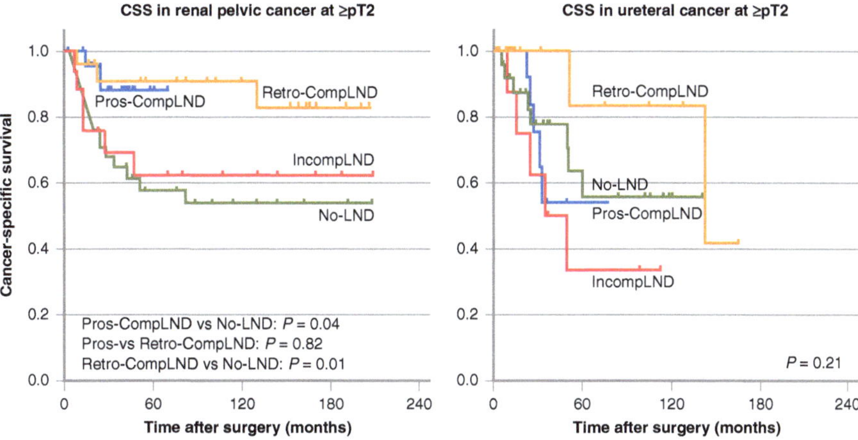

Fig. 7.7 Results from a prospective study on CSS comparing no LND to incomplete and extended LND. Adapted from Kondo T, Hara I, Takagi T, et al. Therapeutic benefit from template-based lymphadenectomy in urothelial carcinoma of the renal pelvis: A prospective study. Int J Urol. 2014: 21:453-9

conducted a single-arm prospective study at two Japanese institutes [26]. Template-based lymphadenectomy was performed according to their previous mapping study. Patients who underwent complete lymphadenectomy in the prospective setting were designated as Pros-CompLND, and complete lymphadenectomy in the retrospective cohort as Retro-CompLND. The control group included patients who underwent lymphadenectomy in the retrospective cohort and those without lymphadenectomy. In patients with renal pelvic cancer stage pT2N0M0 or higher, the 3-year CSS was 90.8 % in Retro-CompLND, 87.9 % in Pros-CompLND, and 64.7 % in No-LND (Fig. 7.7). Patients with Pros-CompLND had significantly higher survival rates than the No-LND groups ($p = 0.04$). Multivariate analysis supported that complete lymphadenectomy is a significant independent factor to reduce the risk of cancer-specific mortality. They concluded that lymphadenectomy is strongly recommended for patients with renal pelvic cancer of ≥ pT2. In addition, their template of lymphadenectomy used for renal pelvic cancer was further validated by this prospective study. On the other hand, this therapeutic benefit could not be observed in patients with ureteral cancer even when limited to muscle-invasive disease (Fig. 7.7), the reason for which is unclear.

A limitation is that those patients without LN dissection are by definition Nx with many N+ in reality and thus falsely classified. These patients may have a worse outcome because they are understaged, and not necessarily because the LN dissection was not completed.

Abe et al. analyzed the micrometastases to LNs by immunohistochemistry using anti-cytokeratin antibody [32]. They showed that micrometastases detected by immunohistochemistry were found in 14 % of patients who were previously diagnosed as pN0. In addition, 5 of 7 patients with lymphatic micrometastases survived a median of 95 months after surgery. Thus, much like bladder and prostate cancers, the removal of micrometastases may be a possible explanation for improving patient survival by lymphadenectomy.

A summary of the results of the above studies examining the therapeutic benefit of lymphadenectomy is described in Table 7.3. Seven retrospective studies and one prospective study favored the benefit of lymphadenectomy in improving the oncological outcome of UCUT, but all were retrospective. The only prospective study demonstrated a therapeutic role for lymphadenectomy in patients with renal pelvic cancer only, not for those with tumors in the ureters. In contrast, 3 multi-institutional studies failed to show an improvement in patient survival undergoing lymphadenectomy. Additional prospective or randomized studies are necessary to confirm the therapeutic role of lymphadenectomy in UCUT.

Does the Number of Lymph Nodes Removed Affect Patient Survival?

In bladder cancer, the number of LNs removed is considered a surrogate of whether a thorough lymphadenectomy has been performed [45–47]. Koppie and colleagues also reported that survival rates continued to rise as the number of resected LNs increased in bladder cancer [48]. One underreported bias regarding the influence of number of nodes removed is the influence of the technicians on lymph node yield as these differences can be obvious when performing an identical procedure with the same surgeon and pathologist but different technicians handling the specimens. A recent study comparing lymph node counts in two institutions performing identical template lymphadenectomy suggested that dissection technique is more important than lymph node count in identifying nodal metastases [49]. Compared to the literature on bladder cancer, the number of reports regarding the benefits and numbers of LNs removed in UCUT is extremely limited.

Roscigno et al. examined 95 patients with ≥ pT2pN0 who underwent lymphadenectomy at a single institute and reported that removal of 7 or more LNs improved survival in these patients [30]. They conducted a similar analysis with more patient data from multiple institutions. When examining 412 patients with ≥ pT1N0, the removal of 8 LNs or more resulted in higher CSS compared to those with less than 8 LNs removed (Fig. 7.6) [44]. They also showed that the number of LNs removed was a significant independent factor predicting both recurrence free and CSS. The results were similar when the number of LNs was assessed as a continuous value or as dichotomized at 8 LNs. In addition, the curve depicting the relationship between the number of LNs removed and cancer-specific mortality did not plateau, but continued to decrease as the number of LNs removed increased (Fig. 7.6).

Kondo et al. have examined which index can be considered more important in the assessment of the benefits of lymphadenectomy, the number of LNs removed or the anatomical boundaries [50]. They showed in a study of 80 patients with ≥ pT2cN0 that the total number of LNs removed did not provide a significant benefit for survival

Table 7.3 Reports on therapeutic benefit of lymphadenectomy in UCUT

Authors	Year	Institute	Subject	No. of pts	Template of LND	Survival results	Independent predictor in multivariate analysis?	Therapeutic benefit?	Minimum No. of LNs required	References
Kondo	2007	Single	All patients	169	Clearly described	CSS: CompLND = IncompLND = No-LND ($p=0.06$)	Yes: CompLND for CSS	Yes In ≥ pT3	Not found	[39]
			≥pT3	88		CSS: CompLND > No-LND ($p=0.01$)				
Kondo	2012	Single	≥pT2	191	Clearly described	5y-CSS: CompLND 77.9 % > IncompLND 54.0 % = No-LND 59.0 % ($p=0.03$)	Not determined	Yes In ≥ pT2	Not examined	[24]
			≥pT3	140		5y-CSS: CompLND 73.2 % > IncompLND 43.7 % = No-LND 47.3 % ($p=0.01$)				
Brausi	2007	Single	≥pT2	82	Described	DFS: RPLN 81.6 % > No-LND 44.8 % ($p=0.007$)	Yes: RPLD for OS	Yes in ≥ pT2	Not examined	[43]
Roscigno	2008	Single	≥pT2	132	Described	5y-CSS: LND 57 % > No-LND 40 % ($p=0.01$) pN0 72 % > pNx 39 % ($p<0.001$)	Yes: LND and pN0 for CSS	Yes in ≥ pT2	–	[30]
			≥pT2pN0	95		7 LNs > less than 7($p<0.001$)	Yes: No. of LNs for CSS	Yes In ≥7 LNs removed	7	
Roscigno	2009	Multi	≥pT2	1130	Not well described	5y-CSS: LND 66 % = No-LND 69 % ($p=0.23$)	Yes: pN0 for CSS	No	Not examined	[31]

(continued)

Table 7.3 (continued)

Authors	Year	Institute	Subject	No. of pts	Template of LND	Survival results	Independent predictor in multivariate analysis?	Therapeutic benefit?	Minimum No. of LNs required	References
Roscigno	2009	Multi	≥pT1pN0	412	Not well described	5y-CSS: 8 LNs or more 84 %>less than 8 73 % (p=0.038)	Yes: No. of LNs for CSS	Yes in ≥8 LNs removed	8	[44]
Abe	2010	Multi	All patients	293	Not well described	RFS: pN0>pNx (p<0.001) >pN+(p=0.004)	Yes: pNx of RFS	Yes	Not examined	[32]
Burger	2011	Multi	Organ-confined	519	Not well described	CSS: pN0=pNx	No	Yes but limited only in locally advanced disease	Not examined	[33]
			Locally advanced	266		CSS: pN0=pNx (p=0.633)	Yes: pN0 for CSS in locally advanced			
Lughezzani	2010	Multi	All patients	2824	Not described	No; CSS is pN0=pNx	No	No	Not examined	[34]
Mason	2012	Multi	All patients	1029	Not described	OS: pN0 66.1 %=pNx 66.0 % (p=0.617)	No	No	Not found	[35]
Ouzzane	2013	Multi	All patients	714	Not described	5y-CSS: pN0 81 %=pNx 85 % (p=0.6) >pN+47 % (p<0.001)	No	No	Not examined	[36]
			≥pT2	337		CSS: pN0=pNx (p=0.44)=pN+(p<0.15)				
Kondo	2013	Multi-Prospective	Renal pelvis at≥pT2	121	Well described	3y-CSS: Retro-CompLND 90.8 %=Pros-CompLND 87.9 %>Lo-LND 64.7 % (p=0.04)	Yes	Yes in renal pelvic cancer at>pT2	Not examined	26
			Ureter at≥pT2	69	Well described	3y-CSS: Retro-CompLND 83.3 %>Pros-Comp 53.9 %=No-LND 77.7 % (p=0.92)	No			

pts patients, *LND* lymphadenectomy, *LNs* lymph nodes, *CompLND* complete lymphadenectomy, *IncompLND* incomplete lymphadenectomy, *DFS* disease-free survival, *RPLD* retroperitoneal lymph node dissection, *RFS* recurrence-free survival, *OS* overall survival

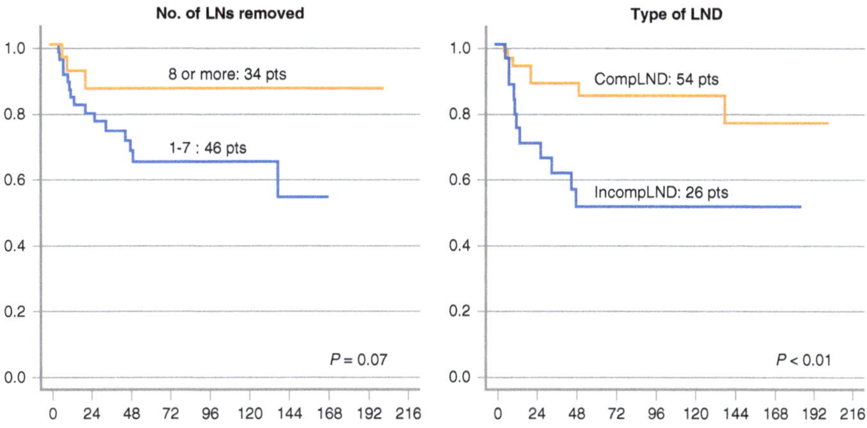

Fig. 7.8 Influence of No. of LNs removed and the extent of lymphadenectomy on patient's survival. Adapted from Kondo. Int J Urol 2010;17: 848

($p=0.07$), although patients who had 8 or more LNs removed were likely to show higher CSS than those in which less than 8 LNs were resected (Fig. 7.8), which is most likely a surrogate for the thoroughness of the lymphadenectomy. On the other hand, CompLND in which all regional LN sites were removed resulted in a higher CSS than IncompLND in which lymphadenectomy did not include all regional sites ($p<0.01$). Their conclusion is that lymphadenectomy should be performed, in high-grade disease, according to anatomical template and the total number of LNs removed can be used only for assessing the quality of lymphadenectomy. It appears reasonable to say that the dissection of all regional nodes when feasible should be encouraged.

The Role of Lymphadenectomy in Patients with Lymph Node Metastases

In muscle-invasive bladder cancer with minimal lymphatic involvement, theoretically surgery including both radical cystectomy and lymphadenectomy alone could provide cure in a limited subset of patients. This benefit is reported to be dependent on the extent of lymphadenectomy [12, 13]. Thus, lymphadenectomy may play a limited therapeutic as well as a staging role for identification in some patients with lymph node metastases [51, 52].

However, the combination of chemotherapy and surgery is the more likely explanation for the survival advantage observed in several radical cystectomy series with extended lymphadenectomy.

Due to the small number of studies, it is still unproven whether lymphadenectomy could cure advanced UCUT disease with lymph node involvement and which patients would truly benefit. The results of multi-institutional studies showed a 5-year CSS range from 10 to 40 % in patients who were found to have pathological metastases in the LNs harvested during lymphadenectomy [31–33, 35, 36]. Although there is a large variability, these results show that radical nephroureterectomy with lymphadenectomy may have some possible potential to cure the disease or prolong survival in a subset of these patients. However, it is difficult to conclude whether the benefit is related to the lymphadenectomy only or more likely to the integrated therapy with systemic chemotherapy.

Lymph node density has been reported to be a good indicator to predict the survival of patients with bladder cancer who have lymph node involvement [53, 54]. Lymph node density is determined as the ratio of the number of LNs positive for metastasis to the total number of nodes removed. A lymph node density of lower than 20 % was associated with higher patient survival in these studies. However other authors have found no real benefit to LN density or other LN parameters [55].

In UCUT, two multi-institutional studies addressed lymph node density. Bolenz et al. showed that patients with lymph node density of ≥30 % were at greater risk of disease recurrence and cancer-specific mortality (HR 1.7 and 1.8, respectively, $p<0.05$) (Fig. 7.9) [56].

The lymphadenectomy template was not standardized and over 40 % of patients received adjuvant chemotherapy [56]. Mason also reported that the cutoff point of ≥20 % was a significant independent factor to predict a worse oncological outcome including recurrence-free, disease-specific, and overall survival (HR 1.94, 2.70, and 2.34, respectively, $p<0.05$) [35]. Thus, lymph node density is possibly a more accurate predictor of the extent of disease than the number of positive nodes itself in UCUT as in bladder cancer, but controversy still surrounds this issue.

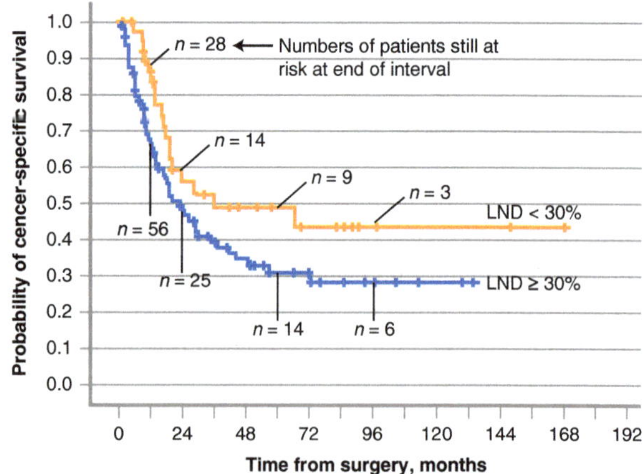

Fig. 7.9 Stratification of cancer-specific survival according to lymph node density (cutoff 30 %). Adapted from Bolenz. *BJU Int*. 2009;103: 30

Who Are Candidates for Lymphadenectomy (Tables 7.2 and 7.3)?

The optimal candidates for LN dissection are those at risk for regional LN involvement. Since the risk of LN involvement is related to primary tumor stage, patients with higher stage lesions (≥T2) would be reasonable candidates for LN dissection. According to the results of Tokyo Women's Medical University, the risk of lymphatic metastases from tumors of pT1 or less is only 1 % (Fig. 7.10). But pT2 tumors and pT3 renal pelvic tumors with renal parenchyma metastasize to lymph nodes in 7 % of cases. Tumors invading surrounding adipose tissue showed a higher incidence of lymphatic metastases at about 40 %. A higher incidence of lymphatic metastases (67 %) was also shown in pT4 tumors. These results support the rationale for a risk-adapted strategy as patients with pT2 or higher appear to be candidates for lymphadenectomy.

However, there is a major difficulty in accurately staging the primary tumor by preoperative imaging studies or biopsy. Although multi-detector computed tomography (MDCT) has been reported to be more than 80 % accurate in staging [57], Kondo reported that 43 % of tumors with a clinical stage of cT1 or lower were up-staged to pT2 or higher [58]. Even in carcinoma in situ, 25 % of patients were ultimately diagnosed as having invasive tumors [59]. Thus, it seems very difficult to exclude patients with clinical T1 or less from being candidates for lymphadenectomy. It appears to be reasonable and justified to consider lymphadenectomy for all patients with high-grade disease undergoing radical surgery, except for those with severe comorbidity [59].

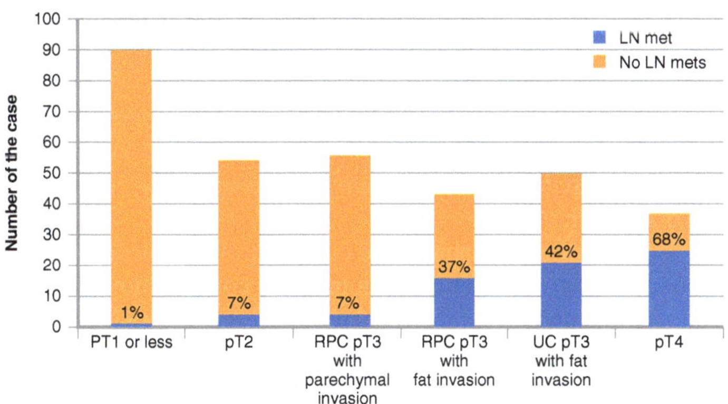

Fig. 7.10 Incidence of lymphatic metastases by pT stage

Lymphadenectomy Procedure: Open, Laparoscopic, or Robotic?

Kondo reported the yield of lymph nodes from complete lymphadenectomy in a retrospective cohort. The mean number of lymph nodes removed was 7.9 in patients who underwent complete lymphadenectomy, and 4.4 in those who underwent incomplete lymphadenectomy [60]. It increased to 13.9 in patients who underwent complete lymphadenectomy in a prospective setting [26]. Lymphadenectomies were performed by open procedure for all patients. The numbers above are considered as the standard for lymphadenectomy in patients with UCUT.

It is still unclear whether laparoscopic and robotic lymphadenectomy show similar efficacy in the yield of lymph nodes although in theory and in the light of data in other urological malignancies, there shouldn't be major differences between the different techniques. Abe reported that laparoscopic retroperitoneal lymphadenectomy yielded a similar number of lymph nodes to that from the open procedure at about 10 [60]. Gerullis and colleagues reported that the average number of lymph nodes removed was only 14 [61]. Thus, the feasibility of laparoscopic lymphadenectomy is controversial, and it has to be performed only by expert laparoscopic surgeons. In contrast, robotic-extended pelvic lymphadenectomy is reported to yield 41 lymph nodes on average [62]. Reports of robotic retroperitoneal lymphadenectomy at the time of UCUT are limited. Hemal et al. reported a low number of lymph node removal at 4–9 [63]. However, when considering the efficiency of robotic-extended pelvic lymphadenectomy that is supported by many studies, robotic retroperitoneal lymphadenectomy may be a feasible approach that can be performed by an increasing number of surgeons.

Disadvantages of Lymphadenectomy in UCUT

In bladder cancer, lymphadenectomy may increase the risk of complications such as lymphocele, lymphedema, or incontinence by disrupting the sympathetic nerve during extensive lymphadenectomy [64]. Brossner et al. reported on side effects of extended lymphadenectomy [65]. Extending the cranial boundary of the template of lymphadenectomy from the bifurcation of the common iliac artery to that of the aortic bifurcation caused no increase in surgical morbidity except when the operation took an extra hour.

Only few reports have documented the complications associated with retroperitoneal lymphadenectomy. Rao et al. examined the complications in a prospective series of patients who underwent radical nephroureterectomy (RNU) with extensive lymphadenectomy [66]. They used a considerably wide template from the retroperitoneum to the pelvis. The morbidity in their study included transfusion (32 %), ileus (5 %), and chylous leakage (10 %). The patients with chylous leakage could be managed conservatively, but one of the other patients required surgical intervention.

They concluded that their super-wide template of lymphadenectomy during RNU is a feasible procedure with acceptable morbidity. Kondo compared the results of RNU in patients with or without complete lymphadenectomy (CompLND) [24]. Compared to the No-LND group, the CompLND group had more intraoperative bleeding and longer operation times (407 versus 321 ml, 323 versus 288 min). The incidence of all complications was also higher in CompLND (17.2 % vs 8.6 %), although the difference was not statistically significant. The incidence of major complications and the length of hospital stay after surgery were very similar. A prospective study of lymphadenectomy in renal cell carcinoma showed that extensive lymphadenectomy did not increase the rate of complications compared to patients without lymphadenectomy (26 % vs 22 %) [6]. Thus, lymphadenectomy at the time of RNU is unlikely to dramatically increase complications. Nevertheless, lymphadenectomy may not be suited for patients with extensive comorbidity or advanced age, unless the benefit of lymphadenectomy is established by further studies.

Description of the Current Guidelines at 2013

Currently, there are three guidelines describing the role of lymphadenectomy. The latest EAU guideline published in 2013 states that lymphadenectomy is recommended for cases of invasive UCUT [38], but the level of recommendation is still low at grade C. The National Cancer Institute (NCI)-Physician Data Query (PDQ) suggests that lymphadenectomy at the time of RNU may offer prognostic information, but little, if any, therapeutic benefit [37]. The National Comprehensive Cancer Network (NCCN) Clinical Practice Guideline in Oncology Version 1.2013 stipulates that lymphadenectomy should be integrated at the time of nephroureterectomy for high-grade tumors or those that are large and invade the renal parenchyma [67]. The International Consultation on Urological Diseases (ICUD)–Société Internationale d'Urologie (SIU) are preparing their guideline on Upper Tract Urothelial Carcinoma, and will recommend lymphadenectomy to some degree.

Conclusions

Although there are limitations in the studies examining the role of lymphadenectomy in UCUT, currently:

1. The extent of the lymphadenectomy is not yet standardized. However, mapping as well as prospective studies supports the rationale of the extent previously reported in renal pelvic cancer.
2. For tumors of the renal pelvis, the templates ideally include the right renal hilum, para-caval, retro-caval, and interaorto-caval nodes. For the left renal pelvis, the left renal hilum and para-aortic nodes are included. The lower boundary is the level of the inferior mesenteric artery.

3. For tumors of the upper 2/3 of the right ureter, the renal hilar, para-caval, retrocaval, and interaorto-caval nodes are considered for the regional lymph nodes. For tumors of the upper 2/3 of the left ureter, the left renal hilar and aortocaval nodes are included. The lower boundary of the template is the level of aortic bifurcation. For tumors of the lower ureter, the ipsilateral common iliac, external iliac, obturator, internal iliac, and presacral nodes were considered as regional nodes.
4. Its role in improving the accuracy of staging is supported by most studies. However, the implication varies among them. Some studies support the role of stratifying both pN0 and pN+from pNx, but others report a limited role for stratifying pN+from PNx.
5. The therapeutic role remains highly controversial. The benefit of combined approaches with systemic chemotherapy especially in node-positive disease is likely to prevent from drawing definitive conclusions outside of randomized controlled trials about the therapeutic value of LND.
6. The number of lymph nodes can be considered as an indicator to assess the quality of LND. Lymphadenectomy, however, should be performed based on the anatomical extent, not on the number of lymph nodes removed.
7. The best candidates for lymphadenectomy are patients with high-grade disease, pT2 or higher. Because of the inaccuracy of preoperative staging, it appears feasible and justified to attempt to perform lymphadenectomy in all patients with high-grade disease. Prospective, randomized trials are clearly needed though. In the meantime, extended lymphadenectomy is recommended at the time of nephroureterectomy for UCUT.
8. Lymphadenectomy is unlikely to be associated with significantly increased complications except an extended operative time.

Acknowledgments The authors thank Ms. Elizabeth Kiritani for the English correction of this manuscript. We also thank and Ms. Noriko Hata for secretarial work.

References

1. Bensalah K, Roupret M, Xylinas E, Shariat S. The survival benefit of lymph node dissection at the time of removal of kidney, prostate and urothelial carcinomas: what is the evidence? World J Urol. 2013;31(6):1369–76.
2. Capitanio U, Becker F, Blute ML, Mulders P, Patard JJ, Russo P, et al. Lymph node dissection in renal cell carcinoma. Eur Urol. 2011;60:1212–20.
3. Miki J, Egawa S. The role of lymph node dissection in the management of prostate cancer. Int J Clin Oncol [Review]. 2011;16:195–202.
4. Kitamura H, Masumori N, Tsukamoto T. Role of lymph node dissection in management of bladder cancer. Int J Clin Oncol [Review]. 2011;16:179–85.
5. Blom JH, van Poppel H, Marechal JM, Jacqmin D, Schroder FH, de Prijck L, et al. Radical nephrectomy with and without lymph-node dissection: Final results of European Organization for Research and Treatment of Cancer (EORTC) Randomized phase 3 trial 30881 Editorial by Urs E. Studer and Frederic D Birkhauser on pp x-y of this issue. Eur Urol. 2009;55:28–34.
6. Crispen PL, Breau RH, Allmer C, Lohse CM, Cheville JC, Leibovich BC, et al. Lymph node dissection at the time of radical nephrectomy for high-risk clear cell renal cell carcinoma: indications and recommendations for surgical templates. Eur Urol. 2011;59:18–23.

7. DiMarco DS, Zincke H, Sebo TJ, Slezak J, Bergstralh EJ, Blute ML. The extent of lymphadenectomy for pTXNO prostate cancer does not affect prostate cancer outcome in the prostate specific antigen era. J Urol. 2005;173:1121–5.
8. Briganti A, Blute ML, Eastham JH, Graefen M, Heidenreich A, Karnes JR, et al. Pelvic lymph node dissection in prostate cancer. Eur Urol [Review]. 2009;55:1251–65.
9. Capitanio U, Jeldres C, Patard JJ, Perrotte P, Zini L, de La Taille A, et al. Stage-specific effect of nodal metastases on survival in patients with non-metastatic renal cell carcinoma. BJU Int [Multicenter Study Research Support, Non-US Gov't]. 2009;103:33–7.
10. Batata MA, Whitmore WF, Hilaris BS, Tokita N, Grabstald H. Primary carcinoma of the ureter: a prognostic study. Cancer. 1975;35:1626–32.
11. Lughezzani G, Jeldres C, Isbarn H, Sun M, Shariat SF, Widmer H, et al. Temporal stage and grade migration in surgically treated patients with upper tract urothelial carcinoma. BJU Int. 2010;105:799–804.
12. Dhar NB, Klein EA, Reuther AM, Thalmann GN, Madersbacher S, Studer UE. Outcome after radical cystectomy with limited or extended pelvic lymph node dissection. J Urol [Comparative Study]. 2008;179:873–8. discussion 8.
13. Abol-Enein H, Tilki D, Mosbah A, El-Baz M, Shokeir A, Nabeeh A, et al. Does the extent of lymphadenectomy in radical cystectomy for bladder cancer influence disease-free survival? A prospective single-center study. Eur Urol. 2011;60:572–7.
14. Stenzl A, Cowan NC, De Santis M, Kuczyk MA, Merseburger AS, Ribal MJ, et al. Treatment of muscle-invasive and metastatic bladder cancer: update of the EAU guidelines. Eur Urol [Practice Guideline Review]. 2011;59:1009–18.
15. Zlotta AR. Limited, extended, superextended, megaextended pelvic lymph node dissection at the time of radical cystectomy: what should we perform? Eur Urol. 2012;61(2):243–4.
16. Grabstald H, Whitmore WF, Melamed MR. Renal pelvic tumors. JAMA. 1971;218:845–54.
17. Skinner DG. Technique of nephroureterectomy with regional lymph node dissection. Urol Clin North Am. 1978;5:252–60.
18. McCarron Jr JP, Chasko SB, Gray Jr GF. Systematic mapping of nephroureterectomy specimens removed for urothelial cancer: pathological findings and clinical correlations. J Urol. 1982;128:243–6.
19. Akaza H, Koiso K, Niijima T. Clinical evaluation of urothelial tumors of the renal pelvis and ureter based on a new classification system. Cancer. 1987;59:1369–75.
20. Komatsu H, Tanabe N, Kubodera S, Maezawa H, Ueno A. The role of lymphadenectomy in the treatment of transitional cell carcinoma of the upper urinary tract. J Urol. 1997;157:1622–4.
21. Miyake H, Hara I, Gohji K, Arakawa S, Kamidono S. The significance of lymphadenectomy in transitional cell carcinoma of the upper urinary tract. Br J Urol. 1998;82:494–8.
22. Sobin LH, Wittekind CH. Renal plevis and ureter (ICD-O C65, C66). TNM classification of malignant tumors. 7th ed. New York: Wiley-Liss; 2009. p. 258–61.
23. Kondo T, Nakazawa H, Ito F, Hashimoto Y, Toma H, Tanabe K. Primary site and incidence of lymph node metastases in urothelial carcinoma of upper urinary tract. Urology. 2007;69:265–9.
24. Kondo T, Tanabe K. Role of lymphadenectomy in the management of urothelial carcinoma of the bladder and the upper urinary tract. Int J Urol. 2012;19:710–21.
25. Assouad J, Riquet M, Foucault C, Hidden G, Delmas V. Renal lymphatic drainage and thoracic duct connections: implications for cancer spread. Lymphology. 2006;39:26–32.
26. Kondo T, Hara I, Takagi T, Kodama Y, Hashimoto Y, Iizuka J, et al. Therapeutic benefit from template-based lymphadenectomy in urothelial carcinoma of the renal pelvis—multi-institutional prospective study. 28th Annual EAU Congress. Milan: European Urological Association; 2013.
27. Bochner BH, Cho D, Herr HW, Donat M, Kattan MW, Dalbagni G. Prospectively packaged lymph node dissections with radical cystectomy: evaluation of node count variability and node mapping. J Urol. 2004;172:1286–90.
28. Stein JP, Penson DF, Cai J, Miranda G, Skinner EC, Dunn MA, et al. Radical cystectomy with extended lymphadenectomy: evaluating separate package versus en bloc submission for node positive bladder cancer. J Urol [Comparative Study Research Support, Non-US Gov't]. 2007;177:876–81. discussion 81-2.

29. Miocinovic R, Gong MC, Ghoneim IA, Fergany AF, Hansel DE, Stephenson AJ. Presacral and retroperitoneal lymph node involvement in urothelial bladder cancer: results of a prospective mapping study. J Urol. 2011;186:1269–73.
30. Roscigno M, Cozzarini C, Bertini R, Scattoni V, Freschi M, Da Pozzo LF, et al. Prognostic value of lymph node dissection in patients with muscle-invasive transitional cell carcinoma of the upper urinary tract. Eur Urol. 2008;53:794–802.
31. Roscigno M, Shariat SF, Margulis V, Karakiewicz P, Remzi M, Kikuchi E, et al. Impact of lymph node dissection on cancer specific survival in patients with upper tract urothelial carcinoma treated with radical nephroureterectomy. J Urol. 2009;181:2482–9.
32. Abe T, Shinohara N, Muranaka M, Sazawa A, Maruyama S, Osawa T, et al. Role of lymph node dissection in the treatment of urothelial carcinoma of the upper urinary tract: multi-institutional relapse analysis and immunohistochemical re-evaluation of negative lymph nodes. Eur J Surg Oncol. 2010;36:1085–91.
33. Burger M, Shariat SF, Fritsche HM, Martinez-Salamanca JI, Matsumoto K, Chromecki TF, et al. No overt influence of lymphadenectomy on cancer-specific survival in organ-confined versus locally advanced upper urinary tract urothelial carcinoma undergoing radical nephroureterectomy: a retrospective international, multi-institutional study. World J Urol. 2011;29:465–72.
34. Lughezzani G, Jeldres C, Isbarn H, Shariat SF, Sun M, Pharand D, et al. A critical appraisal of the value of lymph node dissection at nephroureterectomy for upper tract urothelial carcinoma. Urology. 2010;75:118–24.
35. Mason RJ, Kassouf W, Bell DG, Lacombe L, Kapoor A, Jacobsen N, et al. The contemporary role of lymph node dissection during nephroureterectomy in the management of upper urinary tract urothelial carcinoma: the Canadian experience. Urology [Multicenter Study]. 2012; 79:840–5.
36. Ouzzane A, Colin P, Ghoneim TP, Zerbib M, De La Taille A, Audenet F, et al. The impact of lymph node status and features on oncological outcomes in urothelial carcinoma of the upper urinary tract (UTUC) treated by nephroureterectomy. World J Urol. 2013;31:189–97.
37. Transitional Cell Cancer of the Renal Pelvis and Ureter Treatment (PDQ®) [database on the Internet] 2013 [cited April 11, 2013]. Available from: http://www.cancer.gov/cancertopics/pdq/treatment/transitionalcell/HealthProfessional.
38. Roupret M, Babjuk M, Comperat E, Zigeuner R, Sylvester R, Burger M, et al. European guidelines on upper tract urothelial carcinomas: 2013 Update. Eur Urol. 2013;63:1059–71.
39. Xylinas E, Rink M, Margulis V, Faison T, Comploj E, Novara G, Raman JD, Lotan Y, Guillonneau B, Weizer A, Pycha A, Scherr DS, Seitz C, Sun M, Trinh QD, Karakiewicz PI, Montorsi F, Zerbib M, Gönen M, Shariat SF. Prediction of true nodal status in patients with pathological lymph node negative upper tract urothelial carcinoma at radical nephroureterectomy. J Urol. 2013;189(2):468–73.
40. Gayed BA, Thoreson GR, Margulis V. The role of systemic chemotherapy in management of upper tract urothelial cancer. Curr Urol Rep. 2013;14(2):94–101.
41. Cordier J, Sonpavde G, Stief CG, Tilki D. Oncologic outcomes obtained after neoadjuvant and adjuvant chemotherapy for the treatment of urothelial carcinomas of the upper urinary tract: a review. World J Urol. 2013;31(1):77–82.
42. Kondo T, Nakazawa H, Ito F, Hashimoto Y, Toma H, Tanabe K. Impact of the extent of regional lymphadenectomy on the survival of patients with urothelial carcinoma of the upper urinary tract. J Urol. 2007;178:1212–7. discussion 7.
43. Brausi MA, Gavioli M, De Luca G, Verrini G, Peracchia G, Simonini G, et al. Retroperitoneal lymph node dissection (RPLD) in Conjunction with nephroureterectomy in the treatment of infiltrative transitional cell carcinoma (TCC) of the upper urinary tract: impact on survival. Eur Urol. 2007;52:1414–20.
44. Roscigno M, Shariat SF, Margulis V, Karakiewicz P, Remzi M, Kikuchi E, et al. The extent of lymphadenectomy seems to be associated with better survival in patients with nonmetastatic upper-tract urothelial carcinoma: how many lymph nodes should be removed? Eur Urol. 2009;56:512–8.

45. Stein JP, Skinner DG. The role of lymphadenectomy in high-grade invasive bladder cancer. Urol Clin North Am. 2005;32:187–97.
46. Capitanio U, Suardi N, Shariat SF, Lotan Y, Palapattu GS, Bastian PJ, et al. Assessing the minimum number of lymph nodes needed at radical cystectomy in patients with bladder cancer. BJU Int. 2009;103:1359–62.
47. Dangle PP, Gong MC, Bahnson RR, Pohar KS. How do commonly performed lymphadenectomy templates influence bladder cancer nodal stage? J Urol [Research Support, Non-US Gov't]. 2010;183:499–503.
48. Koppie TM, Vickers AJ, Vora K, Dalbagni G, Bochner BH. Standardization of pelvic lymphadenectomy performed at radical cystectomy: can we establish a minimum number of lymph nodes that should be removed? Cancer. 2006;107:2368–74.
49. Dorin RP, Daneshmand S, Eisenberg MS, Chandrasoma S, Cai J, Miranda G, Nichols PW, Skinner DG, Skinner EC. Lymph node dissection technique is more important than lymph node count in identifying nodal metastases in radical cystectomy patients: a comparative mapping study. Eur Urol. 2011;60(5):946–52.
50. Kondo T, Hashimoto Y, Kobayashi H, Iizuka J, Nakazawa H, Ito F, et al. Template-based lymphadenectomy in urothelial carcinoma of the upper urinary tract: impact on patient survival. Int J Urol. 2010;17:848–54.
51. Steven K, Poulsen AL. Radical cystectomy and extended pelvic lymphadenectomy: survival of patients with lymph node metastasis above the bifurcation of the common iliac vessels treated with surgery only. J Urol. 2007;178:1218–23. discussion 23-4.
52. Karl A, Carroll PR, Gschwend JE, Knuchel R, Montorsi F, Stief CG, et al. The impact of lymphadenectomy and lymph node metastasis on the outcomes of radical cystectomy for bladder cancer. Eur Urol [Review]. 2009;55:826–35.
53. Stein JP, Cai J, Groshen S, Skinner DG. Risk factors for patients with pelvic lymph node metastases following radical cystectomy with en bloc pelvic lymphadenectomy: concept of lymph node density. J Urol. 2003;170:35–41.
54. Masson-Lecomte A, Vordos D, Hoznek A, Yiou R, Allory Y, Abbou CC, de la Taille A. Salomon external validation of extranodal extension and lymph node density as predictors of survival in node-positivebladder cancer after radical cystectomy. Ann Surg Oncol. 2013;20(4):1389–94.
55. Jensen JB, Ulhøi BP, Jensen KM. Evaluation of different lymph node (LN) variables as prognostic markers in patients undergoing radicalcystectomy and extended LN dissection to the level of the inferior mesenteric artery. BJU Int. 2012;109(3):388–93.
56. Bolenz C, Shariat SF, Fernandez MI, Margulis V, Lotan Y, Karakiewicz P, et al. Risk stratification of patients with nodal involvement in upper tract urothelial carcinoma: value of lymph-node density. BJU Int. 2009;103:302–6.
57. Fritz GA, Schoellnast H, Deutschmann HA, Quehenberger F, Tillich M. Multiphasic multidetector-row CT (MDCT) in detection and staging of transitional cell carcinomas of the upper urinary tract. Eur Radiol. 2006;16:1244–52.
58. Kondo T, Tanabe K. The role of lymph node dissection in the management of urothelial carcinoma of the upper urinary tract. Int J Clin Oncol. 2011;16:170–8.
59. Yuasa T, Tsuchiya N, Narita S, Inoue T, Saito M, Kumazawa T, et al. Radical nephroureterectomy as initial treatment for carcinoma in situ of upper urinary tract. Urology. 2006; 68:972–5.
60. Abe T, Harabayashi T, Shinohara N, Sazawa A, Maruyama S, Sasaki H, et al. Outcome of regional lymph node dissection in conjunction with laparoscopic nephroureterectomy for urothelial carcinoma of the upper urinary tract. J Endourol. 2011;25:803–7.
61. Gerullis H, Kuemmel C, Popken G. Laparoscopic cystectomy with extracorporeal-assisted urinary diversion: experience with 34 patients. Eur Urol. 2007;51:193–8.
62. Lavery HJ, Martinez-Suarez HJ, Abaza R. Robotic extended pelvic lymphadenectomy for bladder cancer with increased nodal yield. BJU Int. 2011;107:1802–5.
63. Hemal AK, Stansel I, Babbar P, Patel M. Robotic-assisted nephroureterectomy and bladder cuff excision without intraoperative repositioning. Urology. 2011;78:357–64.

64. Thurairaja R, Studer UE, Burkhard FC. Indications, extent, and benefits of pelvic lymph node dissection for patients with bladder and prostate cancer. Oncologist. 2009;14:40–51.
65. Brossner C, Pycha A, Toth A, Mian C, Kuber W. Does extended lymphadenectomy increase the morbidity of radical cystectomy? BJU Int. 2004;93:64–6.
66. Rao SR, Correa JJ, Sexton WJ, Pow-Sang JM, Dickinson SI, Lin HY, et al. Prospective clinical trial of the feasibility and safety of modified retroperitoneal lymph node dissection at time of nephroureterectomy for upper tract urothelial carcinoma. BJU Int. 2012;110:E475–80.
67. Bladder cancer: NCCN Clinical Practice Guideline in Oncology (NCN GuidelineTM) Version 1.2013 [database on the Internet]. National Comprehensive Cancer Network. 2013 [cited March 7, 2013]. Available from: http://www.nccn.org/professionals/physician_gls/PDF/bladder.pdf.

Chapter 8
Chemotherapy

Arjun Vasant Balar, Matthew D. Galsky, Arlene O. Siefker-Radtke, Scott T. Tagawa, and Matthew I. Milowsky

Abstract Urothelial cancer is a chemotherapy-sensitive pan-urothelial disease that arises from both the upper and lower urinary tract. Due to its rarity, the principles for management of upper tract urothelial cancer are derived from evidence gathered in bladder cancer trials. To date, no definitive evidence has differentiated upper tract from lower tract cancer and both are managed similarly. Epidemiologic observations, tissue-based genetic studies, and recent subset analyses from randomized trials suggest potential differences between upper tract and bladder cancers which will need to be validated in prospective trials. This chapter will review the current role for perioperative chemotherapy in high-grade upper tract urothelial cancer as well as the use of chemotherapy in advanced disease.

Keywords Urothelial cancer • Transitional cell cancer • Upper tract urothelial or transitional cell cancer • Ureter cancer • Renal pelvis cancer • Muscle-invasive bladder cancer

---

A.V. Balar, MD
Division of Hematology and Medical Oncology, NYU Perlmutter Cancer Center, 160 E 34th Street 8th Floor, New York, NY 10016, USA
e-mail: arjun.balar@nyumc.org

M.D. Galsky, MD
Mount Sinai School of Medicine, Tisch Cancer Institute, New York, NY 10029, USA
e-mail: matthew.galsky@mssm.edu

A.O. Siefker-Radtke, MD
The M. D. Anderson Cancer Center, 1155 Pressler, Unit 1374, CPB7.3508, Houston, TX 77030, USA
e-mail: asiefker@mdanderson.org

S.T. Tagawa, MD, MS
Weill Cornell Cancer Center, Weill Cornell Medical College, 525 E 68th Street, New York, NY 10065, USA
e-mail: stt2007@med.cornell.edu

M.I. Milowsky, MD (✉)
UNC Lineberger Comprehensive Cancer Center, 3rd Floor Physicians Office Building, 170 Manning Drive, Chapel Hill, NC 27599, USA
e-mail: matt_milowsky@med.unc.edu

© Springer Science+Business Media New York 2015

S.F. Shariat, E. Xylinas (eds.), *Upper Tract Urothelial Carcinoma*,
DOI 10.1007/978-1-4939-1501-9_8

Introduction

Early clinical trials of chemotherapy in advanced disease conducted in the 1970s identified urothelial cancer as a chemotherapy-sensitive malignancy [1]. These trials included patients with metastatic disease irrespective of the primary site of disease as early research identified urothelial cancer as a single, pan-urothelial disease. Indeed, morphologically, upper and lower tract urothelial cancer is indistinguishable [2] and genetic studies on tumor tissue have suggested no significant differences in oncogenomic events [3–6]. Further, recurrence and survival rates between upper and lower tract urothelial cancers appear to be similar after adjusting for disease stage and grade although upper tract disease is more likely to present with advanced stage [7, 8].

Only recently has progress in the ability to better molecularly characterize tumors led to the notion that these diseases may, in fact, be distinct. Epidemiologic observations provided an initial basis for a distinction. While smoking is overwhelmingly the most common risk factor for both upper and lower tract urothelial cancers, a history of phenacetin abuse, balkan nephropathy, and hereditary non-polyposis colorectal cancer (HPNCC) syndrome are risk factors unique to upper tract urothelial cancer suggesting that at least a subset of cases are clinically distinct. Interestingly, phenacetin abuse is a risk factor shared with renal cell carcinoma.

Outcomes observed in modern trials of combination chemotherapy in advanced urothelial cancer have not been substantially different between cancers originating in the upper versus lower urinary tract [9–14]. In the perioperative setting, neoadjuvant cisplatin-based chemotherapy has been demonstrated definitively to improve survival in muscle-invasive lower urinary tract urothelial cancer when added to radical cystectomy; however no adequately powered prospective trials in upper urinary tract urothelial cancer have been reported. Given the biological and clinical similarities, and the inherent difficulties of administering cisplatin-based chemotherapy in the adjuvant setting with a solitary kidney, a similar approach is recommended prior to nephroureterectomy in high-grade upper tract urothelial cancer. This chapter will review the current role for perioperative chemotherapy in high-grade upper tract urothelial cancer as well as the current status of chemotherapy in advanced disease and potential differences in outcomes between cancers originating in the upper and lower urinary tract.

Neoadjuvant Chemotherapy

In muscle-invasive bladder cancer there is definitive evidence demonstrating a survival benefit with neoadjuvant chemotherapy prior to radical cystectomy. The seminal Southwest Oncology Group (SWOG) 8710 study randomized 317 patients with cT2-T4a N0 muscle-invasive bladder cancer to three cycles of neoadjuvant methotrexate, vinblastine, doxorubicin, and cisplatin (MVAC) followed by radical cystectomy or radical cystectomy alone and demonstrated a survival benefit with neoadjuvant chemotherapy. Patients who were treated with surgery alone had a 33 % increased risk of death compared to those treated with combination therapy (HR 1.33; 95 % CI, 1.00–1.76) [15]. The Medical Research Council (MRC) of the United Kingdom and the European Organization for Research and Treatment of Cancer (EORTC) conducted a phase III trial of neoadjuvant cisplatin, methotrexate, and vinblastine (CMV) versus no therapy prior to surgery or definitive radiotherapy in 976 patients with cT2-T4a N0 muscle-invasive bladder cancer and demonstrated a statistically significant 16 % relative reduction in the risk of death in the 484 patients who underwent radical cystectomy (HR 0.84; 95 % CI, 0.72–0.99; $P<0.037$; median follow-up >8 years) corresponding to an increase in 10-year survival from 30 to 36 % for patients receiving neoadjuvant CMV [16, 17]. Similar outcomes were observed in an additional randomized study of neoadjuvant MVAC as well as a large meta-analysis of 11 randomized trials, and thus neoadjuvant cisplatin-based chemotherapy prior to radical cystectomy is the standard of care in patients with muscle-invasive bladder cancer [18, 19].

In upper tract urothelial cancer, due to anatomic and procedural constraints, accurate clinical staging is often difficult and therefore all patients with upper tract urothelial cancer are considered for extirpative surgery. Neoadjuvant chemotherapy is less well studied in this patient population, but clinical and biological similarities with lower tract disease and the significant increase in mortality associated with T3 or greater or lymph node positive disease at the time of surgery mandate at least the consideration of neoadjuvant chemotherapy [20]. A variety of prognostic factors have been evaluated retrospectively that may assist in identifying patients most appropriate for neoadjuvant therapy. In addition to tumor grade, which correlates strongly (75–90 %) with pathologic stage and grade after nephroureterectomy [21–24], hydronephrosis, sessile architecture on ureteroscopy, and lymphovascular invasion on biopsy are factors associated with a poor prognosis and may serve as basis for treatment with neoadjuvant chemotherapy [25–31]. Retrospective experiences and subset analyses from modern prospective trials of neoadjuvant chemotherapy suggest that this approach is warranted (Table 8.1). The largest retrospective experience was reported by M.D. Anderson Cancer Center in which two cohorts with high-grade upper tract urothelial cancer were compared: 107 patients treated with nephroureterectomy between 1993 and 2004 during which surgery alone was uniformly recommended, and 43 patients treated with neoadjuvant chemotherapy followed by nephrouretectomy between 2004 and 2008 during which time combined modality therapy was recommended [32]. Baseline characteristics were not significantly different between cohorts. The neoadjuvant group experienced a significantly lower rate of pT2 or higher disease (46.5 % vs. 65.4 %; $P=0.043$) and had a 14 % complete response rate (compared to none in the control group) suggesting a pathologic down-staging effect with chemotherapy. While long-term survival data were not included in this initial report due to short follow-up, pathologic down-staging with neoadjuvant chemotherapy has been associated with improved long-term survival in muscle-invasive bladder cancer [15, 33], and thus a similar outcome association could reasonably be expected in upper tract disease as well. Recently reported long-term outcomes demonstrated a 3- and 5-year disease-specific survival

Table 8.1 Select studies of perioperative chemotherapy in upper tract urothelial cancer

	Study	Setting	Inclusion criteria	*N*=	Regimen	Primary outcomes	
						pCR	Survival at 5 years
Prospective	Siefker Radtke et al. ASCO GU 2012 [35]	Neoadjuvant		16	Dose dense MVAC + Bevacizumab	38%	93 % DSS; 93 % OS (2 years)
	Bamias et al. (2004)	Adjuvant	pT2-4N0/+	36	Paclitaxel/Carboplatin	N/A	40 % DFS; 52 % OS
Retrospective	Matin et al. (2010)	Neoadjuvant	cT2-4N0/+	43 107	MVAC, GC, others Surgery alone	14 % (52 % <pT3N0) 0 % (72 % <pT3N0)	NR NR
	Igawa et al. (1995)	Neoadjuvant	cT2-4N0	15	MVAC, MEC, MVEC	13 % (40 % PR)	
	Vassilakopoulou et al. (2011)	Adjuvant	pT3-4N0/+M+ (M1+)	140 (31)	Platinum based	NA	54 % RFS; 43 % OS
	Kawashima et al. (2011)	Adjuvant	pT3N0	38 55	82 % Cisplatin based Surgery alone	NA	74 % RFS; 81 % CSS 57 % RFS; 64 % CSS
	Hellenthal et al. (2009)	Adjuvant	pT3-4N+	121 421	89% Cisplatin based Surgery alone	NA	45 % CSS; 38 % OS 45 % CSS; 38 % OS
	Kwak et al. (2006)	Adjuvant	pT2-3N+	32 7	MVAC, GC, CISCA Surgery Alone	NA	63 % DFS; 78 % OS 36 % DFS; 36 % OS

Abbreviations: *CISCA* cisplatin, cyclophosphamide, and adriamycin, *CSS* cancer-specific survival, *DFS* disease-free survival, *DSS* disease-specific survival, *GC* gemcitabine and cisplatin, *MEC* methotrexate, epirubicin, and cisplatin, *MVAC* methotrexate, vinblastine, adriamycin, and cisplatin, *MVEC* methotrexate, vinblastine, epirubicin, and cisplatin, *NR* not reported, *OS* overall survival, *pCR* pathologic complete response rate, *RFS* recurrence-free survival

Table 8.2 Ongoing perioperative chemotherapy trials in upper tract urothelial cancer

Lead site or sponsor	Setting	*N*=	Regimen	Primary endpoint	Trial identifier
MSKCC	Neoadjuvant	54	GC	pCR	NCT01261728
U. Michigan	Neoadjuvant	55	GC	2 year RFS	NCT01663285
Institute for Cancer Research (UK)	Adjuvant	345	GC or GCa versus Surveillance	3 year DFS	ISRCTN98387754

Abbreviations: *DFS* disease-free survival, *GC* gemcitabine and cisplatin, *GCa* gemcitabine and carboplatin, *MSKCC* Memorial Sloan-Kettering Cancer Center, *pCR* pathologic complete response rate, *RFS* recurrence-free survival

(DSS) of 90 % and 90 %, respectively, for initially clinically lymph node negative patients receiving neoadjuvant chemotherapy (overall survival (OS) 87 % and 80 %, respectively, median follow-up 64 months) compared to the 70 % 3-year DSS and 62 % 5-year OS for the historical group (median follow-up of 87 months) which strongly suggest a survival benefit to neoadjuvant chemotherapy [34]. More recently a phase II clinical trial of neoadjuvant dose-dense MVAC chemotherapy plus bevacizumab in 60 invasive urothelial cancer patients at high risk for recurrence included 16 patients with upper tract disease [35]. Pathologic response rate (<pT2N0) and complete response rate (pT0 N0) were 75 % and 38 %, respectively, for the patients with upper tract disease, which was similar for patients with lower tract disease (45 % and 39 %, respectively). To date, no adequately powered prospective trials of neoadjuvant chemotherapy in upper tract urothelial cancer have been reported, although single arm phase II studies led by Memorial Sloan-Kettering Cancer Center and the University of Michigan are currently under way (Table 8.2).

Adjuvant Chemotherapy

Cisplatin is the only chemotherapeutic agent shown in randomized trials to improve survival in any urothelial cancer disease state; however it carries significant risk for toxicity particularly in the setting of renal impairment. Adjuvant cisplatin-based chemotherapy, in contrast to neoadjuvant, overcomes the inaccuracies of clinical staging [36], and allows for surgical pathology-driven selection of patients at highest risk of recurrence and therefore highest probability of deriving benefit from treatment. However, study of this agent in patients with upper tract urothelial cancer is fraught with challenges in large part due to the high rate of impaired renal function both before and in particular after nephroureterectomy [37]. Combined with the rarity of the disease, it is not surprising that there are no prospective data evaluating cisplatin-based chemotherapy in the adjuvant setting. Limited retrospective data and extrapolation from adjuvant chemotherapy trials in bladder cancer provide some justification for its use in otherwise fit patients at high risk for recurrence.

Two retrospective experiences with cisplatin-based chemotherapy in the adjuvant setting provide conflicting data. Hellenthal et al. reported on 542 patients with pT3-4 N0/+ upper tract urothelial cancer of whom 121 received adjuvant chemotherapy (89 % receiving cisplatin-based chemotherapy) [38]. Cancer-specific survival (CSS) and OS were 45 % and 38 % at 5 years, respectively, for both groups, suggesting no benefit to adjuvant therapy; however baseline factors for both groups were not well balanced. A similar, yet smaller, retrospective experience reported by Kwak et al. included 39 patients with pT2-3 N0/+of whom 32 received adjuvant cisplatin-based chemotherapy [39]. Disease-free survival (DFS) and OS were substantially higher at 5 years for the group receiving chemotherapy (63 % vs. 36 % DFS and 78 % vs. 36 % OS); however the interpretation of the results is limited by the small sample size.

In bladder cancer, similar confusion also exists in the study of adjuvant cisplatin-based chemotherapy. Several studies have attempted to evaluate adjuvant therapy in bladder cancer; however most have suffered from poor accrual and noncompliance with study treatment and have ultimately closed early [40]. Further, a meta-analysis of six trials provides limited evidence for its benefit [41]. However, Spanish Oncology Group Trial 99/01, a randomized trial of adjuvant chemotherapy in patients with invasive urothelial cancer at high risk for recurrence, did provide some evidence that adjuvant chemotherapy can perhaps improve survival in selected patients. With a target enrollment of 340 patients, this trial randomized high-risk patients after radical cystectomy with pT3-T4 or lymph node positive urothelial cancer of the bladder to observation versus adjuvant paclitaxel, gemcitabine, and cisplatin (PGC) for four cycles. Although it was closed early due to poor accrual in 2007, a preliminary analysis at a median follow-up of 51 months for the 142 patients enrolled demonstrated a significant improvement in overall survival at 5 years with adjuvant PGC (60 % vs. 30 %, HR 0.44, $P<0.0009$) [42]. This trial demonstrated a survival benefit with adjuvant chemotherapy despite accruing less than half the target enrollment likely because the trial selected for patients with the highest risk for recurrence, and therefore the highest likelihood of deriving benefit from adjuvant chemotherapy. Small sample size and incomplete accrual limit interpretation of this trial; however it does provide a basis for considering adjuvant chemotherapy in selected high-risk patients. In the absence of prospective data in upper tract urothelial cancer to suggest the contrary, there is no evidence to suggest similar patients with upper tract disease should be treated differently. Therefore, patients with pT3 or greater or lymph node positive upper tract urothelial cancer who are cisplatin eligible should be considered for cisplatin-based adjuvant chemotherapy.

Alternatively, carboplatin-based therapy is a less toxic approach and safer in the setting of renal impairment and has been investigated prospectively. Bamias et al. reported a prospective trial of adjuvant paclitaxel and carboplatin in 36 patients with pT2-4 N0/+upper tract urothelial cancer that demonstrated a 40 % DFS and 52 % OS at 5 years [43]. Thirty-four of these patients had ≥pT3 disease and outcomes reported in this study compare favorably to the poor long-term survival (40 % 5-year survival for pT3 and 6 months median survival for pT4 [44]) typically observed for these patients with surgery alone.

Chemotherapy in Metastatic Disease

Regardless of the primary site of origin, metastatic urothelial cancer is a chemotherapy-sensitive disease. Early clinical trials of single-agent chemotherapy identified doxorubicin, 5-fluorouracil, vinblastine, vincristine, and mitomycin C as active agents with response rates of approximately 15 %. Cisplatin and methotrexate were associated with the highest response rates of approximately 30 %, and thus served as the backbone for the development of older combination strategies such as MVAC, CMV, and CISCA (cisplatin, cyclophosphamide, and adriamycin) and modern regimens that have included ifosfamide [45, 46]. Outcomes reported with cisplatin-based chemotherapy, the only regimens associated with a survival benefit in randomized trials, include response rates of approximately 50–60 % and median survival between 13 and 15 months [10, 46–48]. MVAC represented the standard of care in metastatic urothelial cancer until a seminal phase III trial compared MVAC to the novel regimen of gemcitabine and cisplatin (GC) in 405 patients with metastatic urothelial cancer and found similar efficacy, but improved tolerability with GC, establishing this regimen as a new standard of care for this disease [10].

However, an increased proportion of patients with metastatic urothelial cancer who have previously undergone nephroureterectomy for upper tract disease, as compared to radical cystectomy for bladder cancer, will be ineligible for cisplatin-based therapy due to impaired renal function [37, 49, 50]. Typically, these patients have been treated with carboplatin-based regimens. The EORTC 30986 phase II/III trial compared gemcitabine and carboplatin (GCa) versus methotrexate, carboplatin, and vinblastine (MCAVI) in 238 patients with metastatic urothelial cancer who were ineligible for cisplatin (poor performance status, impaired renal function, or both) and demonstrated a 41.2 % response rate and 9.3 months median survival for GCa. Similar response and survival outcomes were observed for MCAVI; however it was less well tolerated, and thus this trial provided the first level one evidence for a non-cisplatin-based regimen in this patient population. More recently the combination of gemcitabine and paclitaxel with doxorubicin has shown promise in this patient population. In a trial in patients with poor renal function, objective responses rates were approximately 50 %, with a median survival of 15 months [51].

Prospective randomized trials of chemotherapy in metastatic urothelial cancer are not typically stratified by primary site of disease and there are no definitive data to suggest outcomes are different between upper and lower tract urothelial cancer. A retrospective report of 72 patients with upper tract urothelial cancer who underwent nephroureterectomy suggested tumor location (renal pelvis versus ureter) independently impacted on 5-year survival outcomes [8]. More recent evidence includes a post hoc subset analysis from a randomized phase III trial of GC versus paclitaxel, gemcitabine, and cisplatin (PCG) in 626 patients with metastatic urothelial cancer and provides some rationale for separate investigation of tumors that originate from the upper versus lower urinary tract. For the entire study population, median survival for GC and PCG was 12.7 and 15.8 months, respectively, which did not reach statistical significance (HR 0.85; 95 % CI, 0.72–1.02; $P=0.075$);

however when the analysis was limited to the 81 % of patients who had bladder cancer as their primary, median survival with PCG was significantly longer than with GC (15.9 versus 11.9 months, respectively; HR, 0.80; 95 % CI, 0.66–0.97; $P=0.025$). While not definitive, this observation in an unplanned subset analysis could serve as a basis for stratification by primary tumor site in future randomized trials of chemotherapy in metastatic urothelial cancer. Until such evidence is available, metastatic urothelial cancer should be treated similarly irrespective of primary tumor site.

Conclusions

There is emerging evidence for biological and clinical differences between urothelial cancer of the upper and lower urinary tract. The rarity of the disease as well as anatomic and procedural constraints has hampered selective study of upper tract urothelial cancer in prospective trials. In the absence of definitive evidence for alternative treatment, management of upper tract urothelial cancer will continue to be guided by lessons learned in the management of lower tract disease. Prospective trials currently under way in upper tract urothelial cancer will further define the role for systemic chemotherapy in this disease.

Summary Points

- Urothelial cancer has been considered, until recently, a single pan-urothelial disease.
- Cisplatin-based chemotherapy when added to radical surgery has definitively demonstrated improved survival in patients with muscle-invasive urothelial cancer of the bladder
- Due to the difficulty of accurate clinical staging in upper tract urothelial cancer and high rate of impaired renal function after nephroureterectomy, all patients with high-grade upper tract disease should be considered for neoadjuvant cisplatin-based chemotherapy prior to nephroureterectomy.
- Patients with pT3 or greater disease at nephroureterectomy who are still candidates for cisplatin should be considered for adjuvant chemotherapy with a cisplatin-based regimen. Those with high-risk resected disease ineligible for cisplatin should be considered for adjuvant clinical trials.
- Metastatic urothelial cancer is a devastating disease and cisplatin-based combination chemotherapy is the only treatment known to improve survival.
- There are no convincing data to suggest that patients with metastatic urothelial cancer should be treated differently based on the primary site of the tumor.
- Patients ineligible for cisplatin-based chemotherapy should be considered for carboplatin-based therapy such as gemcitabine and carboplatin.

References

1. Yagoda A. Chemotherapy of urothelial tract tumors. Cancer. 1987;60(3 Suppl):574–85.
2. Gupta R, Paner GP, Amin MB. Neoplasms of the upper urinary tract: a review with focus on urothelial carcinoma of the pelvicalyceal system and aspects related to its diagnosis and reporting. Adv Anat Pathol. 2008;15(3):127–39.
3. Tzai TS, et al. Clinical significance of allelotype profiling for urothelial carcinoma. Urology. 2003;62(2):378–84.
4. Hafner C, et al. Clonality of multifocal urothelial carcinomas: 10 years of molecular genetic studies. Int J Cancer. 2002;101(1):1–6.
5. Hafner C, et al. Evidence for oligoclonality and tumor spread by intraluminal seeding in multifocal urothelial carcinomas of the upper and lower urinary tract. Oncogene. 2001; 20(35):4910–5.
6. Jones TD, et al. Molecular evidence supporting field effect in urothelial carcinogenesis. Clin Cancer Res. 2005;11(18):6512–9.
7. Catto JW, et al. Behavior of urothelial carcinoma with respect to anatomical location. J Urol. 2007;177(5):1715–20.
8. Akdogan B, et al. Prognostic significance of bladder tumor history and tumor location in upper tract transitional cell carcinoma. J Urol. 2006;176(1):48–52.
9. Kaufman DS, et al. A multi-institutional phase II trial of gemcitabine plus paclitaxel in patients with locally advanced or metastatic urothelial cancer. Urol Oncol. 2004;22(5):393–7.
10. von der Maase H, et al. Gemcitabine and cisplatin versus methotrexate, vinblastine, doxorubicin, and cisplatin in advanced or metastatic bladder cancer: results of a large, randomized, multinational, multicenter, phase III study. J Clin Oncol. 2000;18(17):3068–77.
11. Sternberg CN, et al. Randomized phase III trial of high-dose-intensity methotrexate, vinblastine, doxorubicin, and cisplatin (MVAC) chemotherapy and recombinant human granulocyte colony-stimulating factor versus classic MVAC in advanced urothelial tract tumors: European Organization for Research and Treatment of Cancer Protocol no. 30924. J Clin Oncol. 2001;19(10):2638–46.
12. Bamias A, et al. Docetaxel and cisplatin with granulocyte colony-stimulating factor (G-CSF) versus MVAC with G-CSF in advanced urothelial carcinoma: a multicenter, randomized, phase III study from the Hellenic Cooperative Oncology Group. J Clin Oncol. 2004;22(2): 220–8.
13. Kaufman D, et al. Phase II trial of gemcitabine plus cisplatin in patients with metastatic urothelial cancer. J Clin Oncol. 2000;18(9):1921–7.
14. Dreicer R, et al. Phase III trial of methotrexate, vinblastine, doxorubicin, and cisplatin versus carboplatin and paclitaxel in patients with advanced carcinoma of the urothelium. Cancer. 2004;100(8):1639–45.
15. Grossman HB, et al. Neoadjuvant chemotherapy plus cystectomy compared with cystectomy alone for locally advanced bladder cancer. N Engl J Med. 2003;349(9):859–66.
16. Griffiths G, et al. International phase III trial assessing neoadjuvant cisplatin, methotrexate, and vinblastine chemotherapy for muscle-invasive bladder cancer: long-term results of the BA06 30894 trial. J Clin Oncol. 2011;29(16):2171–7.
17. Neoadjuvant cisplatin, methotrexate, and vinblastine chemotherapy for muscle-invasive bladder cancer: a randomised controlled trial. International collaboration of trialists. Lancet. 1999;354(9178):533–40.
18. Neoadjuvant chemotherapy in invasive bladder cancer: a systematic review and meta-analysis. Lancet. 2003;361(9373):1927–34.
19. Kitamura H et al. Randomized phase III trial of neoadjuvant chemotherapy (NAC) with methotrexate, doxorubicin, vinblastine, and cisplatin (MVAC) followed by radical cystectomy (RC) compared with RC alone for invasive bladder cancer (BC): Japan Clinical Oncology Group Study, JCOG0209. J Clin Oncol. 2013;31(suppl 6; abstr 249).

20. Margulis V, et al. Outcomes of radical nephroureterectomy: a series from the Upper Tract Urothelial Carcinoma Collaboration. Cancer. 2009;115(6):1224–33.
21. Keeley FX, et al. Diagnostic accuracy of ureteroscopic biopsy in upper tract transitional cellcarcinoma. J Urol. 1997;157(1):33–7.
22. Williams SK, et al. Correlation of upper-tract cytology, retrograde pyelography, ureteroscopic appearance, and ureteroscopic biopsy with histologic examination of upper-tract transitional cell carcinoma. J Endourol. 2008;22(1):71–6.
23. Brown GA, et al. Ability of clinical grade to predict final pathologic stage in upper urinary tract transitional cell carcinoma: implications for therapy. Urology. 2007;70(2):252–6.
24. Skolarikos A, et al. Cytologic analysis of ureteral washings is informative in patients with grade 2 upper tract TCC considering endoscopic treatment. Urology. 2003;61(6):1146–50.
25. Fritsche HM, et al. Macroscopic sessile tumor architecture is a pathologic feature of biologically aggressive upper tract urothelial carcinoma. Urol Oncol. 2012;30(5):666–72.
26. Remzi M, et al. Tumour architecture is an independent predictor of outcomes after nephroureterectomy: a multi-institutional analysis of 1363 patients. BJU Int. 2009;103(3):307–11.
27. Kikuchi E, et al. Lymphovascular invasion predicts clinical outcomes in patients with node-negative upper tract urothelial carcinoma. J Clin Oncol. 2009;27(4):612–8.
28. Bolenz C, et al. Lymphovascular invasion and pathologic tumor stage are significant outcome predictors for patients with upper tract urothelial carcinoma. Urology. 2008;72(2):364–9.
29. Kim DS, et al. Lymphovascular invasion and pT stage are prognostic factors in patients treated with radical nephroureterectomy for localized upper urinary tract transitional cell carcinoma. Urology. 2010;75(2):328–32.
30. Hurel S, et al. Impact of lymphovascular invasion on oncological outcomes in patients with upper tract urothelial carcinoma after radical nephroureterectomy. BJU Int. 2013;111(8):1199–207.
31. Ito Y, et al. Preoperative hydronephrosis grade independently predicts worse pathological outcomes in patients undergoing nephroureterectomy for upper tract urothelial carcinoma. J Urol. 2011;185(5):1621–6.
32. Matin SF, et al. Incidence of downstaging and complete remission after neoadjuvant chemotherapy for high-risk upper tract transitional cell carcinoma. Cancer. 2010;116(13):3127–34.
33. Splinter TA, et al. A European Organization for Research and Treatment of Cancer–Genitourinary Group phase 2 study of chemotherapy in stage T3–4N0–XM0 transitional cell cancer of the bladder: evaluation of clinical response. J Urol. 1992;148(6):1793–6.
34. Porten SP, et al. Survival outcomes in patients undergoing neoadjuvant chemotherapy for upper tract urothelial cell carcinoma. J Clin Oncol. 2013;31(suppl 6; abstr 311).
35. Siefker-Radtke A, et al. Neoadjuvant chemotherapy with DD-MVAC and bevacizumab in high-risk urothelial cancer: results from a phase II trial at the University of Texas M. D. Anderson Cancer Center. J Clin Oncol. 2012;30(suppl; abstr 4523).
36. Gray P, et al. Clinical-pathologic stage discrepancy in patients with bladder cancer treated with radical cystectomy: associations with clinical variables and survival. J Clin Oncol. 2013; 31(suppl 6; abstr 248).
37. Kaag MG, et al. Changes in renal function following nephroureterectomy may affect the use of perioperative chemotherapy. Eur Urol. 2010;58(4):581–7.
38. Hellenthal NJ, et al. Adjuvant chemotherapy for high risk upper tract urothelial carcinoma: results from the Upper Tract Urothelial Carcinoma Collaboration. J Urol. 2009;182(3): 900–6.
39. Kwak C, et al. Adjuvant systemic chemotherapy in the treatment of patients with invasive transitional cell carcinoma of the upper urinary tract. Urology. 2006;68(1):53–7.
40. Stadler WM, et al. Phase III study of molecularly targeted adjuvant therapy in locally advanced urothelial cancer of the bladder based on p53 status. J Clin Oncol. 2011;29(25):3443–9.
41. Adjuvant chemotherapy in invasive bladder cancer: a systematic review and meta-analysis of individual patient data Advanced Bladder Cancer (ABC) Meta-analysis Collaboration. Eur Urol. 2005;48(2):89–199. discussion 199–201.
42. Paz-Ares LG et al. Randomized phase III trial comparing adjuvant paclitaxel/gemcitabine/cisplatin (PGC) to observation in patients with resected invasive bladder cancer: Results of the

Spanish Oncology Genitourinary Group (SOGUG) 99/01 study. J Clin Oncol. 2008;28:18s, 2010 (suppl; abstr LBA4518).
43. Bamias A, et al. Adjuvant chemotherapy with paclitaxel and carboplatin in patients with advanced carcinoma of the upper urinary tract: a study by the Hellenic Cooperative Oncology Group. J Clin Oncol. 2004;22(11):2150–4.
44. Hall MC, et al. Prognostic factors, recurrence, and survival in transitional cell carcinoma of the upper urinary tract: a 30-year experience in 252 patients. Urology. 1998;52(4):594–601.
45. Siefker-Radtke AO, et al. A phase 2 clinical trial of sequential neoadjuvant chemotherapy with ifosfamide, doxorubicin, and gemcitabine followed by cisplatin, gemcitabine, and ifosfamide in locally advanced urothelial cancer: final results. Cancer. 2013;119(3):540–7.
46. Bajorin DF, et al. Ifosfamide, paclitaxel, and cisplatin for patients with advanced transitional cell carcinoma of the urothelial tract: final report of a phase II trial evaluating two dosing schedules. Cancer. 2000;88(7):1671–8.
47. Bellmunt J, et al. Randomized phase III study comparing paclitaxel/cisplatin/gemcitabine and gemcitabine/cisplatin in patients with locally advanced or metastatic urothelial cancer without prior systemic therapy: EORTC Intergroup Study 30987. J Clin Oncol. 2012;30(10): 1107–13.
48. Logothetis CJ, et al. A prospective randomized trial comparing MVAC and CISCA chemotherapy for patients with metastatic urothelial tumors. J Clin Oncol. 1990;8(6):1050–5.
49. Balar AV, et al. Phase II study of gemcitabine, carboplatin, and bevacizumab in patients with advanced unresectable or metastatic urothelial cancer. J Clin Oncol. 2013;31(6):724–30.
50. Galsky MD, et al. A consensus definition of patients with metastatic urothelial carcinoma who are unfit for cisplatin-based chemotherapy. Lancet Oncol. 2011;12(3):211–4.
51. Pagliaro L, et al. Gemcitabine, paclitaxel, and doxorubicin for patients (pts) with urothelial carcinoma (UC) and renal insufficiency: Preliminary results of a multicenter phase II study. J Clin Oncol. 2011;29(suppl 7; abstr 246).

Index

© Springer Science+Business Media New York 2015

S.F. Shariat, E. Xylinas (eds.), *Upper Tract Urothelial Carcinoma*,
DOI 10.1007/978-1-4939-1501-9

C

D

M

V

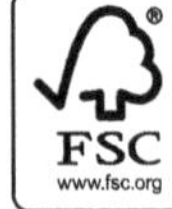

MIX
Papier aus verantwortungsvollen Quellen
Paper from responsible sources
FSC® C105338

If you have any concerns about our products,
you can contact us on
ProductSafety@springernature.com

In case Publisher is established outside the EU,
the EU authorized representative is:
Springer Nature Customer Service Center GmbH
Europaplatz 3, 69115 Heidelberg, Germany

Printed by Libri Plureos GmbH
in Hamburg, Germany